International classification in psychiatry

International classification in psychiatry

Unity and diversity

Edited by
JUAN E. MEZZICH, M.D., PH.D.
Professor of Psychiatry
University of Pittsburgh

MICHAEL VON CRANACH, M.D.
Director
Bezirkskrankenhaus Kaufbeuren

SECTION ON NOMENCLATURE AND CLASSIFICATION
WORLD PSYCHIATRIC ASSOCIATION

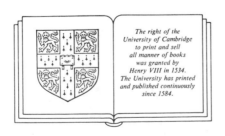

The right of the
University of Cambridge
to print and sell
all manner of books
was granted by
Henry VIII in 1534.
The University has printed
and published continuously
since 1584.

CAMBRIDGE UNIVERSITY PRESS
Cambridge
New York   New Rochelle   Melbourne   Sydney

Published by the Press Syndicate of the University of Cambridge
The Pitt Building, Trumpington Street, Cambridge CB2 1RP
32 East 57th Street, New York, NY 10022, USA
10 Stamford Road, Oakleigh, Melbourne 3166, Australia

First published 1988

Printed in the United States of America

Library of Congress Cataloging-in-Publication Data
International classification in psychiatry.
Based on the Conference on International Classification
in Psychiatry, organized by the Section on Nomenclature
and Classification of the World Psychiatric Association,
and held in Montréal, June 26–29, 1985.
Includes index.
1. Mental illness – Classification – Congresses.
2. Psychiatry – Classification – Congresses. I. Mezzich,
Juan E. II. Cranach, Michael von. III. Conference on
International Classification in Psychiatry (1985:
Montréal, Québec) IV. World Psychiatric Association.
Section on Nomenclature and Classification. [DNLM:
1. Mental Disorders – classification – congresses.
2. Mental Disorders – diagnosis – congresses. 3. Psychiatry
– classification – congresses. WM 15 161 1985]
RC455.2.C4155 1988 616.89'0012 87–25618

British Library Cataloguing in Publication Data
International classification in psychiatry:
unity and diversity.
1. Mental illness – Classification
I. Mezzich, Juan E. II. Von Cranach, Michael
616.89'0012 RC455.2.C4

ISBN 0 521 32754 7

Contents

v

Foreword

As we all know, classification in psychiatry existed long before psychiatry as a discipline was established. In fact, psychiatry itself was born out of classification. Europe was its birthplace, and European nosologists were its founding fathers. About a century of keen observation and detailed phenomenological description passed before a diagnostic system that provided the new discipline with the right to claim an equal stance among the other medical specialties was established at the turn of the century. Within the frame of this classification system, mechanisms were explored, theories of causation were developed, and treatment modalities were tried that either failed or have survived to this day. Worth keeping in mind is the fact that even theories and practices disputing the validity of the nosological system grew out of it, and although on extreme occasions they attempted to negate its usefulness, they failed to propose a substantive and survivable alternative. The dispute continued though, on both epistemological and empirical grounds, and was accompanied by an increasing shift in emphasis from symptoms to mechanisms, resulting in a gradual neglect of diagnostic issues.

The latter trend took place primarily in North America during the post–World War II era, but had a pervasive influence on psychiatric thinking all over the world. Combined with an expansion of professional concern toward psychosocial aspects of human behavior, it gradually transformed psychiatry from a medical specialty to a discipline with vague boundaries, inspired by paradigms that reduced the complexity of psychopathology to either psychological abstractions or sociological speculations. Empiricism gave way to theorizing and based its appeal on antimedical rhetoric rather than on the validity of its propositions.

Whereas in the prewar years psychiatry, because of the zeal of nosologists to secure a place in posterity, was plagued by an inflow of new descriptive categories, in the following years the field was flooded by innumerable causation theories and schools of thought, each one inventing its own vocabulary and code. This babel could not last long. Psychiatry in the meantime acquired considerable empirical information on its subject matter, an unprecedented ability to modify states of mind by chemical intervention, an increased commitment to expand its scientific frontiers, and too much social power for which it had to be accountable. To meet the challenges posed by these developments and to answer their critics more comprehensibly and factually, psychiatrists and their professional societies realized that they had to renew their efforts to create a common frame of reference and a common language to deal with treatment and research issues. All this meant that diagnosis had to be reinstated as the pivotal element in psychiatric theory and practice. The recent worldwide upsurge of interest in the diagnosis and classification of mental disorders culminated with the publication of DSM-III in 1980 in the United States, perhaps the country in which diagnosis had been most widely disregarded. The first edition of DSM-III marked a turning point in contemporary psychiatry. It had been preceded by years of long, laborious groundwork, collective bargaining, and empirical investigation, and it provided psychiatry with a conceptual framework in which isolated pieces of knowledge could be compared and interpreted.

DSM-III has certainly been subject to criticism, for example, for its failure to define mental disorders adequately, arbitrariness in its operational criteria for differential diagnosis, haste in introducing new categories with poor empirical foundation, and atheoreticism that inhibits creative thinking. On the other hand, DSM-III reopened the door to a rational approach to mental disorders by establishing diagnosis as an essential part of psychiatry's scientific basis and as a necessary condition for accountable and justifiable therapeutic intervention. In the years that have passed since its publication, DSM-III, despite its many limitations and cultural biases, has become not only a national but also an international guidebook for psychiatrists and mental-health professionals at large. This development demonstrates the need for a truly international system based on the widest consensus possible among professionals from all over the world.

As the applicability of DSM-III to settings other than certain Western countries is increasingly questioned, the construction of an international system becomes an imperative task. Against the background of ICD-9, the currently official World Health Organization (WHO) system, ICD-10 is now in preparation. Aimed at revising old notions, it has been inspired to a considerable extent by DSM-III, and it is an attempt to incorporate new knowledge and recent developments in mental-health care in diverse sociocultural settings around the world.

The Conference on International Classification in Psychiatry, organized by the Section on Nomenclature and Classification of the World Psychiatric Association (WPA), was held at the opportune moment: halfway between the publication of DSM-III and the eventual approval of ICD-10 by the WHO General Assembly. It furnished an opportunity to reflect on the consequences of DSM-III while there was still time to influence the development of ICD-10.

In order to contribute substantially to the construction of an international system of classification that aspires to receiving ecumenical acceptance as well as effective implementation, as an instrument of international communication, we must be aware of pertinent constraints at both theoretical and pragmatic levels. The fundamental issues are conceptual. We have to clarify what we diagnose and classify, by which criteria, for whom, and for what purposes. These questions are inherently linked to the difficult task of drawing sharp and universally valid boundaries between normality and mental disorder. For a diagnostic system to demonstrate conceptual clarity, it has to distinguish convincingly between the two.

At our present stage of knowledge in psychiatry and general medicine, the above-mentioned goal appears hard to attain. Although we should apply ourselves diligently to advancing the conceptual framework and empirical infrastructure of our discipline, it seems unlikely that we will soon be able to diagnose the highly complex mental disorders by their nature rather than by their describable manifestations. This would be particularly true for marginal conditions that are closely linked to personality traits and maladaptive reactions to life events. All that may be feasible at the present stage in the development of psychiatry is to be able to test empirically its propositions. This is becoming possible now, at least for what we consider the major mental disorders.

In addition to the basic conceptual issues, questions on categorization models, definitional criteria, and the subject and purpose of classification remain formidable challenges. In the process of developing a classification system, we often face unforeseen difficulties and the need to accommodate conflicting demands. To illustrate this situation, some common dilemmas may be cited. To be compelling, a diagnostic category has to be both reliable and valid, but reliability does not guarantee validity. With overinclusive definitions, we may gain reliability but lose validity, as happened in the past with broader definitions of schizophrenia. Similarly, by using improved standardization techniques and very strict diagnostic criteria, we may again end up with increased diagnostic concordance, but it may be applicable only to a limited number of cases and not cover the broad spectrum of clinical reality. Such a procrustean approach leaves out many undiagnosed conditions and overlooks dimensions of psychopathology that may be of value in elucidating underlying mechanisms.

The inclination of psychiatry to strive for universal laws and nomothetic approaches, although commendable and legitimate, does not meet the present requirements of clinical reality, in which the attributes of an individual have to be considered in the context of the relevant sociocultural environment.

Admittedly, a diagnostic system is not an end in itself. It is an instrument to be used for a variety of purposes, such as promoting communication among practitioners and facilitating more rational and effective treatment. The science of psychiatry, however, does not reach for the known or the established. It strives to elucidate the unknown. For this reason the system of classification has to be flexible and capable of assimilating new information. Further, it has to be based on logical thinking and the generation of new empirical data, testable hypotheses, and interesting ideas that can raise the level of our understanding of clinical reality. The issues involved in the construction of an international classification system for mental disorders that is intended to serve both clinical care and scientific research are highly complex. They require penetrating study and balancing of conflicting demands. A system that is simple, clear in its definitions, and closely connected with familiar nosological concepts would best serve international communicability and practical use. In contrast, a system that incorporates available knowledge in a thorough, rigorous, polyaxial, and innovative way would be more intellectually satisfying and more fitting for research purposes.

The meeting organized by the Section Committee on Nomenclature and Classification of the World Psychiatric Association marked a very important development in our field by addressing the crucial issues involved in constructing an updated international system for the classification of mental disorders. It offered a unique opportunity for comprehensively overviewing and appraising the principal lines of thought and current trends in the theory and practice of psychiatric diagnosis. It also provided a forum for an informative and inspiring exchange of views among scientists currently involved in the development of forthcoming standard diagnostic systems (ICD-10, DSM-IV) and other international experts in the field of nosology and classification. The present volume is composed of contributions based on presentations made at that conference. It covers a wide range of theoretical and methodological topics and offers stimulating reading for psychiatrists and mental-health professionals in general. It is through commonly applied diagnostic concepts that a worldwide framework can be obtained for both scientific research and patient-care activities. Conversely, it is to a large extent the collective experience of clinicians across the world that should constitute the empirical basis for the construction of a universally acceptable and valid diagnostic system. The need for such contributions from the world psychiatric community has increasingly been recognized and has been attested recently by the establishment of a collaborative agreement between the WHO and the WPA for the development of ICD-10. Following guidelines jointly prepared by the WPA Executive Committee and Section on Nomenclature and Classification, the rank and file of psychiatrists and their national societies are thus able to present their views, comments, and suggestions on proposals for the forthcoming edition of the International Classification of Diseases. The present volume will undoubtedly help to promote the goals of this WHO–WPA effort.

The WPA Section on Nomenclature and Classification deserves all our gratitude and appreciation for organizing such an important conference, for editing this volume, and for undertaking a major role in the WPA collaborative project with the WHO.

COSTAS N. STEFANIS
President, World Psychiatric Association

Editors' preface

This is an exciting time for both psychiatric diagnosis and international psychiatry. Innovative models and procedures are coming to light, and new challenges and opportunities for worldwide communication are appearing before us.

In recent decades, diagnosis and classification have experienced considerable methodological advancement along several lines. One notable change is that greater rigor is now applied in data gathering. This has led to the vigorous development of structured and semistructured evaluation procedures. Structured evaluation procedures are usually used in community surveys conducted according to strict schedules and algorithms that lead to the assignment of categories from a subset of categories covering the psychopathological domain. Semistructured evaluation procedures are more often used by clinicians relying on their experience to conduct a flexible interview and using all informational sources available to arrive at a diagnostic formulation within the time constraints imposed by clinical decision making.

Another significant methodological development is that rules have been established for defining and assigning diagnostic categories. Here we see, for example, more explicit and specific criteria for including and excluding given categories in the differential diagnosis process. These guidelines, with perhaps different degrees of specificity, are pertinent to both research and patient-care purposes. In addition, we note the use of prototypical models of categorization, particularly in the field of personality disorders. These probabilistic models require that a certain number (but not all) of the attributes of a category be present for making a given diagnosis.

Third, major strides have been made in developing more comprehensive diagnostic formulations. Such formulations, usually known as multiaxial, are attempts to describe the patient's condition in terms of aspects exemplified by psychiatric syndromes, personality conditions, concomitant physical problems, abnormal psychosocial situations, and disabilities. This architectural approach has attracted considerable interest, but its most appropriate content and scaling, as well as its lasting impact, remain to be seen.

These developments are making psychiatric diagnosis not only more precise and systematic but also potentially more useful for clinical description, treatment decisions, prognosis, public-health planning, and scientific research. Another important point is that these current diagnostic developments have international roots. In the nosological arena, the work of Emil Kraepelin in Germany, formulating the concept of disease entity and delineating dementia praecox (or schizophrenia) and manic-depressive illness as major endogenous psychoses, has been of paramount importance. Illustrating related nosological topics, we find the work of S. S. Korsakov on organic psychoses and the systematic description of longitudinal disease patterns (continuous, shiftlike, progressive, and periodic) in Soviet psychiatry, and the concepts of *bouffée délirante* in France, psychogenic psychosis in Scandinavia, and acute transient psychoses in the developing countries. Also pertinent to the fundamentals of nosology have been the Latin American contributions of Seguín in 1946 formulating psychiatric illness as reaction to stress, and more recently the contributions of both Horacio Fábrega and Javier Mariátegui toward an ethnohistorical understanding of disease and social responses to it. Explicit diagnostic criteria, the need for which was cogently pointed out by Edward Stengel from England in 1959, were first used and published by Peter Berner in Austria in 1969. Multiaxial thinking had its early antecedents in the holistic approach inaugurated by Hippocrates on the Greek island of Cos and in the need for conceptual clarity and structural logic epitomized by the Platonic tradition. Specific diagnostic systems of this kind were originally developed around 1950 by E. Essen-Möller and S. Wolfahrt in Sweden and José Leme Lopes in Brazil. In the early 1970s, they were implemented into a successful approach for child psychiatry by Michael Rutter and his colleagues at the Institute of Psychiatry in London. DSM-III, published by the American Psychiatric Association in 1980 and highlighted by specific diagnostic criteria, a multiaxial approach, and an innovative grouping of diagnostic categories, has attracted wide international interest.

In addition to the enriching perspective afforded by considering our roots, the need for an international psychiatry is compellingly pointed out by the fact that 75 percent of the psychiatric population lives in the developing nations. Therefore, greater and broader international input is required in refining the standard tools of our field, among which classification systems have a central position.

Leading the way in the construction of an international classification is the World Health Organization (WHO). Continuing the tradition begun by the International Statistical Institute in 1893, it assumed in the late 1940s the responsibility for the decennial revisions of the ICD and through many international seminars and collaborative projects sought to enhance the soundness of the mental-disorders component. The WHO is now embarked on preparing the tenth revision, for which, at least in its psychiatric section, it will attempt to complement traditional statistical and public-health purposes with utility for clinical care and research.

The World Psychiatric Association (WPA), through a formal collaborative agreement, is joining the WHO in an endeavor to produce an effective and broadly based ICD-10. To this end, it is inviting comments and critical reports of experience on ICD-10 proposals from psychiatrists and psychiatric associations across the world. A significant role in this collaborative effort has been assumed by the WPA Section Committee on Nomenclature and Classification. Its membership, which is steadily growing in international representation, includes key contributors to the major transcultural diagnostic projects of recent times.

The Conference on International Classification in Psychiatry organized by this WPA section took place in Montreal on June 26–9, 1985. It was intended to further the section's aim of enhancing the development of improved diagnostic and nosological models and procedures within a worldwide framework. The present volume is composed of further elaborations of the core conference presentations. Some of the chapters correspond to invited contributions that for logistical reasons were not orally presented.

The volume contains thirty essays organized into five parts. It starts with a review of international and representative national diagnostic systems; continues with a discussion of specific syndromes, recent terminological and assessment instruments, and critical nosological issues; and ends with a panel on ICD-10. The authors are among the leading contributors to diagnosis and classification, representing about twenty (Eastern and Western, developed and developing) countries.

Part I opens with a historical overview of the International Classification of Diseases, including the gradual shift of its focus from mortality to morbidity, the evolution of its taxonomic principles, and the relatively recent growth of its mental-disorders component. The first national approach presented is the Brazilian, which shows the influence of various European schools, as well as the development in Rio de Janeiro in 1954 of one of the first multiaxial systems in the world, composed of a syndrome, premorbid personality, and etiological constellation. A presentation of the French school outlines the historical trajectory of such interesting diagnostic entities as *bouffée délirante* and *état délirant chronique* and reports on an attempt to operationalize these concepts in order to compare them empirically with those of other international systems. Scandinavia, where Carolus Linnaeus established the principles of biological taxonomy, has also offered several pioneering developments in psychiatric nosology, such as the concepts of psychogenic and cycloid psychoses, Henrik Sjöbring's personality patterns, and some of the earliest multiaxial classifications. Presented next is the Egyptian Diagnostic System, along with its historical and cultural background, the influences it received from Anglo-Saxon, French, and Soviet psychiatries, and the particular attention given to the connections between physical problems and psychiatric nosology. The chapter on psychiatric classification in Nigeria identifies an ethnocentric position on the part of official (predominantly European) psychiatry vis-à-vis African reality, considers the influences of culture on psychopathology, and reviews major syndromes, particularly non-readily classifiable excitement states encompassing affective, psychotic, and trancelike features highlighted by an outpouring of verbiage and energy. The presentation of the Chinese Classification of Mental Disorders describes its use of etiological understanding (particularly for organic brain syndromes) and the concepts of psychosis and neurosis (descriptively considered) as important clas-sificatory principles, and points out the validity of neurasthenia based both on clinical practice and on empirical studies showing its reliability and its usefulness for describing 59 percent of neurotic patients in China. Completing this part, the fundamentals of DSM-III are outlined, particularly its consensual devel-opment, commitment to patient care and research, descriptive approach, specific diagnostic criteria, hierarchical organization, and multiaxial system.

Part II considers international views on specific syndromes, starting with schizophrenia and related psychotic disorders. Their bases on a hierarchical organization of psychopathology, a dichotomy of endogenous psychoses, and the role of prognosis are discussed, along with a comparison of defini-tions corresponding to German-speaking, French, Scandinavian, and English-speaking approaches, and the value of explicit diagnostic criteria for clarifying relationships among various concepts of schizophrenia. In a related chapter, the intricacies of the nosology of childhood psychoses, particularly those of autism, are discussed, with an emphasis on biopsychosocial empirical studies and the current need to base their diagnosis on phenomenology and natural history. The clinical features and favorable outcome of acute and transient psychoses as often described in developing countries are outlined next, along with some recom-mendations for covering them more adequately in future international classifi-cations. The controversial nosological position of schizoaffective psychosis is then examined by empirically comparing contemporary concepts of this con-dition with cycloid psychosis, *bouffée délirante*, and ICD-9 schizophrenic and affective psychoses. A prospective classification of affective and anxiety disorders is the subject of a chapter that traces their roots to "emotional" conditions and emphasizes the classificatory pertinence of descriptive phenomenology, on which basis it proposes specific diagnostic groupings such as the subdivision of phobias into isolated, social, and agoraphobic types. International views on somatoform and dissociative disorders are then reviewed, with an emphasis on the history of hysteria, current controversies on the linkage among conditions of this general type, and the need for a balanced biopsychological approach and more empirical studies on this intriguing area. Next, a cultural analysis of adjustment disorder as a transitional category of illness is presented, after a discussion of traditional and biomedical theories of illness, behavioral changes as basic indicators of morbidity, and the role of clinicians in interpreting presenting complaints. This part closes with a review of problems and perspectives with regard to the di-agnosis of personality disorders and includes an examination of the historical consistency of standard types, cultural variability as exemplified by the *shin-keishitsu* condition, and the value of both considering severity in the assessment of personality disorders and placing these on an axis different from that of other psychiatric syndromes.

Part III, which focuses on nomenclature and assessment developments, begins with a discussion of translating psychopathological concepts and terms as crucial to international communication and the preparation of the WHO's Lexicon in Arabic, Chinese, English, French, Russian, and Spanish. Several chapters review various standardized approaches to psychiatric evaluation, starting with the European Association for Methodology and Documentation in Psychiatry (AMDP) procedure for systematically recording psychiatric history, psychopathological symptoms, and somatic data, and the results of its ingenious use within a comprehensive diagnostic framework. Presented next are the Diagnostic Interview Schedule (DIS) and the Composite International Diagnostic Interview (CIDI), two fully structured interview procedures designed primarily for community surveys conducted by laymen, the algorithmic organization of which allows the computerized assignment of diagnoses from a subset of those included in standard diagnostic systems. This is followed by a report on the reliability of the German version of the CIDI, which was found to be adequate for the majority of the included diagnostic categories. The final chapter in Part III discusses the Initial Evaluation Form, a semistructured evaluation procedure involving a format with standardized and narrative components complementing each other and, in contrast to rigidly structured instruments, using all informational sources available and covering all categories of a standard diagnostic system. A report is also included on the reliability and clinical utility of English and Spanish versions of this instrument, as used in Pittsburgh and Lima.

Part IV deals with critical nosological issues and opens with an examination of the use of standard diagnostic systems in national admission statistics by focusing on cases of schizophrenic, affective, and "intermediate" psychoses and pointing out the importance of an appropriate hierarchical organization of major diagnostic classes to optimize the informativeness of national and international statistical reports. The presentation of the principles for revising a standard diagnostic system such as DSM-III highlights the role of a broad panel of advisory committees and the use of the experience gained with the basic diagnostic system to formulate changes in it. Diagnosis and classification issues in child psychiatry are considered next, with attention given to both developmental unfolding and environmental influences as key classificatory principles, the pertinence of the so-called comprehensive clinical formulation model, and the impact of multiaxial diagnostic systems for dealing with the complexities of children's conditions. The structure of diagnostic systems and methodological aspects pertinent to their design are reviewed, with particular focus on the scaling of psychopathology, the definition of syndromes, the hierarchical organization of the whole classification, and the architecture of a comprehensive diagnostic formulation. The contribution of epidemiology to the furtherance of nosology is discussed by using as an example a large community survey project and its impact on clarifying the hierarchical organization of a standard diagnostic system and the delineation of specific categories such as panic disorder and agoraphobia. Using as an illustration a real case history from Tanzania, cultural requirements for nosological understanding and development are considered next, and recommendations are offered for a diagnostic system simple enough to be used by front-line workers and to have a multiaxial structure to accommodate information on acute psychopathology, personality, physical conditions, and sociocultural factors. The next chapter examines issues pertaining to the presentation and documentation of a standard psychiatric classification, with particular attention given to what is classified (disorders versus patients), the need to explain the conceptual bases of a classification, and the organization of the manual to facilitate its effectiveness for different types of users. This part ends with a chapter that outlines recent critical advances in diagnostic methodology and discusses the need for an international lingua franca on psychiatric morbidity, the prospective relationship between ICD-10 and DSM-IV, and some outstanding nosological issues, such as the definition of a mental disorder.

Part V presents an overview and a discussion of the prospects for ICD-10. It starts with an authoritative review of the historical background of ICD-10; pertinent epistemological, cognitive, and utility requirements; the principal features of ICD-10 in general and its mental-disorders component in particular; its expanded objectives encompassing patient care and scientific research in addition to public-health planning; and its combining of a core nosological classification with a family of documents serving a number of purposes. An ensuing panel discussion considers diverse key issues, including the concept of a nosological spectrum, particularly as it applies to affective and schizophreniform syndromes; the importance of hierarchically organizing a classification, for example, the number of major classes of psychiatric conditions; and the question of the conceptualization of mental disorder. Several controversial or intricate categories not classified elsewhere, such as schizoaffective disorder, delirium tremens, conversive and dissociative hysterical neuroses, anorexia nervosa, and conduct disorder, are discussed. The need for adequate attention to developmental factors and comprehensive diagnostic formulations in child psychiatry is pointed out. Also discussed are issues related to cultural demands, such as Western and non-Western culture-bound syndromes, and ways of adapting international classifications to national realities, as exemplified by the remarkable Second Cuban Glossary for ICD-9. Furthermore, attention is given to the presentation of a psychiatric classification, its basic concepts, the specificity of its diagnostic criteria, and its overall architecture.

We hope this volume will stimulate productive work on diagnostic models and procedures. The international roots of many of these developments and the scope of the population we serve demand increasing worldwide cooperation in these endeavors.

JUAN E. MEZZICH
MICHAEL VON CRANACH

Contributors

Carlos Acosta, M.D.
Professor of Psychiatry
Hospital Docente "Calixto Garcia"
Instituto Superior de Ciencias Medicas
Universidad de La Habana
Havana, Cuba

Federico Allodi, M.D.
Head, Transcultural Psychiatry Unit
Toronto Western Hospital
Toronto, Ontario, Canada

Peter Berner, M.D.
Professor of Psychiatry
Universität Wien
Vienna, Austria

Ayo Binitie, M.D.
Professor of Mental Health
University of Benin
Benin, Nigeria

Jeffrey H. Boyd, M.D., M.P.H.
Deputy Chief, Center for Epidemiological
Studies
National Institute of Mental Health
Rockville, Maryland, USA

Jack D. Burke, Jr., M.D., M.P.H.
Deputy Chief, Clinical Research Division
National Institute of Mental Health
Rockville, Maryland, USA

Jorge Castro, M.D.
Head, Department of Child and Adolescent
Psychiatry
Instituto Nacional de Salud Mental
"Honorio Delgado-Hideyo Noguchi"
Lima, Peru

Chen Changhui, M.D.
Associate Professor and Chief
Department of Social Psychiatry

Institute of Mental Health
Beijing, People's Republic of China

Donald J. Cohen, M.D.
Professor of Pediatrics, Psychiatry and
Psychology
Director, Yale University Child Study
Center
New Haven, Connecticut, USA

John E. Cooper, M.B., FRCP, FRC
Psych. DPM
Professor of Psychiatry
University of Nottingham
Nottingham, England

Michael von Cranach, M.D.
Director
Bezirkskrankenhaus Kaufbeuren
Kaufbeuren, Federal Republic of Germany

Maurice Dongier, M.D.
Professor and Chairman of Psychiatry
McGill University
Montreal, Quebec, Canada

Horacio Fabrega, Jr., M.D.
Professor of Psychiatry and Anthropology
University of Pittsburgh
Pittsburgh, Pennsylvania, USA

E. Fähndrich, M.D.
Privatdozent, Psychiatrische Klinik
Freie Universität Berlin
Berlin (West), Federal Republic of
Germany

Michael Göpfert, M.D., MRC Psych
Abteilung für Psychotherapie
Psych. Landeskrankenhaus Reichenau
Konstanz, Federal Republic of Germany

xix

Hanfried Helmchen, M.D.
Professor of Psychiatry
Freie Universität Berlin
Berlin (West), Federal Republic of
  Germany

Assen Jablensky, M.D.
Senior Medical Officer
Division of Mental Health
World Health Organization
Geneva, Switzerland

Masaaki Kato, M.D.
Professor of Psychiatry
Tokyo Medical College
Tokyo, Japan

Robert E. Kendell, M.D., FRCP, FRC
  Psych
Professor of Psychiatry
University of Edinburgh
Edinburgh, Scotland

Dr. William Kieffer
Universität Wien
Vienna, Austria

Gerald L. Klerman, M.D.
Professor of Psychiatry
Cornell University Medical College
New York, New York, USA

Morton Kramer, Sc.D.
Professor of Mental Hygiene
Johns Hopkins University
Baltimore, Maryland, USA

James F. Leckman, M.D.
Associate Professor of Psychiatry and
  Pediatrics
Associate Director, Children's Research
  Center
Yale University
New Haven, Connecticut, USA

José Leme Lopes, M.D.
Professor of Psychiatry
Universidade Federal Do Rio de Janeiro
Rio de Janeiro, Brazil

Ignacio López-Merino, M.D.
Head, Department of Adult and Geriatric
  Psychiatry
Instituto Nacional de Salud Mental
"Honorio Delgado-Hideyo Noguchi"
Lima, Peru

Ada C. Mezzich, Ph.D.
Clinical Assistant Professor of Psychiatry
University of Pittsburgh
Pittsburgh, Pennsylvania, USA

Juan E. Mezzich, M.D., Ph.D.
Professor of Psychiatry
University of Pittsburgh
Pittsburgh, Pennsylvania, USA
Visiting Professor of Psychiatry
Universidad Peruana Cayetano Heredia
Lima, Peru

P. Chr. Mussert, M.D.
Chairman, Commission for Classification
  and Documentation
European Society for Child and Adolescent
  Psychiatry
Clinic for Child and Adolescent Psychiatry
  FORNHESE
Amersfoort, The Netherlands

Ahmed Okasha, M.D.
Professor of Psychiatry
Ain Shams University
Cairo, Egypt

R. Parhee, M.D.
Senior Research Officer in Psychiatry
Indian Council of Medical Research
New Delhi, India

Rhea Paul, Ph.D.
Assistant Professor
Speech and Hearing Sciences Program
Portland State University
Portland, Oregon, USA

Pierre Pichot, M.D.
Professor of Psychiatry
Clinique des Maladies Mentals et de
  l'Encephale
Paris, France

Charles B. Pull, M.D.
Professor of Psychiatry
Centre Hospitalier de Luxembourg
Luxembourg, Luxembourg

Dr. M. C. Pull
Psychologist
Centre Hospitalier de Luxembourg
Luxembourg, Luxembourg

Darrel A. Regier, M.D., M.P.H.
Chief, Clinical Research Division
National Institute of Mental Health
Rockville, Maryland, USA

Lee N. Robins, Ph.D.
Professor of Psychiatry and Sociology
Washington University
St. Louis, Missouri, USA

Letten Saugstad, M.D.
National Case Register
Gaustad Hospital
Oslo, Norway

Fini Schulsinger, M.D.
Secretary General, World Psychiatric
  Association
Professor of Psychiatry
University of Copenhagen
Copenhagen, Denmark

Gert Semler, Dipl. Psych.
Research Psychologist
Max Planck Institut für Psychiatrie
Munich, Federal Republic of Germany

Shen Yu-cun, M.D.
Professor and Director
Institute of Mental Health
Beijing, People's Republic of China

Cecilia Sogi, M.D.
Research Psychiatrist
Instituto Nacional de Salud Mental
"Honorio Delgado-Hideyo Noguchi"
Lima, Peru

Robert L. Spitzer, M.D.
Professor of Psychiatry
Columbia University
New York, New York, USA

Costas N. Stefanis, M.D.
President, World Psychiatric Association
Professor and Chairman of Psychiatry
University of Athens
Athens, Greece

Herbert Steinböck, M.D.
Research Psychiatrist
Bezirkskrankenhaus Kaufbeuren
Kaufbeuren, Federal Republic of Germany

R.-D. Stieglitz, Dipl. Psych.
Research Psychologist
Psychiatrische Klinik
Freie Universität Berlin
Berlin (West), Federal Republic of
  Germany

Erik Strömgren, M.D.
Professor of Psychiatry
Aarhus University
Aarhus, Denmark

Fred R. Volkmar, M.D., Ph.D.
Assistant Professor of Pediatrics and
  Psychiatry
Yale University
New Haven, Connecticut, USA

Dante Warthon, M.D.
Chief, Emergency Psychiatry Service
Instituto Nacional de Salud Mental
"Honorio Delgado-Hideyo Noguchi"
Lima, Peru

Narendra N. Wig, M.D., DPM, FRC
  Psych, FAMS
Regional Adviser in Mental Health
Eastern Mediterranean Regional Office
World Health Organization
Alexandria, Egypt

Janet B. W. Williams, D.S.W.
Associate Professor of Clinical Psychiatric
  Social Work
Columbia University
New York, New York, USA

Hans-Ulrich Wittchen, Ph.D., Dipl.
  Psych.
Professor of Psychology
Max Planck Institut für Psychiatrie
Munich, Federal Republic of Germany

Michael Zaudig, M.D.
Research Psychiatrist
Bezirkskrankenhaus Kaufbeuren
Kaufbeuren, Federal Republic of Germany

PART I

Recent international and national classification systems

1 Historical roots and structural bases of the International Classification of Diseases

MORTON KRAMER (USA)

INTRODUCTION

The Tenth Revision Conference of the International Classification of Diseases (ICD) is planned for 1989, forty-one years after the Sixth Revision Conference, which approved the first ICD to contain a separate section (Section V) devoted to "Mental, Psychoneurotic and Personality Disorders." I would also like to call attention to the year of the Tenth Revision Conference, 1989. That conference will take place a few years short of a century since the adoption in 1893 of the International Statistical Classification of Causes of Death, which established the basic framework for what is now the International Statistical Classification of Diseases, Injuries, and Causes of Death.

The revisions of these classifications during the past century reflect the extraordinary advances in knowledge of the causes of diseases, injuries, and death; the changing and increasing needs of governments for morbidity and mortality statistics for monitoring, planning, and evaluating programs for the prevention and control of specific diseases and disabling conditions; and the needs of many nongovernmental professional and lay organizations for morbidity and mortality statistics for varied purposes. I also wish to emphasize that these continuous revisions are a tribute to the persistent efforts of nosologists, clinicians, epidemiologists, statisticians, and members of many other professions from many different countries, political systems, languages, and cultures to create an instrument that facilitates communication across national and international boundaries on matters relating to human health.

BASIC CONCEPTS

As background for the sections of this chapter, I should like to review two basic concepts: the definition of a classification of diseases and the distinction between a classification of diseases and a nomenclature.

Definition of a classification of diseases

As stated in the introduction to ICD-6 (World Health Organization, 1948):

3

Classification is fundamental to the quantitative study of any phenomenon. It is recognized as the basis of all scientific generalizations and is therefore an essential element in statistical methodology. Uniform definition and uniform systems of classification are prerequisites in the advancement of scientific knowledge. In the study of illness and death, therefore, a standard classification of disease and injury for statistical purposes is essential.

A classification of diseases may be defined as a system of categories to which morbid entities are assigned according to some established criteria (World Health Organization, 1977). The particular axis of classification depends upon the purpose for which the classification has been designed. Since the ICD has been designed to serve multiple purposes, there is no single axis of classification in its various sections. The axes in the various sections are discussed in a later chapter.

Distinction between a statistical classification and nomenclature of diseases

WHO issues regulations regarding nomenclature with respect to diseases and causes of death. The Nomenclature Regulations of 1967 state that the International Statistical Classification of Diseases, Injuries, and Causes of Death may be cited as the International Classification of Diseases (World Health Organization, 1977). The abridged title and its abbreviation – ICD – are used much more frequently than the complete one, and this tends to obscure the fact that the ICD is a *statistical classification of diseases and not a nomenclature of diseases*. It is essential for users of the ICD to be aware of this distinction. The introduction to ICD-6 spells out the distinction quite clearly:

The purpose of a statistical classification is often confused with that of a nomenclature. Basically, a medical nomenclature is a list or catalogue of approved terms for describing and recording clinical and pathological observations. To serve its full function it should be extensive, so that any pathological condition can be accurately recorded. As medical science advances, a nomenclature must expand to include new terms necessary to record new observations. Any morbid condition that can be specifically described will need a specific designation in a nomenclature.

This complete specificity of a nomenclature prevents it from serving satisfactorily as a statistical classification. When one speaks of statistics it is at once inferred that interest is in a group of cases and not in individual occurrences. The purpose of a statistical compilation of disease data is primarily to furnish quantitative data that will answer questions about groups of cases. . . .

A statistical classification of disease must be confined to a limited number of categories which will encompass the entire range of morbid conditions. The categories should be chosen so that they will facilitate the statistical study of disease phenomena. A specific disease entity should have a separate title in the classification only when its separation is warranted because the frequency of its occurrence, or its importance as a morbid condition, justifies its isolation as a separate category. On the other hand, many titles in the classification will refer to groups of separate but usually related morbid conditions. Every disease or morbid condition, however, must have a definite and appropriate place as an inclusion in one of the categories of the statistical classification. A few items of the statistical list will be residual titles for other and miscellaneous conditions which cannot be classified under the more specific titles. These miscellaneous categories must be kept to a minimum.

It is essential for users of ICD to be aware of the distinction between a nomenclature and a classification since clinicians, medical record librarians, and other users have expressed dissatisfaction with the ICD because it does not provide a unique code for each morbid condition. The complete ICD consists of two main volumes: Volume I, the detailed statistical classification and the codes for each rubric and its subdivisions; Volume II, an alphabetical index of all morbid conditions that provides the ICD code to which each condition should be assigned.

The concepts of a classification and nomenclature are closely related in the sense that some classifications are so detailed that they become a nomenclature. Such classifications are not generally suited for statistical analysis. More will be said about this later in the chapter.

BRIEF HISTORY OF THE DEVELOPMENT OF THE ICD AND ITS PERIODIC REVISIONS

The ICD had its roots in the International Classification of Causes of Death (also referred to as the Bertillon Classification), which was adopted by the International Statistical Institute (ISI) in Chicago in 1893 (World Health Organization, 1977). The actions that resulted in this classification started with a resolution of the International Statistical Congress in 1853, which requested William Farr, the first medical statistician of the Registrar General's Office of England and Wales, and Marc d'Espine of Geneva to prepare a uniform nomenclature of the causes of death applicable in all countries. The lists so developed were revised at four succeeding congresses. The final classification was prepared in 1891 by a committee under the chairmanship of Jacques Bertillon, chief of statistical activities of the city of Paris, and adopted by the ISI at its meeting in Chicago in 1893.

In 1899 the International Statistical Congress adopted a resolution recommending a system of decennial revisions of the International Classification of Causes of Death. This classification and its successor, the International Statistical Classification of Diseases, Injuries, and Causes of Death (ICD), have been revised regularly at approximately 10-year intervals. The First Revision Conference was held in Paris in 1900 and the Ninth in Geneva in 1975.

The revisions incorporate changes in disease classification resulting from new discoveries, the correction of errors and inconsistencies, and attempts to meet the changing and expanding needs of health and social agencies, clinicians, research workers, and consumers of health statistics for improved classifications of diseases. The Sixth Revision, in 1946, marked the beginning of a new era in international vital and health statistics (World Health Organization, 1948). This revision brought about sweeping changes in the International List of Causes of

Death and produced a single classification to serve the dual purposes of coding morbidity and mortality data. The Eighth Revision in 1967, and the Ninth in 1975, incorporated major changes in the classification of many of the major disease categories, particularly of mental disorders (World Health Organization, 1967, 1977). These changes made the organization and contents of several chapters more compatible with modern clinical concepts.

The next Revision Conference is planned for 1989 with the World Health Assembly voting to approve ICD-10 in 1990. The new classification will come into use in member states of the World Health Organization (WHO) in 1992 or 1993 (World Health Organization, 1984).

CONTENTS AND USES OF ICD

The ICD is a statistical classification not only of mental disorders but of the following conditions: Infectious, parasitic, and noninfectious diseases; complications of pregnancy, childbirth, and the puerperium; congenital abnormalities; causes of perinatal morbidity and mortality; accidents, poisonings, and violence; and symptoms, signs, and ill-defined conditions.

The principal use of the ICD is in the classification of morbidity and mortality information for statistical purposes. This use of the ICD is mandated by the Nomenclature Regulations of the World Health Organization to which member states of the WHO are party (World Health Organization, 1977): "Members compiling mortality and morbidity statistics shall do so in accordance with the current revision of the International Statistical Classification of Diseases, Injuries, and Causes of Death as adopted from time to time by the World Health Assembly."

This regulation also requires that the member states in course of compiling and publishing mortality and morbidity statistics "shall comply as far as possible with recommendations made by the World Health Assembly as to classification, coding procedures, age groupings, territorial areas to be identified, and other relevant definitions and standards" (World Health Organization, 1977).

The ICD has also been adapted for use in indexing medical records and as a nomenclature for various medical specialties. The WHO has prepared adaptations of the ICD for specific specialties (e.g., oncology, dentistry, and stomatology). The Clinical Modification of ICD-9 in the United States (ICD-9-CM) was developed to meet needs expressed by the professional medical and psychiatric associations of the United States. As stated in introduction to ICD-9-CM (Commission on Professional and Hospital Activities, 1978):

The term "clinical" is used to emphasize the modification's intent: to serve as a useful tool in the area of classification of morbidity data for indexing of medical records, medical care review, and ambulatory and other medical care programs, as well as for basic health statistics. To describe the clinical picture of the patient, the codes must be more precise than those needed only for statistical groupings and trends analysis.

Another example of the adaptation of the various revisions of the ICD is the manner in which it has been modified to accommodate the diagnostic concepts

Table 1.1. *Distribution of the three-digit categories of ICD-9 by the number of digits allocated to each chapter*

Major chapters	Digits allocated to category	No. of three-digit categories
I Infectious and parasitic disease	001–139	139
II Neoplasms	140–239	100
III Endocrine, nutritional and metabolic disorders	240–279	40
IV Diseases of blood and blood forming organs	280–289	10
V Mental disorders	290–319	30
VI Diseases of the nervous system and sense organs	320–389	70
VII Diseases of the circulatory system	390–459	70
VIII Diseases of the respiratory system	460–519	60
IX Diseases of the digestive system	520–579	60
X Diseases of the genitourinary system	580–629	50
XI Complications of pregnancy, childbirth and puerperium	630–679	50
XII Diseases of the skin and subcutaneous tissue	680–709	30
XIII Diseases of the musculoskeletal system and connective tissue	710–739	30
XIV Congenital abnormalities	740–759	20
XV Certain conditions originating in the prenatal period	760–779	20
XVI Symptoms, signs and ill-defined conditions	780–799	20
XVII Injury and poisoning	800–999	200
	Total	999

and terms of American psychiatry used in the three editions of the *Diagnostic and Statistical Manual* (American Psychiatric Association, 1952, 1968, 1980).

STRUCTURE OF THE ICD

The ICD is organized into 17 major sections, each of which is devoted to a specific set of conditions (Table 1.1). Each of these major sections is subdivided into a defined set of categories, identified by three digits ranging from 001 to 999. To provide greater detail, each such category is further divided into additional subcategories by a fourth digit (.0 to 0.9). Table 1.1 also shows the number of three-digit categories allotted to each major section. There is a considerable imbalance in these categories, as they range from 10 for diseases of the blood and blood-forming organs to 200 for injuries and poisonings. Only 30 of these three-digit categories are allotted to mental disorders, so all mental disorders must be classified within these categories and their fourth-digit subdivisions.

The structure of the classification is eclectic in that the axes of classification are not consistent within each of its 17 major sections. The primary axis is topographical in some sections (e.g., diseases of the respiratory system); less frequently, it is etiological (e.g., infectious diseases) or situational (e.g., complications of pregnancy). In other sections, still other primary axes are used, reflecting the fact that the ICD is a compromise that provides a pragmatic classification that can be used for a variety of purposes. To illustrate, the section on mental disorders of ICD-9 subdivides these disorders into the following major categories: organic conditions; other psychoses; neurotic disorders, personality disorders, and other nonpsychotic mental disorders; and mental retardation.

There are also two supplementary chapters: one for classifying external causes of injury and poisoning (the E code) and the other for classifying factors influencing health status and contact with health services (the V code). Both of these classifications contain rubrics with relevant items for agencies and facilities that provide psychiatric and mental-health services.

REVISIONS OF THE ICD

The ICD is revised regularly, at approximately 10-year intervals. This pattern was initiated with the First Revision Conference of the International List of Causes of Death held in Paris in 1900. Indeed, the revision of ICD is a continuous process. As soon as one revision is completed, and, even before, work starts on the next.

The original classification, as indicated by its title, was used solely for coding causes of death and did not provide a separate section for the mental disorders. To illustrate, in the Fifth Revision of the International List of Causes of Death (1938), the classification of mental disorders consisted of only a single three-digit rubric with four subcategories in the section "Diseases of the Nervous System and Sense Organs": (a) mental deficiency, (b) schizophrenia, (c) manic depressive psychosis, and (d) all other mental disorders. Deaths due to or associated with other mental disorders were classified elsewhere; for example, general paralysis of the insane in the section "Infectious and Parasitic Diseases"; insanity of pellagra under the section "Rheumatism, Diseases of Nutrition and of the Endocrine Glands," and so forth; alcoholic psychosis, chronic alcoholism including delirium tremens under "Chronic Poisoning and Intoxication."

The Fifth Revision Conference (1938) recognized the growing need for a classification of diseases among widely differing organizations that require morbidity statistics. Indeed, many countries were developing such lists. Accordingly, this conference recommended that a committee be formed to undertake the preparation of an International List of Diseases and, as far as possible, to bring various national lists of diseases that had already been developed into line with the detailed International List of Causes of Death. In compliance with this resolution, the U.S. State Department in 1945 appointed a U.S. Committee on Joint Causes of Death, under the chairmanship of the late Lowell J. Reed, vice-president and professor of biostatistics of the Johns Hopkins University. This

. *List of three-digit categories in Section V, mental disorders of ICD-8*

(290–299)

 and pre-senile dementia

olic psychosis

osis associated with intracranial infection

osis associated with other cerebral condition

osis associated with other physical condition

ophrenia

ive psychoses

oid states

 psychoses

ecified psychosis

ersonality disorders and other non-psychotic mental disorders (300–309)

ses

nality disorders

l deviation

lism

dependence

al disorders of presumably psychogenic origin

l symptoms not elsewhere classified

ient situational disturbances

ior disorders of childhood

l disorders not specified as psychotic associated with physical conditions

rdation (310–315)

line mental retardation

mental retardation

ate mental retardation

 mental retardation

nd mental retardation

cified mental retardation

HE ICD-8 GLOSSARY OF MENTAL DISORDERS

lthough agreement had been reached on the content and form of ICD-

fully recognized that the use of the classification per se would not

mparable international data on the mental disorders. To accomplish

 essential for the diagnostic terms allocated to each category in the

on to be used in a uniform and consistent way by the international

y of psychiatrists. Comparisons of mortality and morbidity rates may

ing and, indeed, meaningless unless the basic diagnostic data from

 rates are derived are reliable, comparable, and accurately recorded.

, communication among psychiatrists would become increasingly

 was apparent that action had to be taken to encourage uniform usage

ive and diagnostic terms in psychiatry.

committee prepared a Proposed Statistical Classification of Diseases, Injuries and Causes of Death, which was reviewed and revised by the Expert Committee for the Preparation of the Sixth Decennial Revision of the International Lists of Diseases and Causes of Death. The Conference for the Sixth Revision, convened in 1948, approved the classification prepared by this Expert Committee. ICD-6 contained the first separate section on mental disorders (Section V).

The Classification of Mental Disorders in ICD-6 was essentially the one developed for the classification of the psychiatric casualties experienced by the members of the armed forces of the United States during World War II. At the beginning of World War II, American psychiatry – civilian and military – was using the nomenclature in a diagnostic system developed primarily for the caseload of public mental hospitals. As stated in the first edition of the *Diagnostic and Statistical Manual of Mental Disorders* the American Psychiatric Association (DSM-1) (1952):

Only about 10% of the total cases seen fell into any of the categories ordinarily seen in public mental hospitals. Military psychiatrists, station psychiatrists, and Veterans Administration psychiatrists found themselves operating within the limits of a nomenclature specifically not designed for 90% of the cases handled. Relatively minor personality disturbances which became of importance only in the military setting had to be classified as "Psychopathic Personality."

Psychosomatic disorders turned up in the nomenclature under the various organ systems by whatever name gastroenterologists or cardiologists had devised for them. The psychoneurotic label had to be applied to men reacting briefly with neurotic symptoms to considerable stress; individuals who, as subsequent studies have shown, were not ordinarily psychoneurotic in the usual meaning of the term. No provision existed for diagnosing psychological reactions to the stress of combat and terms had to be invented to meet this need. The official system of nomenclature rapidly became untenable.

To meet their needs, the army abandoned the basic classification found in the Standard Nomenclature of Diseases (American Medical Association, 1938) and developed a diagnostic nomenclature and classification to cover the types of mental disorders it was encountering (Menninger, Mayman & Pryser, 1963). This nomenclature provided the basis for the U.S. revision proposals for the mental disorders section of ICD-6. At the Seventh International Revision Conference in 1955, no major revisions were made in the ICD-6 section of mental disorders.

A comparison of the classification of mental disorders in the Fifth Revision of the International List of Causes of Death (ICD-5) with the three-digit list of Mental Disorders in ICD-6 and ICD-7 is given in Table 1.2.

DEVELOPMENT OF SECTION ON MENTAL DISORDERS OF ICD-8

As part of the preparatory work for ICD-8, the WHO commissioned Professor E. Stengel to study classifications of mental disorders used in different countries and to conduct a survey to determine the acceptability and use of the

Table 1.2. *Comparison of the list of mental disorders in the Fifth Revision of the International List of Causes of Death with the corresponding list of the Sixth and Seventh Revisions of the International Classification of Diseases, Injuries, and Causes of Death*

ICD-5 (1938), Section VI, Diseases of the nervous system and sense organs	ICD-6 (1948) and ICD-7 (1955), Section V, Mental, psychoneurotic, and personality disorders
List of three-digit categories	*List of three-digit categories*
84. Mental disorders and deficiency (excluding general paralysis of the insane)	Psychoses (300–309)
a. Mental deficiency	300 Schizophrenic disorders (dementia praecox)
b. Schizophrenia (dementia praecox)	301 Manic-depressive reaction
c. Manic-depressive psychosis	302 Involutional melancholia
d. Other mental disorders	303 Paranoia and paranoid states
	304 Senile psychosis
Examples of other categories in ICD-5 that included mental disorders are:	305 Presenile psychosis
56. Alcoholism (acute or chronic)	306 Psychosis with cerebral arteriosclerosis
57. Chronic lead poisoning	307 Alcoholic psychosis
67. General paralysis of insane	308 Psychosis of other demonstrable aetiology
68. Insanity of pellagra	309 Other and unspecified psychoses
	Psychoneurotic disorders (310–318)
	310 Anxiety reaction without mention of somatic symptoms
	311 Hysterical reaction without mention of anxiety reaction
	312 Phobic reaction
	313 Obsessive-compulsive reaction
	314 Neurotic-depressive reaction
	315 Psychoneurosis with somatic symptoms (somatization reaction) affecting circulatory system
	316 Psychoneurosis with somatic symptoms (somatization reaction) affecting digestive system
	317 Psychoneurosis with somatic symptoms (somatization reactions) affecting other systems
	318 Psychoneurotic disorders, other, mixed, and unspecified types)
	Disorders of character, behaviour, and intelligence (320–326)
	320 Pathological personality
	321 Immature personality
	322 Alcoholism
	323 Other drug addiction

Table 1.2. (*continued*)

ICD-5 (1938), Section VI, Diseases of the nervous system and sense organs	ICD-6 (1... V, Ment... personal...
	324 P... d
	325 M...
	326 C... b... c...

ICD-6 Classification of Mental Disorders (Steng... sifications then in use: 11 official, semi-official... 27 other classifications that had been develop... countries of the world for use in their respective... This study revealed general dissatisfaction with... sification in all member countries of the WHO... the growing recognition that mental disorders... problem, led the WHO to make a strong app... sistance in developing a classification of mental... the ICD's shortcomings and gain general inter... sification was recognized as indispensable for i... scientific work on the mental disorders.

The response was excellent, and quite a fe... laborate with the WHO in an intensive progr... the development of revision proposals by natio... and vital statistics; bipartite or mutipartite m... developing joint proposals; the coordination o... in different regions with the programs of the... of Diseases; the convening of expert committ... matters related to specific classification proble... carry out special studies. Of particular impo... of mental disorders prepared by a Preparat... Mental Disorders. A detailed account of th... (Kramer, 1968).

The ICD-8 revision, approved by the Inte... 1965, was a considerable improvement over... product of an international effort that starte... a comprehensive classification of mental dis... disorders associated with organic and physica... in ICD. Also, a series of categories that did... mental disorders not specified as psychotic,... physical disorders of presumably psychogen... disturbances. The three-digit categories of m... in Table 1.3.

Table 1.4. *Location and subject of seminars held in conjunction with the WHO program, on Standardization of Psychiatric Diagnosis and Statistics*

Place	Year	Subject
London	1965	Functional psychoses, with emphasis on schizophrenia
Oslo	1966	Borderline psychosis, reactive psychosis
Paris	1967	Psychiatric disorders of childhood
Moscow	1968	Mental disorders of old age
Washington	1969	Mental retardation
Basle	1970	Neurotic and psychosomatic disorders
Tokyo	1971	Personality disorder and drug addiction
Geneva	1972	Summary, conclusions, recommendations, and proposals for further research

As a first step, the Mental Health Unit of the WHO appointed a working group, chaired by the late Sir Aubrey Lewis, to prepare a glossary. The draft was reviewed by leading clinicians in different countries and tested on an experimental basis. It was finalized and published in 1974 as the *Glossary of Mental Disorders and Guide to Their Classification for Use in Conjunction with ICD-8* (World Health Organization, 1974). The main purpose of the glossary was

... to ensure as far as possible that those who apply it will arrive at a uniform use of principal diagnostic terms current in psychiatry. In addition to helping to minimize discrepancies among the diagnostic concepts used by psychiatrists in different countries for statistical reporting of mental illness, use of the Glossary in publications dealing with either clinical work or research work will also assist psychiatrists from different countries and schools of thought in understanding each other's work and concepts. (World Health Organization, 1974)

DEVELOPMENT OF SECTION ON MENTAL DISORDERS OF ICD-9

Although the classification of mental disorders in ICD-8 was a considerable improvement over that in ICD-6 and ICD-7, various aspects of it were still unsatisfactory (Kramer, 1968). Therefore, in 1965 the Mental Health Unit of the WHO embarked on an intensive program to acquire systematic data on variations in diagnostic practice and the use of diagnostic terms among psychiatrists from a large number of countries representing different schools of psychiatric thought and practice (Lin, 1967; Sartorius, 1971). This program consisted of eight annual seminars on psychiatric diagnosis, classification, and statistics held annually between 1965 and 1972 (Kramer et al., 1979). Each seminar was held in a different part of the world and concentrated on a specific group of disorders (Table 1.4).

Experts from nearly forty countries took part in this program. The information gained in these seminars provided the basis for recommending that the classification be included in ICD-9. As stated by the WHO (1978):

Changes and new categories in the International Classification of Diseases (ICD-9) have been introduced only for sound reasons and after much consideration. As far as possible, the changes in chapter 5 have been based upon evidence that the new codes function better than the old ones. Some of this evidence and a large proportion of other changes based upon discussion and consideration of different viewpoints emanated from the World Health Organization's program on the Standardization of Psychiatric Diagnosis, Classification and Statistics. A central feature of this program was the series of eight international seminars held annually between 1965 and 1972, each of which focused upon a recognized problem area in psychiatric diagnosis. Psychiatrists from more than 35 countries participated, and the documents and proposals that were used to produce the recommendation for ICD-9 in the eighth and final seminar were seen and commented on by many more.

A list of the three-digit categories of mental disorders in ICD-9 is given in Table 1.5. Quite a few of the categories presented in Table 1.3 were recast and several new categories added. A detailed discussion of the differences between these classifications may be found in Kramer et al. (1979).

THE ICD-9 GLOSSARY OF MENTAL DISORDERS

A major innovation in ICD-9 was the incorporation of the glossary in the printed text of its section of mental disorders. It is the only section in the entire ICD that contains such a glossary. The reason stated in the introduction to Section V reemphasizes the points made in the introduction to the ICD-8 Glossary (1978):

This section of the Classification differs from the others in that it includes a glossary, prepared after consultation with experts from many different countries, defining the contents of the rubrics. This difference is considered to be justified because of the special problems posed for psychiatrists by the relative lack of independent laboratory information upon which to base their diagnoses. The diagnosis of many of the most important mental disorders still relies largely upon descriptions of abnormal experience and behavior, and without some guidance in the form of a glossary that can serve as a common frame of reference, psychiatric communications easily become unsatisfactory at both clinical and statistical levels.

Many well-known terms have different meanings in current use, and it is important for the user to use the glossary descriptions and not merely the category titles when searching for the best fit for the condition he is trying to code. This is particularly important if a separate national glossary also exists.

ELIMINATION OF COMBINATION CATEGORIES
FROM ICD-9

ICD-9 also differs from ICD-8 in that it does not include the so-called combination categories. These are categories for coding combined mental and

Table 1.5. *List of three-digit categories of mental disorders in ICD-9*

Organic psychotic conditions (290–294)
290 Senile and presenile organic psychotic conditions[a]
291 Alcoholic psychoses[a]
292 Drug psychoses[a]
293 Transient organic psychotic conditions[a]
294 Other organic psychotic conditions (chronic)[a]

Other psychoses (295–299)
295 Schizophrenic psychoses
296 Affective psychoses[a]
297 Paranoid states
298 Other nonorganic psychoses
299 Psychoses with organic specific to childhood[a]

Neurotic disorders, personality disorders and other nonpsychotic mental disorders (300–316)
300 Neurotic disorders
301 Personality disorders
302 Sexual deviations and disorders
303 Alcohol dependence syndrome
304 Drug dependence
305 Nondependent abuse of drugs[b]
306 Physiological malfunction arising from mental factors
307 Special symptoms or syndromes not elsewhere classified
308 Acute reaction to stress
309 Adjustment reaction[b]
310 Specific nonpsychotic mental disorders following organic brain damage
311 Depressive disorder, not elsewhere classified[b]
312 Disturbance of conduct not elsewhere classified[b]
313 Disturbance of emotions specific to childhood[b]
314 Hyperkinetic syndrome of childhood[b]
315 Specific delays in development[b]
316 Psychic factors associated with diseases classified elsewhere[b]

Mental Retardation (317–319)
317 Mild mental retardation
318 Other specified mental retardation
319 Unspecified mental retardation

[a]Categories that were recast.
[b]New categories.

physical disorders such as organic mental disorders and mental retardation. To illustrate, in certain instances in ICD-8 category designated a mental disorder associated with a specific physical condition (e.g., psychosis with cerebral arteriosclerosis). In other instances, the category consisted of a specified mental condition and a general class of associated physical disorders (e.g., moderate mental retardation following infections and intoxications). Combination cate-

Table 1.6. *Examples of coding of combination categories of mental disorders in ICD-9*

Diagnosis	Code from ICD–9	Associated condition
Organic psychosis (dementia) in general paralysis of the insane	294.1	094.1
Organic psychosis with arteriosclerosis (arteriosclerotic dementia)	290.4	437.0
Organic psychosis (dementia) with multiple sclerosis	294.1	340
Organic psychosis (dementia) with epilepsy (convulsive)	294.1	345.1
Nonpsychotic mental disorders (e.g., personality changes with convulsive epilepsy)	310.1	345.1
Psychogenic duodenal ulcer	316	532
Mental retardation, moderate, associated with rubella, congenital	318.0	771.0
Mental retardation, severe, associated with lead poisoning	318.1	984
Suicide attempt, barbiturate poisoning, as a result of neurotic depression	300.4	E950.1

Source: World Health Organization (1978).

gories such as these have been eliminated from ICD-9 and replaced by categories that require coding on two independent axes. Thus, a psychotic condition arising from a physical disorder would be classified by using two code numbers: one for the mental disorder and one for the underlying physical disease. The following are categories that require multiple coding:

Disorder	ICD–9 Codes
Senile and presenile organic psychotic conditions	290
Transient organic psychotic conditions	293
Other organic psychotic mental conditions (chronic)	294
Specific nonpsychotic mental disorder following organic brain damage	310
Physiological malfunction arising from mental factors	306
Psychic factors associated with diseases classified elsewhere	316
Mental retardation	317, 318, 319

The use of the second code requires the psychiatrist to become familiar with all of the sections of the ICD and its alphabetical index (World Health Organization, 1977a,b). The index assists in locating the code number for the associated condition. Table 1.6 provides some illustrations of how the dual codes are used.

OTHER DETAILS OF ICD-9

Several other features of the revision were also important:

1. There were several instances in which a given code number in ICD-8, when used in ICD-9, applies to quite a different condition. For example:

ICD-8		ICD-9	
Code	Condition	Code	Condition
312	Moderate mental retardation	312	Disturbance of conduct NEC
314	Profound mental retardation	314	Hyperkinetic syndrome of childhood
296.0	Involutional melancholia	296.0	Manic-depressive psychosis, depressed type
296.1	Manic-depressive manic type	296.1	Manic-depressive psychosis, manic type

It is essential for statisticians, medical record librarians, computer programmers and clinicians to be aware of these differences, particularly when comparing diagnostic distributions based on ICD-8 with those based on ICD-9.

2. There was a change in assignment of a code for a given rubric or inclusion term. For example, in ICD-8, psychosis with cerebral arteriosclerosis was included under psychosis with other cerebral conditions (ICD-8: 293.0). In ICD-9 it is coded under senile and presenile organic psychotic condition as arteriosclerotic dementia (ICD-9: 290.4); a second code is used to identify cerebral arteriosclerosis (437.0). In ICD-8, infantile autism was coded under 295.8 (schizophrenia, other).

In ICD-9, it is a subcategory of 299, a three-digit category specifically for psychoses with origin specific to childhood (299.0). In ICD-8, frigidity and impotence were coded as 305.6 (physical disorders of presumably psychogenic origin: genitourinary). In ICD-9, they are coded as 302.7 (sexual deviations and disorders: frigidity and impotence).

3. Personality disorders (ICD-9: 301) is a major category that remained exactly the same in ICD-9 and ICD-8. The WHO seminar that reviewed this condition concluded that there was insufficient new knowledge on which to base a modification of this category of disorders (Jablensky, 1976; Shepherd & Sartorius, 1974).

4. Certain changes were made in nomenclature; for example:

	ICD-8	ICD-9
290	Senile and presenile dementia	Senile and presenile *organic psychotic conditions*
291	Alcoholic psychosis	Alcoholic *psychoses*
295	Schizophrenia	Schizophrenic *psychoses*
300	Neuroses	*Neurotic disorders*

Some of these changes reflect the effort to make the categories in Chapter V of ICD-9 descriptive so that conditions showing the same symptoms are grouped together as far as possible, regardless of their etiology.

Table 1.7. *Supplementary classification of factors influencing health status and contact with health services (82 categories, including subdivisions under each of the V categories)*

Persons with potential health hazards related to communicable diseases (V01–V07)

Persons with potential health hazards related to personal and family history (V10–V19)

Persons encountering health services in circumstances related to reproduction and development (V20–V28)

Healthy liveborn infants according to type of birth (V30–V39)

Persons with a condition influencing their health status (V40–V49)

Persons encountering health services for specific procedures and aftercare (V50–V59)

Persons encountering health services in other circumstances (V60–V68)

Persons without reported diagnosis encountered during examination and investigation of individuals and populations (V70–V82)

Other changes in nomenclature were made to reflect clinical usage in the late 1970s and to allow multiple coding wherever a symptom pattern accompanies another condition without causal connections between them (e.g., transient organic psychotic conditions of different types [293] in an individual with a personality disorder [301] and of low intelligence [317]).

However, a number of terms now included in the ICD-9 Chapter V are neither defined nor described in the glossary. These terms, as well as some others in the ICD index, are under discussion in a new WHO project carried out jointly with the Council for International Organizations of Medical Sciences and the Alcohol Drug Abuse and Mental Health Administration of the United States. One part of this project will be to prepare a *Lexicon of Psychiatric and Mental Health Terms* that will serve as a companion volume to ICD-9 Section V. Its objective is to facilitate the use of synonyms, recommended terms, and inclusion terms and to discourage the use of obsolete and ambiguous terms and eponyms (World Health Organization, 1983).

THE ICD-9 SECTION ON SUPPLEMENTARY CLASSIFICATION OF FACTORS INFLUENCING HEALTH STATUS AND CONTACT WITH HEALTH SERVICES (V-CODES)

Another part of ICD-9 that is receiving increasing attention in the mental health field is the supplementary classification of factors influencing health status and contact with the health services. The codes in this section of ICD-9 – the V-codes – are particularly important in obtaining information on relevant psychosocial and environmental factors related to the problem of psychiatric morbidity and primary health care and factors that lead a person to enter the health service system. The eight major categories of this classification are shown in Table 1.7.

More will be heard about these and other classifications of psychosocial factors and environments because the WHO emphasizes the need for such classifications in primary health care, particularly in the less developed areas of the world, and the need for classifications that can be used to plan and evaluate the services provided (Gulbinat, 1985).

SUPPLEMENTARY CLASSIFICATION OF EXTERNAL CAUSES OF INJURY AND POISONING (E CODES)

This section is provided to permit the classification of environmental events, circumstances, and conditions as the cause of injury, poisoning, and other adverse effects. It contains many rubrics highly relevant to the mental health area, such as motor vehicle accidents, falls, suicide and attempted suicide, homicide, accidental poisoning, utilization of psychotropic drugs, soporifics, and other drugs that affect central nervous system function and may cause brain damage. The major categories of this section are listed in Table 1.8.

MULTIAXIAL CLASSIFICATION

A multiaxial classification system for the Mental Disorders section of the ICD was first proposed at the WHO Seminar, "Mental Disorders of Childhood," held in Paris in 1967 (Rutter et al., 1969). The condition of the child was to be recorded on three axes: clinical syndrome, intellectual level, and etiologic factors. Two years later, during a seminar in Washington on the problems in classifying mental retardation, another axis was suggested for coding associated social and cultural factors (Tarjan, Tizard, & Rutter 1972).

A number of studies initiated by the WHO have demonstrated the usefulness of the multiaxial classification internationally (Rutter, Shaffer & Shepherd, 1975). The concept of the multiaxial classification exerted a strong influence on the development of DSM-III's 5 axes of classification (American Psychiatric Association, 1980).

As mentioned earlier, in ICD-8 and ICD-9 associated physical conditions are now coded on a separate axis for organic mental disorders and several other conditions. Research is currently under way on triaxial recording of health problems present in primary care settings and on associated psychosocial environmental factors (World Health Organization, 1981, 1984).

HISTORICAL DEVELOPMENT OF CAUSAL CLASSIFICATIONS AND CLASSIFICATIONS OF PSYCHOSOCIAL FACTORS

Of particular interest is the recent emphasis on causal classifications for mental disorders. There is a long tradition in the development of such classifications, dating back to classic investigations of causes of insanity published in the nineteenth century.

Table 1.8. *Supplementary classification of external causes of injury and poisoning (1,000 categories, including subcategories under each of the major E categories)*

Railway accidents (E800–E807)
Motor vehicle traffic accidents (E810–E819)
Motor vehicle nontraffic accidents (E820–E825)
Other road vehicle accidents (E826–E829)
Water transport accidents (E830–E838)
Air and space transport accidents (E840–E845)
Vehicle accidents not elsewhere classifiable (E846–E848)
Accidental poisoning by drugs, medicaments, and biologicals (E850–E858)
Accidental poisoning by other solid and liquid substances, gases, and vapors (E860–E869)
Misadventures to patients during surgical and medical care (E870–E876)
Surgical and medical procedures as the cause of abnormal reaction of patient or later complication, without mention of misadventure at the time of procedure (E878–E879)
Accidental falls (E880–E888)
Accidents caused by fire and flames (E890–E899)
Accidents due to natural and environmental factors (E900–E909)
Accidents caused by submersion, suffocation, and foreign bodies (E910–E915)
Other accidents (E916–E928)
Late effects of accidental injury (E929)
Drugs, medicaments and biological substances causing adverse effects in therapeutic use (E930–E949)
Suicide and self-inflicted injury (E950–E959)
Homicide and injury purposely inflicted by other persons (E960–E969)
Legal intervention (E970–E978)
Injury undetermined, whether accidentally or purposely inflicted (E980–E989)
Injury resulting from operations of war (E990–E999)

Bucknill and Tuke have a fascinating chapter in their *Manual of Psychological Medicine (1858)* that reviews some of the early classifications of mental disorders and the factors believed to be associated with their causation – currently called risk factors. Table 1.9 shows several of these early classifications: that of Pinel, 1745–1826; of Esquirol, 1782–1840; of Parchappe, 1846, (Bucknill & Tuke, 1858) and one used by the British Metropolitan Commission in Lunacy, 1844 (Thurnam, 1845). These classifications contained a limited number of categories, but they represented the result of careful consideration of how to characterize types of insanity manifested by patients admitted to the asylums where these pioneers in psychiatric nosology worked.

Considerable effort was also made to determine the causes of insanity. It is interesting to note the classification of causes of insanity as presented during the early 1800s in the writings of two famous French alienists – Esquirol and Parchappe (Bucknill & Tuke, 1858). Causes were subdivided into two major categories: predisposing and exciting. Among the predisposing causes were

Table 1.9. *Comparisons of several early classifications of mental disorders*

Pinel (1745–1826)	Esquirol (1782–1840)	England Metropolitan Commission in Lunacy (1844)	Parchappe (1846)
Melancholia	Lypemania	Partial insanity (so-called)	Acute mania
Mania	Monomania	I. Moral insanity	Acute melancholia
Dementia	Mania	II. Monomania	Acute monomania
Idiocy	Dementia	III. Melancholia	Chronic insanity
	Imbecility	General insanity	Insanity with paralysis
		IV. Mania	Insanity with epilepsy
		1. Acute mania (raving madness)	Idiocy
		2. Ordinary mania (chronic madness) (with comparatively lucid intervals)	Idiocy, epileptic
		3. Periodical or remitment mania (with comparatively lucid intervals)	
		V. Dementia (decay and obliteration of the intellectual faculties)	
		1. Imbecility (acquired)	
		2. fatuity (confirmed dementia)	
		VI. Amentia	
		1. idiocy (congenital)	
		2. imbecility (congenital)	
		VII. Delirium tremens (where, as in the U.S., this is regarded as a form of insanity and is treated in hospitals for the insane)	

Table 1.10. *Distribution of admissions to Parchappe's institution (about 1830) as rearranged by Bucknill and Tuke (1858)*

Physical causes		Moral causes	
Epilepsy	68	Disappointed affections	53
Intemperance	164	Domestic troubles	241
Vice and immorality	40	Domestic grief	88
Injuries to head and spine	4	Religious anxiety and excitement	56
Disease of brain	14	Political and other excitement	34
Other diseases	18	Wounded feelings	84
Uterine and childbearing	45	Fright	48
Old age	8	Overstudy	8
Mercury	3		
	364		612

hereditary disposition, sex, age, seasons, life-style, occupation, and marriage. The exciting causes were subdivided into moral and physical. Among the moral were disappointed affections, domestic troubles, and grief; and among the physical were epilepsy, intemperance, and diseases of the brain. Table 1.10 provides a distribution of physical and moral causes of insanity among admissions to the asylum where Parchappe gathered his data about 1830 (Bucknill & Tuke, 1858).

Moral causes were considerably more frequent than physical. The leading moral cause was domestic troubles; the leading physical cause, intemperance. When both moral and physical causes were combined, the following rank order resulted:

Among males	Among females
1. Abuse of alcoholic drinks	1. Domestic troubles
2. Reverse of fortune	2. Loss of friends
3. Domestic troubles	3. Reverse of fortune
4. Loss of friends	4. Abuse of alcoholic drinks

Tabulations were also made to demonstrate the relative importance of each cause for each type of disorder. There was so much interest in the subject of physical and moral causes that Bucknill and Tuke carried out an international study analyzing about 30,000 cases admitted into a large number of asylums in England, France, and America. They reported (Bucknill & Tuke, 1858):

On the whole, we have found a very marked agreement between the gross results of the asylums whose statistics we have consulted. . . .

In the first place, we find that, among moral causes, domestic troubles or grief, stand first on the list in every instance; next in order stands religious anxiety or excitement; then disappointed affections; fourthly, political and other excitement; fifthly, fear and fright; and lastly we have excess of study; and wounded feelings (as wounded self, love, etc.).

Secondly, as regards physical causes, we observe that, with one exception, intemperance ranks first in the scale; while in the second, epilepsy and disorders more or less connected with the uterus are equally productive of insanity; in the third rank are other diseases than those just mentioned; vicious indulgences follow in order of frequency; lastly, succeed affections of the head and spine, whether ideopathic or traumatic.

These early classifications exerted considerable influence on the types of statistics published on patients admitted to mental institutions, and their use persisted for a considerable period of time. Examples may be found in the early reports of the English Commissioners in Lunacy on causes of insanity in patients admitted to the asylums in England and Wales during 1878 and 1887 (Tuke, 1892) and in tables in the annual reports of the State of New York Department of Mental Hygiene on causes of mental disease among first admissions to the Civil State Hospitals of New York as late as 1951 (New York State, 1952) (Tables 1.11 and 1.12).

Contemporary studies of factors that account for high utilization rates of mental health services and epidemiologic studies of factors associated with high prevalence rates of mental disorders still point to "abuse of alcohol, loss of fortune, loss of friends and domestic problems" as major risk factors for mental disorders (Kramer et al., 1983; Pollack, 1975; World Health Organization, 1976).

The classifications of moral and physical causes of insanity developed in the early 1800s are the "roots" of classifications of psychosocial factors and life events that investigators are still endeavoring to develop in the quest for causes of mental disorder and social and behavioral factors that influence an individual's health status, his or her decision to obtain health and mental health care, and the outcome of treatment received (Deliege-Rott, 1983; World Health Organization, 1981, 1984).

COMPUTER-GENERATED DIAGNOSES OF SPECIFIC MENTAL DISORDERS FROM STRUCTURED INTERVIEWS

One of the important developments in the continuing effort to obtain uniform and consistent diagnostic data has been the use of the computer to generate diagnoses of specific mental disorders from responses to a structured interview administered by a lay interviewer. A current example of this procedure is the use of the Diagnostic Interview Schedule in the surveys of the Epidemiologic Catchment Area Program of the National Institute of Mental Health (Robins et al., 1984; Regier et al., 1984). This instrument operationalized the diagnostic criteria for a set of specific disorders as given in the DSM-III. A well-trained lay interviewer administers a questionnaire that contains questions relevant to each diagnosis. The responses are analyzed by a computer programmed with algorithms that determine whether a subject fulfills the operationalized criteria for a set of DSM-III diagnoses. These include major affective disorders (major depressive disorders, bipolar disorders, and dysthymia); panic

Table 1.11. *Causes of insanity in patients admitted into the asylums and registered hospitals in England and Wales, 1878–87*

Cases of insanity	Proportions percent to the admissions		
	Male	Female	Total
Moral:			
Domestic trouble (including loss of relatives and friends)	4.2	9.7	7.0
Adverse circumstances (including business anxieties and pecuniary difficulties)	8.2	3.7	5.9
Mental anxiety and "worry" (not included under the above two heads) and overwork	6.6	5.5	6.0
Religious excitement	2.5	2.9	2.7
Love affairs (including seduction)	0.7	2.5	1.6
Fright and nervous shock	0.9	1.9	1.4
Physical:			
Intemperance in drink	19.8	7.2	13.4
Intemperance (sexual)	1.0	0.6	0.7
Venereal disease	0.8	0.2	0.5
Self-abuse (sexual)	2.1	0.2	1.2
Overexertion	0.7	0.4	0.5
Sunstroke	2.3	0.2	1.2
Accident or injury	5.2	1.0	3.0
Pregnancy	—	1.0	0.5
Parturition and the puerperal state	—	6.7	3.4
Lactation	—	2.2	1.1
Uterine and ovarian diseases	—	2.3	1.2
Puberty	0.2	0.6	0.4
Change of life	—	4.0	2.0
Fevers	0.7	0.5	0.6
Privations and starvation	1.7	2.1	1.9
Old age	3.8	4.6	4.2
Other bodily diseases or disorders	11.1	10.5	10.8
Previous attacks	14.3	18.9	16.6
Hereditary influence ascertained	19.0	22.1	20.5
Congenital defect ascertained	5.1	3.5	4.3
Other ascertained causes	2.3	1.0	1.7
Unknown	21.3	20.1	20.7

Note: The above table is based upon 136,478 admissions (male, 66,918; female, 69,560). These totals represent the entire number of instances in which the several causes (either alone or in combination with other causes) were stated to have produced the mental disorder. The aggregate of these totals (including "unknown") exceeds the total number of patients admitted. The excess is due to combinations (see *Forty-third Report of the Commissioners*, 1889, p. 67).

Source: Tuke (1892).

Table 1.12. *Causes of mental disease among first admissions to the civil state hospitals in New York, 1951*

Causes	Number of Cases			Percent		
	Males	Females	Total	Males	Females	Total
Alcohol[a]	1,232	364	1,596	16.0	4.7	10.3
Syphilis	306	128	434	4.0	1.6	2.8
Drugs	48	56	104	0.6	0.7	0.7
Temperamentally abnormal makeup[a]	2,513	2,511	5,024	32.7	32.2	32.4
Injury to head[a]	142	40	182	1.8	0.5	1.2
Physical illness[a]	427	393	820	5.6	5.0	5.3
Senility	1,214	1,925	3,139	15.8	24.7	20.3
Arteriosclerosis	2,145	2,209	4,354	27.9	28.3	28.1
Epilepsy[a]	152	111	263	2.0	1.4	1.7
Death in family[a]	56	172	228	0.7	2.2	1.4
Loss of employment or financial loss[a]	69	49	118	0.9	0.6	0.8
Disappointment in love[a]	27	124	151	0.4	1.6	1.0
Pregnancy[a]	—	20	20	—	0.3	0.1
Childbirth[a]	—	90	90	—	1.2	0.6
Involution[a]	389	836	1,225	5.1	10.7	7.9
Other specified causes	111	93	204	1.4	1.2	1.3
Unascertained	605	745	1,350	7.9	9.6	8.7
Total first admissions[a]	7,678	7,801	15,479	—	—	—

[a]As one or more etiological factors may be reported in a given case, the total of such factors exceeds the number of first admissions.

Source: New York Department of Mental Hygiene, 1952.

disorder; phobic disorders; schizophrenic disorders (schizophrenia and schizophreniform disorders); alcohol use disorder (alcohol abuse/dependence); substance use disorder (substance abuse/dependence); antisocial personality; obsessive compulsive disorder; anorexia nervosa; and somatization disorder.

The data so generated have been used to obtain prevalence rates of specific mental disorders by age, sex, and other sociodemographic factors. To emphasize that these diagnoses were not obtained by a clinical examination of the subject by a psychiatrist using DSM-III criteria, they have been characterized as DIS/DSM-III disorders. A major contribution of the use of the DIS in the ECA surveys is that they have yielded a set of prevalence and utilization rates that are based on diagnostic data derived in a uniform and comparable way in five different sites in the United States, a major achievement in its own right (Meyers et al., 1984; Robins et al., 1981; Shapiro et al., 1984). There is, however, ongoing debate as to the meaning of DIS/DSM-III diagnoses in comparison with diagnoses obtained on samples of the same subjects when interviewed by a psychiatrist (Burke, 1986). Several major studies have demonstrated that the degree of agreement between clinicians' DSM-III diagnoses and the DIS/DSM-II diagnoses are not particularly high (Anthony et al., 1985; Helzer et al., 1985).

Important questions remain to be answered about computer-derived diagnoses such as DIS/DSM-III diagnoses. Has the use of the DIS procedure produced a set of new psychiatric diagnoses? Should a DIS/DSM-III diagnosis of a specific disorder (e.g., schizophrenia, a major affective disorder) be allocated to the section of the ICD designed for classifying that diagnosis? Should separate rubrics be developed for classifying diagnoses generated by computer analyses of responses to structured interviews?

These are questions that need to be given careful consideration by the World Psychiatric Association Section on Nomenclature and Classification and the Committee developing the proposals for the Mental Disorder Section of ICD-10 and its accompanying glossary.

DISCUSSION AND SUMMARY

This chapter has reviewed the events and activities that were involved in the development of the first International Classification of Mental Disorders in ICD-6, approved by the World Health Assembly in 1948, and its subsequent decennial revisions, the last being ICD-9, approved in 1975.

Activities are now under way to revise ICD-9. The revision of ICD-9 is responding to pressures exerted over the years by the international community of psychiatrists to produce a more detailed classification that will be essentially a nomenclature of mental disorders within the framework of the ICD and reflect modern clinical concepts. This will satisfy the needs of clinicians, medical record librarians, medical care programs, statisticians, epidemiologists, and others for a detailed listing of terms used in clinical psychiatry. The advantage of developing this nomenclature within the framework of the ICD is that the detailed listings can be collapsed into broader groups for statistical purposes.

Activities have also been initiated to develop classifications of psychosocial and behavioral factors that influence an individual's health status and his or her decision to obtain health and mental health care and the outcome of treatment. Illustrations of the roots of such classifications are provided in the research of Esquirol and Parchappe during the early 1800s.

Computers are now being used in epidemiologic surveys to generate uniform and consistent diagnostic data from responses to structured interviews administered by trained lay interviewers. An example is the use of the Diagnostic Interview Schedule in the Epidemiologic Catchment Area Surveys of the U.S. National Institute of Mental Health (NIMH). This instrument operationalized the criteria for selected diagnoses given in the DSM-III. Questions are raised as to whether the classification of diagnoses so generated requires special consideration in the forthcoming ICD-10.

All of the activities that have been developed and implemented over the years and those that are continuing to improve the International Classification of Mental Disorders are a model of international collaboration. To adapt a sentence in the report of the Copenhagen Conference to the activities that WHO has initiated and implemented to achieve an internationally acceptable nomenclature and classification of mental disorders (WHO/ADAMHA, 1983) – these activities have demonstrated that "international collaboration on a worldwide scale in the mental health field can be both feasible and fruitful when geared to a topic of universal concern and scientific importance."

REFERENCES

American Medical Association. 1938. Standard Nomenclature of Disease. Edited by E. P. Jordon. Chicago: American Medical Association.

American Psychiatric Association. 1952. *Diagnostic and Statistical Manual (DSM-I)*. Washington, D.C.

American Psychiatric Association. 1968. *Diagnostic and Statistical Manual*, 2nd ed. *(DSM-II)*. Washington, D.C.

American Psychiatric Association. 1980. *Diagnostic and Statistical Manual of Mental Disorders*, 3rd ed., *DSM-III*. Washington, D.C.

Anthony, J. C., Folstein, M., Romanoski, A. J., Von Korff, M. R., Mestadt, G. R., Chahal, R., Merchant, A., Brown, C. H., Shapiro, W., Kramer, M., and Gruenberg, E. M. 1985. Comparison of the lay Diagnostic Interview Schedule and a standardized psychiatric diagnosis: Experience in eastern Baltimore. *Archives of General Psychiatry* 42: 667–675.

Bucknill, J. C., and Tuke, D. H. 1858. *A manual of psychological medicine: A facsimile of the 1858 edition published under the auspices of the Library of the New York Academy of Medicine*. New York: Hafner.

Burke, J. 1986. Diagnostic categorization by the Diagnostic Interview Schedule (DIS): A comparison with other methods of assessment. In *The Community: Findings from Psychiatric Epidemiology*, ed. J. Barrett and R. Rose. New York: Guilford Press.

Commission on Professional Hospital Activities. 1978. *ICD-9-CM: International Classification of Diseases Ninth Revision Clinical Modification (Volume 1)*. Michigan: Edward Brothers.

Deliege-Rott, D. 1983. Indicators of physical, mental and social well being. Technical Report MNH/82.5. Geneva: World Health Organization.

Esquirol, J. E. D. 1845. *Mental Maladies: A Treatise on Insanity*. New York: Hafner.

Gulbinat, W. 1985. Mental Health Problem Assessment and Information Support: Directions of WHO's Work. *World Health Statistics Quarterly* 36: 224–233.

Helzer, J. E., McEvay, L. T., Robins, L. N., Spitznagel, E., Stoltzman, R. K., Farmer, A., and Brockington, I. F. 1985. Results of the St. Louis ECA Physician Reexamination Study of the DIS Interview. *Archives of General Psychiatry* 42: 657–666.

Jablensky, A. 1976. Personality disorders and their relationship to illness and social deviance. *Psychiatric Annals* 8: 375–386.

Kramer, M. 1968. The historical background of ICD-8. Introduction in *American Psychiatric Association: DSM-III Diagnostic and Statistical Manual*, pp. xi–xvi. Washington, D.C.: American Psychiatric Association.

Kramer, M., Pollack, E. S., Redick, R., and Locke, B. Z. 1972. *Mental Disorders/Suicide*. Vital and Health Statistics Monographs, American Public Health Association. Cambridge, Mass.: Harvard University Press.

Kramer, M., Sartorius, N., Jablensky, A., and Gulbinat, W. 1979. The ICD-9 classification of mental disorders: A review of its development and contents. *Acta Psychiatrica Scandinavica* 59: 241–262.

Kramer, M., Skinner, E. A., German, P. S., and Anthony, J. C. 1983. Marital status, household composition and living arrangements as predictors of mental disorder prevalence. Presented at Annual Meeting of the American Public Health Association, Dallas, Texas.

Lin, T.-Y. 1967. The epidemiological study of mental disorders. *WHO Chronicle* 21: 509–516.

Menninger, K., Mayman, M., and Pryser, P. 1963. *The Vital Balance: Life Processes in Mental Health and Illness*. New York: Viking Press.

Myers, J. K., Weissman, M. M., Tischler, G. L., Holzer, C. E., Leaf, P. J., Orvaschel, H., Anthony, J. C., Boyd, J. H., Burke, J. E., Kramer, M., and Stoltzman, R. 1984. Six-month prevalence of psychiatric disorders in three communities: 1980 to 1982. *Archives of General Psychiatry* 41: 959–967.

New York State, Department of Mental Hygiene. 1952. Sixty-third Annual Report for the year ended March 31, 1951. Legislative Document (1952) No. 86. Albany.

Parchappe, M. 1893. *Recherches statistiques sur les causes de l'alienation mentale*. Roven: D. Briere.

Pollack, E. S. 1975. Mental health indices of family health. *World Health Statistics Report* 28: 278–294.

Regier, D. A., Myers, J. K., Kramer, M., Robins, L. N., Blazer, D. G., Hough, R. L., Eaton, W. W., and Locke, B. Z. 1984. The NIMH Epidemiologic Catchment Area Program: Historical context, major objectives, and study population characteristics. *Archives of General Psychiatry* 41: 934–941.

Robins, L. N., Helzer, J. E., Croughan, J., and Ratcliff, K. S. 1981. National Institute of Mental Health Diagnostic Interview Schedule: Its history, characteristics, and validity. *Archives of General Psychiatry* 38: 381–389.

Rutter, M., Lebovici, S., Eisenberg, L., Sneznevsky, A. V., Sadoun, R., Brooke, E., and Lin, T.-Y. 1969. A tri-axial classification of mental disorders in childhood. *Journal of Child Psychology and Psychiatry* 10: 41–61.

Rutter, M., Shaffer, D., and Shepherd, M. 1975. *A Multiaxial Classification of Child Psychiatric Disorders*. Geneva: World Health Organization.

Sartorius, N. 1971. The epidemiological approach to psychiatric disorders. *Acta Paedopsychiatrica* 38: 335–345.

Shapiro, S., Skinner, E. A., Kessler, L. G., Von Korff, M., German, P. S., Tischler, G. L., Leaf, P. J., Benham, L., Cottier, L., and Regier, D. A. 1984. Utilization of health and mental health services: Three epidemiologic catchment area sites. *Archives of General Psychiatry* 41: 971–978.

Shepherd, M., and Sartorius, N. 1974. Personality disorders and the ICD. *Psychological Medicine*. 4: 141–146.

Stengel, E. 1959. Classification of Mental Disorders. *Bulletin of the WHO* 21: 601–663.

Tarjan, G., Tizard J., and Rutter, M. 1972. Classification and mental retardation: Issues arising in the Fifth WHO Seminar on Psychiatric Diagnosis, Classification and Statistics. *American Journal of Psychiatry* 128 (Suppl.): 34–35.

Thurnam, J. 1845. *Statistics of Insanity*. Reprint Edition, 1976. New York: Arno Press.

Tuke, D. H. 1982. Statistics of Insanity. In *A Dictionary of Psychological Medicine*, ed. D. H. Tuke (Reprint Edition 1976). New York: Arno Press. (Available from Ayer Publishing Co.).

WHO/ADAMHA. 1983. Research report: Diagnosis and classification of mental disorders and alcohol-drug-related problems: A research agenda for the 1980's. *Psychological Medicine* 13: 907–921.

World Health Organization. 1948. *Manual of the International Statistical Classification of Diseases, Injuries and Causes of Death* (6th Revision). Geneva: World Health Organization.

World Health Organization. 1967. *Manual of the International Statistical Classification of Diseases, Injuries and Causes of Death*. Based on the recommendations of the Eighth Revision Conference, 1965 and adopted by the Nineteenth World Health Assembly.

World Health Organization. 1974. *Glossary of Mental Disorders and Guide to Their Classification*. For use in conjunction with the International Classification of Diseases (8th Revision). Geneva: World Health Organization.

World Health Organization. 1975. *Mental Health Indices of Family Health. World Health Statistics Report*. No. 28. Geneva: World Health Organization.

World Health Organization. 1977. *International Classification of Diseases: Manual of the International Statistical Classification of Diseases, Injuries and Causes of Death* (9th Revision). Geneva: World Health Organization.

World Health Organization. 1978. *Mental Disorders: Glossary and Guide to Their Classification in Accordance with the Ninth Revision of the International Classification of Diseases*. Geneva: World Health Organization.

World Health Organization. 1981. *Current State of Diagnosis and Classification in the Mental Health Field*. WHO Publication MNH/81. Geneva: World Health Organization.

World Health Organization. 1983. *Lexicon of Psychiatric and Mental Health Terms: A Companion to the ICD-9 Classification and Glossary of Mental Disorders*. WHO Publication MNH/83.9 Draft. Geneva: World Health Organization.

World Health Organization. 1984. *Informal Consultation on Proposals for the Classification of Mental Disorders and Psychosocial Factors in ICD-10*. WHO/MNH/MEP/84.1. Geneva: World Health Organization.

2 Brazilian contributions to diagnostic systems in psychiatry

JOSÉ LEME LOPES (Brazil)

During its early development, Brazilian psychiatry was strongly influenced by the French school. In 1852, when the Hospicio (Asylum) Pedro II was opened, its director, Dr. Pereira das Neves, traveled to France intending to specialize in the treatment of mental diseases. A few years later Dr. Manuel Fernandes Eiras, founder of a private sanitarium in Rio de Janeiro in 1864, also visited Paris for the purpose of enriching his psychiatric knowledge. His son Dr. Carlos Eiras stayed in Paris, working with Magnan in Sainte Anne (Leme Lopes, 1965).

In 1887 João Carlos Teixeira Brandão was appointed as the first chairman of a psychiatric department at a medical school in Rio de Janeiro (Brandão, 1897). He, too, was a follower of the French school of psychiatry. His diagnostic system entailed comparing the patient's mental status with recognized patterns of mental disease. This diagnostic approach was continued by his successor, Henrique Roxo (Roxo, 1938). Their "decision tree" method was an early system of differential diagnosis, similar to that now outlined in the DSM-III (American Psychiatric Association, 1980).

In 1904, Dr. Juliano Moreira was appointed director of the National Asylum in Rio de Janeiro. Owing to his efforts, the Kraepelinian psychiatric system was introduced into Brazil. In 1905 Moreira and Peixoto wrote the first Brazilian papers on manic-depressive psychosis and paranoia (Leme Lopes, 1961, 1980).

In 1908 the Brazilian Society of Neurology, Psychiatry, and Legal Medicine was founded. One of its first tasks was to elaborate a classification of mental diseases (Leme Lopes, 1949). Although not well systematized, this classification included the following 14 categories:

1. Infectious psychoses
2. Autotoxic psychoses
3. Heterotoxic psychoses (alcoholism, morphinism, cocainism, etc.)
4. Dementia praecox
5. Chronic, systematized delusions and paraphrenia
6. Paranoia
7. Manic-depressive (or periodical) psychosis, one form predominantly manic, one predominantly depressive, and one mixed
8. Involutional psychosis
9. Cerebral injury psychoses and final dementias (arteriosclerosis and cerebral lues)

10. General paresis
11. Epileptic psychosis
12. "Neurotic" psychosis (hysteria, neurasthenia, chorea)
13. Constitutional psychopathies (degenerative atypical states)
14. Imbecility and idiocy

This remained the official classification system until 1935, when the National Service of Mental Diseases introduced some modifications. Despite the revision, however, the old designation "dementia praecox" was preserved in lieu of the newer term "schizophrenia."

In 1948 the Brazilian Society of Neurology, Psychiatry, and Legal Medicine reformed the national classification system and proposed a table with 13 categories and 37 forms of mental disorder (Leme Lopes, 1949). This new nosological scheme included the following:

  I. Infectious psychoses
     A. Psychoses due to infections
     B. Postinfection mental deterioration
  II. Autotoxic psychoses
     A. Metabolic
     B. Endogenic
     C. Associated
  III. Heterotoxic psychoses
     A. Alcoholism
     B. Toxicomanias
     C. Professional
     D. Other
  IV. Schizophrenias
     A. Schizophrenic forms
     B. Paraphrenic forms
     C. Chronic hallucinatory forms
  V. Manic-depressive psychosis
     A. Manic states
     B. Depressive states
     C. Mixed states
     D. Cyclothymic states
  VI. Aging psychoses
     A. Involutional psychosis
     B. Senile psychosis
     C. Special forms of senile dementia
  VII. Lesional cerebral psychoses
     A. Commotion
     B. Cerebral arteriosclerosis
     C. Cerebral syphilis
     D. Mental disorders in the course of neurological diseases
  VIII. General Paresis
     A. Typical forms
     B. Atypical forms
  IX. Epilepsy

        A. Genuine epilepsy
        B. Symptomatic epilepsy
   X. Psychoneuroses
        A. Hysteria
        B. Compulsive states
        C. Neurasthenic states
        D. Psychogenic reactions
  XI. Psychopathic personalities
        A. Disharmonious types
        B. Parahedonic types
        C. Complex psychopathic types
  XII. Oligophrenias
        A. Endogenous mental deficiency
        B. Special forms
 XIII. Without diagnosis
        A. Not diagnosed
        B. In observation

This classification system was adopted with few modifications by the National Service of Mental Diseases and retained until a chapter including the mental disorders was incorporated into the International Classification of Diseases. Subsequently, both ICD-8 and ICD-9 were adopted as the official diagnostic system for Brazilian psychiatry.

Thus, from its inception the psychiatric classification system in Brazil emphasized differential diagnoses. In most instances, the patient was forced to fit into a single diagnostic pattern. Such a process made it possible to assign a label, but this did not adequately describe the complexities of the patient's condition.

I expounded on this dilemma by affirming that in psychiatry it is almost impossible to make a unidirectional diagnosis. The results of this work were brought together in a monograph, "The Dimensions of Psychiatric Diagnosis" (Leme Lopes, 1954).

The starting point of this approach was the discrimination of those elements that are integrated in one diagnosis and can be obtained either in a clinical interview (mental examination) or by objective anamnesis. The patient's mental state (psychopathology) was considered to be primordial information. This was to be complemented by information on other elements – constitution (physical makeup) and somatic state (organic and functional condition) – and by psychological test results. Finally, the anamnesis, involving both personal and family history, could be investigated by the social service.

These two main sources of information were used to develop and propose three dimensions: syndrome, premorbid personality, and etiological constellation.

First, mental disorders are manifested by syndromes, for example, mania depression, delusions, and anxiety attacks. Syndrome is the immediate expression of the psychopathology, in other words, the psychopathology itself. Mental disorder is expressed through a syndromic face.

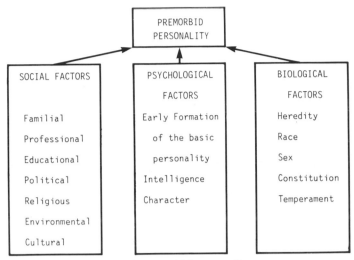

Figure 2.1. The roots of premorbid personality

At present, the psychiatrist works not with diseases but with syndromes, for which many classifications exist. It is not my intention to review this subject here, but the reader should recognize that the combination of signs and symptoms, the syndromic exteriorization, must be carefully evaluated to achieve a proper diagnosis.

The second dimension, which focuses on the premorbid personality, includes all of those biological, psychological, and social factors that contribute to the development of a personality. This dimension must also be evaluated thoroughly and completely. Genetics, sex, age, physical constitution, health conditions (particularly neurological problems, which can be assessed with either an EEG, CAT, or PET), and all other potentially noxious factors in the background of the individual – from conception until the moment of the interview – must be taken into consideration. Such forces, with their reciprocal interaction, constitute the biological basis of personality.

Included in this dimension are all the psychological factors resulting from influences during the period of nursing and early maternal care: house, neighborhood, and school influences occurring during childhood and all the experiences surrounding the individual during adolescence and early adulthood. The patient's intellectual quotient, psychological skills, handicaps, and character traits must all be considered facets of the premorbid personality. Social, familial, educational, professional, economic, political, and religious factors must also be included and analyzed within the context of a particular environment (rural, suburban, urban).

Thus, the premorbid personality results from the sum of these many interrelated factors (see Figure 2.1).

The third dimension – the etiological constellation – has been classically divided into endogenous and exogenous factors. But the concept of endogeneity

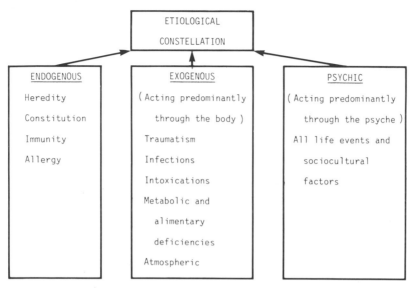

Figure 2.2. The elements of the etiological constellation

is not well formulated. Such antecedents as genetic, gestational, birth, and early childhood events do not appear to sufficiently explain the endogenous element. Tellenbach (1961) has proposed an *Endon* as a biological element underlying the innate condition.

The exogenous factor acts on the mind through the body. Trauma (especially of a cranio-encephalic type), infectious diseases, intoxication (with an emphasis on alcoholism and drug addictions), metabolic disorders, visceral decompensations, and nutritional or alimentary deficiencies are the major etiological factors of an exogenous type (see Figure 2.2).

Three levels of diagnostic evaluation are involved in arriving at a psychiatric diagnosis. Contributing to these levels are the following clinical items:

    0. Chief complaint
    1. Present state history
    2. Personal history
    3. Family history
    4. Psychiatric examination
    5. Medical examination
    6. Constitution
    7. Laboratory tests
    8. Psychological tests

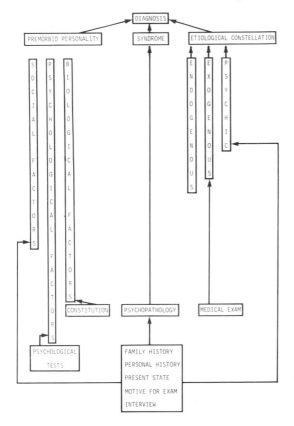

Figure 2.3 The diagnostic process

The organization of these three levels is illustrated below. Clinical procedures contributing to each level are indicated by the numbered items.

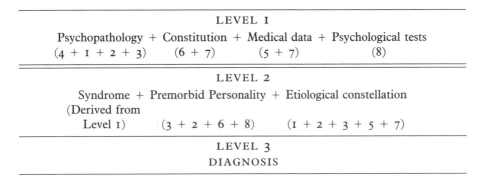

LEVEL 1			
Psychopathology +	Constitution +	Medical data +	Psychological tests
(4 + 1 + 2 + 3)	(6 + 7)	(5 + 7)	(8)

LEVEL 2		
Syndrome +	Premorbid Personality +	Etiological constellation
(Derived from		
Level 1)	(3 + 2 + 6 + 8)	(1 + 2 + 3 + 5 + 7)

LEVEL 3
DIAGNOSIS

A diagnostic evaluation proceeds through the three levels in the following manner: The first step is the result of integrating existent psychopathology with the physical constitution and information from the medical record (including the results of laboratory and psychological tests). In the second step, the premorbid personality and the etiological constellation are considered together with the syndrome derived from the first level. This produces the third level, the diagnosis. The model in Figure 2.3 demonstrates the dynamics of this process.

As indicated at the bottom of Figure 2.3, the interview initially consists of the motive examination, the present mental state, and the personal and family histories. Those elements constituting the premorbid personality are illustrated to the left in Figure 2.3. To the right are the etiological factors: endogenous, exogenous, and psychological. The syndrome, which is deduced from the psychopathology, is in the center. All of these factors interrelate to produce the diagnosis, as presented in the model.

Numeric codes have not been proposed for any dimensions. Rather, my intention was to arrive at a multidimensional diagnostic framework that could be compared with the items of current international classifications.

SUMMARY

Brazilian contributions to the field of psychiatric diagnosis are reviewed, and a three-dimensional system of diagnosis is proposed. The dimensions or axes presented include the syndrome, the premorbid personality, and the etiological constellation.

REFERENCES

American Psychiatric Association. 1980. *Diagnostic and Statistical Manual of Mental Disorders*. 3rd ed. (DSM-III). Washington, D.C.

Brandão, J. C. T. 1897. *Os alienados no Brasil*. Rio de Janeiro: Imprensa Nacional.

Leme Lopes, J. 1949. Subsídio à revisão da Classificação brasileira das doenças mentais. *Arq. Ass. Psicopatas Estado de São Paulo*. 143: 70–78.

Leme Lopes, J. 1954. *As dimensões do diagnóstico psiquiátrico*. Rio de Janeiro: Agir.

Leme Lopes, J. 1965. A psiquiatria e o velho Hospício. *J. Bras. Psiq*. 14: 117–130.

Roxo, H. 1938. *Manual de Psychiatria*. Rio de Janeiro: Liv. Francisco Alves.

Tellenbach, H. 1961. *Melancholie*. Berlin: Springer.

3 The French approach to psychiatric classification

CHARLES B. PULL (Luxembourg), M. C. PULL
(Luxembourg), AND PIERRE PICHOT (France)

INTRODUCTION

The French approach to psychiatric classification cannot be understood without some knowledge of developments in both German and French psychiatry between 1880 and World War I (e.g., Pichot, 1982, 1983, 1984). By 1880 the clinical approach, with its emphasis on evolution, was becoming the basic principle on which Magnan and Serieux (1893) in France and Kraepelin (1896) in Germany were beginning to build psychiatric classifications. For reasons that are too complex to discuss in this chapter, the Kraepelinian system eventually came to be accepted throughout the world, whereas Magnan's nosology survived exclusively in those few, although important, peculiarities that have continued to differentiate French psychiatric thinking from other standard national or international concepts and terminology since the beginning of this century.

Although Kraepelinian psychiatry gradually established its position, even in France, the shift from Magnan's nosology to Kraepelin's system was slow and difficult. The concept of "manic-depressive insanity" was the first to be accepted, obviously because it was already implicit in the constructions of Falret (1854) and Baillarger (1854). In contrast, the concept of "dementia praecox" could not be accommodated within the conceptual system of French nosology. The French reluctantly accepted Kraepelin's terminology, but at the same time they kept dementia praecox separate from not only the bulk of acute delusional states (*bouffées délirantes*) but also a number of chronic delusional states (*délires chroniques*) that had been incorporated by Kraepelin in the paranoid form. From 1910 onward, those chronic delusional states were redivided in terms of their *mécanism* into "chronic interpretative delusional state" (*délire chronique d'interprétation*), "chronic hallucinatory delusional state" (*psychose hallucinatoire chronique*), and "chronic imaginative delusional state" (*délire chronique d'imagination*).

Some clinicians have argued that these historical developments made French approaches to diagnosis and classification of mental disorders difficult to understand. Be that as it may, opposition to Kraepelin's system has, without doubt, given French psychiatry a unique stance in the field of nonaffective psychoses.

37

The striking outcome is that traditional French nosology reflects trends that have only recently begun to appear in other classifications outside of France.

THE OFFICIAL FRENCH CLASSIFICATION

The official French classification of mental disorders was published in 1969 by the Institut de la Santé et de la Recherche Médicale (INSERM, 1969). The INSERM classification is the result of a national inquiry and as such corresponds closely to common diagnostic practices of French psychiatrists. It is organized into 20 major categories, which are subdivided by a third and, in some instances, a fourth digit. With a few, although important, exceptions concerning the boundaries of schizophrenia, it is compatible with the Ninth Revision of the International Classification of Mental Diseases (ICD-9) (World Health Organization, 1978). It has not been revised since 1968.

The INSERM classification is merely a list of terms in outline form. It contains no glossary, and therefore its diagnostic criteria cannot be reliably ascertained. As a recent investigation has shown, there is nevertheless a surprising consensus among French clinicians about diagnostic concepts and practices (Pull, Pichot & Overall, 1979). In particular, French clinicians remain attached to the differentiation of schizophrenia from the nonschizophrenic delusional states (Pichot, 1979).

The present report is part of a global attempt initiated by the authors to translate essential elements of French nosology into internationally recognizable criteria and to facilitate direct comparisons between French diagnostic practices and those emerging from other classification schemes. The following survey of contemporary French approaches to psychiatric diagnosis and classification is based upon an empirical investigation in the field of nonaffective psychoses. A second investigation concerning French diagnostic practices in the field of depression has just been completed and will be published elsewhere.

THE FRENCH APPROACH TO NONAFFECTIVE PSYCHOSES

French psychiatry divides the nonaffective psychoses into three major groups: the chronic schizophrenias, the transitory delusional states, and the chronic delusional states. The three groups are conceived as fundamentally independent.

In the INSERM classification, schizophrenia is listed only in connection with the term *chronic*. The chronic schizophrenias (INSERM 02) are subdivided into eight types reflecting cross-sectional clinical syndromes and two types based on psychoses with an origin specific to childhood. The eight types of clinical syndromes are simple (020); hebephernic (021); catatonic (022); paranoid (023); with disturbance of mood (024); residual (025); pseudo-psychopathic, heboidophrenic, or pseudo-neurotic (026); and unspecified (029).

The transitory delusional states (INSERM 04) are subdivided into three subcategories: acute or subacute delusional state presumed to be a prodromal episode of schizophrenia, acute schizophrenia (040); acute reactive delusional psychosis, reactive *bouffée délirante* (041); and acute delusional psychosis, *bouffée délirante* (042).

The chronic delusional states (INSERM 03) are subdivided into interpretive delusional states (030 and 031), chronic hallucinatory psychosis (032), chronic imaginative psychosis (033), chronic delusional states arising in the senium (034), and unspecified (039).

This chapter focuses on schizophrenia and those transitory or chronic delusional states that are unique to French nosology, namely, reactive and nonreactive *bouffée délirante*, interpretive delusional state, and chronic hallucinatory psychosis.

Results from a recent empirical investigation (Pull, Pull & Pichot, 1981c, 1984) have enabled us to develop diagnostic criteria for each of the five categories under discussion. As a consequence, it has become possible, for the first time, to compare directly the French classification of mental diseases and the conditions described in the Ninth Revision of the International Classification of Diseases (ICD-9), as well as disorders defined in the third edition of the *Diagnostic and Statistical Manual of Mental Disorders* (DSM-III) (Pull, Pull & Pichot, 1985a,b).

In 1981, a survey was carried out with a representative sample of French psychiatrists. The group consisted of 87 qualified psychiatrists who had previously collaborated in similar studies. The participants were invited to provide several cases of psychotic conditions, excluding the purely affective psychoses. No criteria were imposed to make a diagnosis. The only requests were that the clinicians (1) should be reasonably positive about their diagnoses and (2) should document their diagnoses using a set of internationally understandable criteria.

The instrument used in the investigation was a List of Integrated Criteria for the Evaluation of Taxonomy in the field of nonaffective psychoses or LICET-S (Pull, Pull & Pichot, 1981a, b), which presents a total of 70 criteria for schizophrenia and schizophrenia-related categories. LICET-S is a polydiagnostic instrument that assembles all specific criteria for schizophrenia proposed by several prominent authors in the past (Kraepelin, 1896; Bleuler, 1911; Schneider, 1950; Langfeldt, 1937) or more recently by different North American authors (Feighner, Robins & Guze, 1972; Taylor, 1972; Astrachan et al., 1972). It also includes the "discriminant" symptoms for schizophrenia emerging from the International Pilot Study of Schizophrenia (World Health Organization, 1973), as well as DSM-III inclusion and exclusion criteria for schizophrenic disorder, paranoid disorder, and psychotic disorders not elsewhere classified.

With regard to the five categories under discussion, the description of cases provided through LICET-S was of remarkable homogeneity. The results were highly consistent for age of onset, duration, symptom pattern, and exclusions. Moreover, the data relevant to a definition of the concepts consisted of objective observable behaviors and reported feelings for which there is no need for in-

Table 3.1. *French diagnostic criteria for schizophrenia*

A. Age of onset: before age 40
B. Onset: acute (a first acute episode would be given a diagnosis of *bouffée délirante*)
   or progressive
C. Chronicity: active phases are followed by a residual phase characterized by at least
   some signs of the illness
D. Characteristic symptoms, at least two of the following:
   1. Marked illogicality: patently unrealistic, bizarre or magical thinking
   2. Inappropriate effect: blunted and/or discordant affect and/or ambivalence
   3. Major formal thought disorder: loosening of associations, inefficient thinking,
      incoherence
   4. Unsystematized delusional ideas having no apparent relation to depression or
      elation
E. Not due to any organic mental disorder

ference. As a consequence, the major elements required to operationalize diagnostic concepts could be elucidated, which in turn made it possible to define
the corresponding diagnostic criteria.

Schizophrenia

For French psychiatrists, schizophrenia is a disease whose first symptoms appear before the age of 40. Its beginning can be either acute or progressive.
It is considered chronic. The diagnosis is based primarily on the symptomatology, the symptoms given most weight being those proposed by Bleuler, that
is, alterations of logical thinking and inadequacy of affectivity. Delusional ideas
are usually present, but they are never organized in a coherent system. The
main symptoms are generally subsumed by French psychiatrists under the terms
dissociation and *discordance*. Schneider's first-rank symptoms are considered of
secondary importance.

Diagnostic criteria. The diagnostic criteria for schizophrenia elucidated through
the above-mentioned survey of French psychiatrists are presented in Table 3.1.

Comparison with ICD-9. ICD-9 requires the presence, at some time during
the illness, of characteristic disturbances of thought, perception, mood, conduct,
or personality – preferably in at least two of these areas. This symptom definition
seems broader than the French one. There is, moreover, no threshold for age
at onset in ICD-9, nor is chronicity postulated. As a consequence, the French
concept appears to be narrower.

Comparison with DSM-III. DSM-III includes a criterion requiring the presence
of at least one of six specific symptoms. The French definition is largely restricted
to the last of these symptoms. The DSM-III upper limit for age at onset is

Table 3.2. *French diagnostic criteria for* bouffée délirante

A. Onset: acute, without any prior psychiatric history (other than identical episodes)
B. Duration: active phases fade away completely in several weeks or months, possibly recurring under the same form, but with the patient remaining devoid of any psychopathology in the interval
C. Characteristic symptoms, all of the following:
  1. Delusions and/or hallucinations of any form
  2. Depersonalization/derealization and/or confusion
  3. Depression and/or elation
  4. Symptoms vary from day to day, even from hour to hour
D. Not due to any organic mental disorder
E. *Bouffée délirante* without other specification (or "genuine" *bouffée délirante*) occurs in the absence of any identifiable psychosocial stressor; *bouffée délirante* occurring in temporal relation with stress is termed "reactive"

higher than the French upper limit. In contrast to the French definition, chronicity is not a requirement in DSM-III, although full recovery is considered exceptional. Owing to the preceding differences, the French concept would be narrower. There is, however, an exclusion criterion in DSM-III, concerning absence of a history of full depression or mania, which is not found in the French definition.

Bouffée délirante

Two major forms of *bouffée délirante* are considered here: the "genuine" form, which occurs without a pertinent psychosocial stressor, and the "reactive" form, which develops in response to such a stressor. In any case, *bouffée délirante* is a transitory disorder. Its beginning is always acute, the patient having no previous psychiatric history, although *bouffées délirantes* may themselves recur. The symptoms disappear completely in a few weeks or months, leaving absolutely no residual anomalies. The symptoms are characterized by their polymorphism: delusions with multiple themes, without any coherence, with or without hallucinations of any type; depersonalization and/or derealization, with or without confusion; depression or euphoria. All symptoms vary from day to day and even from hour to hour.

Diagnostic criteria. Diagnostic criteria for *bouffée délirante* are presented in Table 3.2.

Comparison with ICD-9. The definition of acute schizophrenic episode provided in the ICD-9 glossary is quite similar to the French definition of "genuine" *bouffée délirante*. The ICD-9 definition of acute paranoid reaction obviously corresponds to reactive *bouffée délirante*, and not, as stated in the ICD glossary, to *bouffée délirante* without specification.

Table 3.3. *French diagnostic criteria for chronic hallucinatory psychosis*

A. Age at onset: after age 30
B. Onset: acute or progressive
C. Chronicity: active phases are followed by a residual phase with at least some signs of the illness
D. Characteristic symptoms, all of the following:
   1. Auditory hallucinations
   2. Delusions, having no apparent relation to depression or elation tend to form a delusional system
   3. Delusions of being controlled, thought broadcasting, thought insertion, thought withdrawal
   4. Formal thought disorder, if present, does not dominate the clinical picture
E. Not due to any organic mental disorder

Comparison with DSM-III. DSM-III lists at least two categories that would be covered by *bouffée délirante*: (1) schizophreniform disorder corresponds to "genuine" *bouffée délirante* but is less specific with regard to onset and characteristic symptoms, and (2) brief reactive psychosis corresponds to reactive *bouffée délirante*. In addition, a number of patients with a DSM-III diagnosis of atypical psychosis or acute paranoid disorder would probably be given a diagnosis of *bouffée délirante* in France.

Chronic hallucinatory psychosis

Chronic hallucinatory psychosis, as now defined in France, is a disease beginning after age 30, either progressively or acutely. Its course is chronic. The diagnosis is based primarily on specific symptomatology, with an emphasis on Schneider's first-rank symptoms. A delusional system is always present, and is characterized by its systematization. Intellectual functioning and affectivity are generally well preserved: Bleuler's basic symptoms are absent or not obvious.

Diagnostic criteria. Diagnostic criteria for chronic hallucinatory psychosis are presented in Table 3.3.

Comparison with ICD-9. Chronic hallucinatory psychosis corresponds closely to the description provided in the ICD-9 glossary for paraphrenia. There is, however, no comment in ICD-9 for age at onset.

Comparison with DSM-III. No category in DSM-III corresponds directly to chronic hallucinatory psychosis. Chronic hallucinatory psychosis with onset before age 45 meets the DSM-III criteria for schizophrenic disorder. For chronic hallucinatory psychosis with onset after age 45, the only possible DSM-III category would be atypical psychosis. This is, however, a residual category

Table 3.4. *French diagnostic criteria for chronic interpretive delusional psychosis*

A. Age of onset: between 25 and 50
B. Onset: acute or (as a rule) progressive
C. Chronicity: acute phases are followed by a residual phase characterized by the presence of at least some signs of the illness
D. Characteristic symptoms, all of the following:
    1. Delusional interpretations
    2. Delusional references
    3. Persistent delusional ideas of either persecution, prejudice, grandeur, love, or delusional jealousy
    4. Delusions are coherent and form a delusional system
E. No formal thought disorder
F. Not due to any organic mental disorder

---

encompassing a number of other disturbances that do not meet the criteria for any specific mental disorder.

The diagnosis of chronic hallucinatory psychosis implies the presence of "automatic mental activity" (*automatisme mental*). This specific French syndrome corresponds basically to a constellation of Schneiderian first-rank symptoms, and, in DSM-III, to symptoms 1 and 4 of criterion A for schizophrenic disorder.

Chronic interpretive delusional state

Chronic interpretive delusional state is a disorder beginning between the ages of 25 and 50, either progressively or acutely. Its course is chronic.

The diagnosis is based primarily on the presence of coherent (logical) delusions, developing into a permanent delusional system. The delusional "mechanism" is interpretive. Hallucinations are absent or insignificant. Intellectual functioning and affectivity are generally well preserved. Bleuler's basic symptoms are absent.

Diagnostic criteria. Diagnostic criteria for chronic interpretive delusional state are presented in Table 3.4.

Comparison with ICD-9. Cases meeting the criteria for paranoia (ICD-9 297.1) would all be diagnosed in France as chronic interpretive psychosis, as would, in addition, most cases meeting the diagnostic criteria for paranoid state, simple (ICD-9 297.0). In France induced psychosis (ICD-9 297.3) is perceived merely as a special aspect of chronic interpretive psychosis.

Comparison with DSM-III. Cases meeting the criteria for paranoia (DSM-III–297.10) would all be diagnosed in France as chronic interpretive psychosis. Shared paranoid disorder (DSM-III–297.30) would be considered a special case of chronic interpretive psychosis. Acute paranoid disorder (DSM-III–298.30) corresponds, to a certain degree, to reactive *bouffée délirante*.

The general diagnostic criteria provided in DSM-III for paranoid disorder corresponds to the French usage of paranoid-paranoiac. In the French edition of DSM-III, paranoid disorders could thus be translated accurately as *troubles paranoïaques*.

DISCUSSION

As noted earlier, this report is part of a global attempt initiated by the authors to develop diagnostic criteria for essential French diagnostic concepts. The experience obtained up to now in this field can be summarized as follows:

1. The French position on schizophrenia, *bouffée délirante*, paranoia, and other paranoid states is in fact more complex than indicated here. Theoretical considerations and subtle subdivisions have been glossed over in the operationalization process. The definition of chronic hallucinatory psychosis does not, for instance, reflect all of the highly complex implications of "automatic mental activity," a term under which the hallucinations of this disorder were classified in the 1920s by De Clerambault (1942). Similarly, the definition provided for chronic delusional psychosis omits time-honored references to focused or non-focused delusions, and a bewildering number of additional subdivisions. On the other hand, it would make little sense to analyze the finer distinctions of French nosology at a time when French positions on diagnosis and classification are, on the whole, viewed as unique and impossible to understand outside of France.

2. Basic French diagnostic concepts are amenable to translation into diagnostic criteria and terminology that do not impede international understanding. In comparison with the St-Louis criteria (Feighner et al., 1972), the Research Diagnostic Criteria (Spitzer et al., 1978) or the DSM-III criteria, however, the definitions presented in this report are less rigorous or operational.

Reasons for this should be sought in the fact that the criteria for French concepts have been derived from empirical data describing actual diagnostic practices of French clinicians. A more complete operationalization of the concepts would have required some arbitrary decisions concerning criteria on which there is no consensus. Duration of genuine *bouffée délirante*, for example, is less than three months in most cases, but for some clinicians it may be as long as six months.

3. French diagnostic concepts defined in this way are directly comparable to concepts that are included in other nomenclatures. This is true even for those concepts that have been considered as "exotic" or "typically French." Genuine *bouffée délirante*, for example, may be related to acute schizophrenic episode in ICD-9 and schizophreniform disorder in DSM-III. In the same way, chronic hallucinatory psychosis would appear to correspond to paraphrenia in ICD-9.

4. A final point to note concerns traditional French nosology as it compares with the new North American concept of schizophrenia presented in DSM-III. The hallmark of traditional French psychiatric nosology consists in restricting

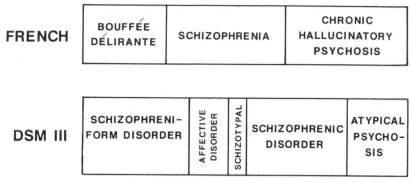

Figure 3.1. Preliminary diagram comparing traditional French and the new American positions on schizophrenia

Table 3.5. *Cross-tabulation of French clinical diagnoses versus DSM-III diagnoses*

	DSM-III Criteria					
French criteria	Schizo-phrenia	Schizo-phreniform[a]	Atypical psychosis	Affective disorder	Other	Total
Schizophrenia	164			15	12	191
Chronic hallucinatory psychosis	21		14	5	1	41
Acute delusional states[b]	12	25	1	8	4	50
Total	197	25	15	28	17	282

[a]Includes brief reactive psychosis.
[b]Includes genuine *bouffée délirante*, reactive *bouffée délirante* and acute delusional state presumed to be a prodromal episode of schizophrenia.

the diagnosis of schizophrenia by (1) separating a number of nonschizophrenic delusional states, acute or chronic, and (2) insisting on the chronicity of the disorder. Until recently, North American nosology has used much broader criteria for the concept. As shown in a comparison of French and American diagnostic practices – based on DSM-II – American clinicians diagnosed schizophrenia approximately three times more often than French psychiatrists. In the same comparison, chronic hallucinatory psychosis and *bouffée délirante* could be identified as the primary basis for the more frequent use of the diagnosis of schizophrenia by American psychiatrists, although they did not account for all the differences (Pull, Pichot & Overall, 1980).

From the comparisons in the present report, it would appear that the new American concept of schizophrenia, as defined in DSM-III, is similar, in some important respects, to the traditional French position. Initial evidence supporting this proposition emerges when French clinical diagnoses are compared with DSM-III criteria on the same cases (Pull, Pull & Pichot, 1985a,b).

A cross-tabulation of French clinical diagnoses for schizophrenia, chronic hallucinatory psychosis and acute delusional states against DSM-III criteria for schizophrenic disorder, schizophreniform disorder and atypical psychosis is presented in Table 3.5.

Although further investigation is needed to establish the correspondence between the traditional French and the new American positions on schizophrenia, Figure 3.1 may serve as a preliminary illustration of the similarities and differences between these two sets of concepts.

REFERENCES

American Psychiatric Association. 1980. *Diagnostic and Statistical Manual of Mental Disorders*. 3rd ed., (DSM-III).Washington, D.C.

Astrachan, B. M. et al. 1972. A checklist for the diagnosis of schizophrenia. *British Journal of Psychiatry* 121: 529–539.

Baillarger, J. 1854. De la folie à double forme. *Annales Médico- Psychologiques* 6: 369–384.

Bleuler, E. 1911. Dementia Praecox oder Gruppe der Schizophrenien. In *Handbuch der Psychiatrie*, ed. G. Aschaffenburg. Leipzig and Vienna: Deuticke.

Clerambault, G. de. 1942. *Ouevre psychiatrique*. Paris: Presses Universitaires de France.

Falret, J. P. 1854. De la folie circulaire. *Bulletin de l'Académie de Médecine* 19: 382–395.

Feighner, J. P., Robins, E., and Guze, S. B. et al. 1972. Diagnostic criteria for use in psychiatric research. *Archives of General Psychiatry* 26: 57–63.

Institut National de la Santé et de la Recherche Médicale. Section Psychiatrie. 1969. Classification française des troubles mentaux. *Bulletin de l'Institut National de la Santé et de la Recherche Médicale* 24, Supplement to no. 2.

Kraepelin, E. 1896. *Psychiatrie. Ein Lehrbuch für Studierende und Aerzte*. 5th ed. Leipzig: A. Abel.

Langfeldt, G. 1937. *The Prognosis in Schizophrenia and the Factors Influencing the Course of the Disease*. Copenhagen: Munksgaard.

Magnan, V., and Serieux, P. 1893. *Le délire chronique à évolution systématique*. Paris: Gauthier Villars/Georges Masson.

Pichot, P. 1979. Definition of the limits of the schizophrenia in France. In *World Issues in the Problems of Schizophrenic Psychoses*, ed. T. Fukuda and H. Mitsuda, pp. 65–72. Tokyo, New York: Igaku-Shoin.

Pichot, P. 1982. The diagnosis and classification of mental disorders in French-speaking countries: background, current views and comparison with other nomenclature. *Psychological Medicine* 12: 475–492.

Pichot, P. 1983. *A Century of Psychiatry*. Paris: Roche.

Pichot, P. 1984. The French approach to psychiatric classification. *British Journal of Psychiatry* 144: 113–118.

Pull, C. B., Pichot, P., and Overall, J. E. 1979. A statistical model of psychiatric diagnostic practices in France. *Comprehensive Psychiatry* 20: 27–39.

Pull, C. B., Pichot, P., and Overall, J. E. 1980. Comparison of French and American diagnostic practices for schizophrenia and depression. *Psychopharmacology Bulletin* 16: 43–46.

Pull, C. B., Pull, M. C., and Pichot, P. 1981a. Des critères cliniques pour le diagnostic de schizophrénie. In *Actualités de la Schizophrénie*, ed. P. Pichot, pp. 23–34. Paris: Masson.

Pull, C. B., Pull, M. C., and Pichot, P. 1981b. L.I.C.E.T.-S: Une Liste Intégrée de Critères d'Evaluation Taxonomiques pour les Psychoses Non-Affectives. *Journal de Psychiatrie Biologique et Thérapeutique* 1: 33–39.

Pull, C. B., Pull, M. C., and Pichot, P. 1981c. Etude Nationale sur les critères de diagnostic des psychiatres français dans les psychoses non-affectives: Premiers Résultats. In *Comptes-Rendus du Congrès des Psychiatres et Neurologues de Langue Française*, ed. P. Sizaret, pp. 244–252. Paris: Masson.

Pull, C. B., Pull, M. C., and Pichot, P. 1984. Des critères empiriques français pour les psychoses. I. Position du problème et méthodologie. *Encéphale* 10: 119–123.

Pull, C. B., Pull, M. C., and Pichot, P. 1985a. Comparing French and international classification systems. I. Schizophrenia. In *Psychiatry: The State of the Art*, ed. P. Berner. London: Plenum Press.

Pull, C. B., Pull, M. C., and Pichot, P. 1985b. Comparing French and international classification systems. III. Paranoid states. In *Psychiatry: the State of the Art*, ed. P. Berner. London: Plenum Press.

Schneider, K. 1950. *Klinische Psychopathologie*. Stuttgart: Georg Thieme.

Spitzer, R. L., Endicott, J., and Robins, E. 1978. Research diagnostic criteria: rationale and reliability. *Archives of General Psychiatry*, 35: 773–782.

Taylor, M. A. 1972. Schneiderian first-rank symptoms and clinical prognostic features in schizophrenia. *Archives of General Psychiatry* 26: 64–67.

World Health Organization. 1973. *The International Pilot Study of Schizophrenia*. Geneva.

World Health Organization. 1978. *Mental Disorders: Glossary and Guide to Their Classification in Accordance with the Ninth Revision of the International Classification of Diseases*. Geneva.

4   Scandinavian approaches to psychiatric diagnosis

ERIK STRÖMGREN (Denmark)

During the nineteenth century, psychiatry in the Scandinavian (or Nordic) countries was equally influenced by English, French, and German psychiatry, but from the beginning of the twentieth century, the influence of the German-speaking countries became dominant as a consequence of the teachings of Kraepelin and Bleuler. The concept of schizophrenia, however, never became as widely accepted in Scandinavia as in the German and, especially, the Swiss schools of psychiatry. One reason for this difference was the wide use in Nordic countries of the concept of psychogenic or reactive psychoses. Greatly influenced by French psychiatry, and in accordance with the teachings of Karl Jaspers (1913) in Germany, August Wimmer, a Danish psychiatrist, in 1916 wrote a monograph on psychogenic psychoses that had great impact on psychiatrists in all the Nordic countries. This impact was not felt beyond Scandinavia because the monograph was written in Danish.

Another distinctive feature of Nordic psychiatry is that it was slow in adopting psychoanalytic concepts. Some of the leading psychiatrists who were interested in the psychological origin of mental disorders felt that Freud had not contributed much beyond what was already commonplace in French psychiatry in the era of Charcot and especially Janet. Psychoanalysis had to make a detour across the Atlantic Ocean before it finally came back from the United States after World War II and settled in Northern Europe.

With regard to psychiatric classification and nomenclature, the Nordic countries kept their own national systems until the appearance of the eighth edition of the International Classification of Diseases. Attempts had been made to accept earlier editions of the ICD, which had been officially accepted by the Nordic countries, but the psychiatrists in these countries refused to use the section on mental disorders. It may be remembered that of all member states of the United Nations only five agreed to use this section of the ICD-7 (World Health Organization, 1957). When ICD-8 was in preparation, the WHO made great efforts to reshape the section on mental disorders in the hope that it could be accepted by the majority of countries. During the preparatory work it became clear that one of the most difficult points was the concept of "psychogenic psychosis," a category that seemed incomprehensible and unacceptable to English-speaking psychiatrists. On the other hand, representatives of a number of other countries

48

indicated that the classification would be unacceptable to them if there was no room for the psychogenic psychoses. Finally, a compromise was reached, and the reactive psychoses were introduced, although under disguise, namely under the heading "other psychoses." These were defined as *including* "psychotic conditions attributable to recent life experience," but in fact included *only* psychogenic subgroups. In ICD-9 the reactive psychoses have retained their position.

The problems surrounding the psychogenic or reactive psychoses indicate some of the basic difficulties in psychiatric classification, especially in its international application. Experience has shown that it is not enough to have international agreement on certain nomenclatures and classifications. The concepts and terms must also be used in a uniform way by all subscribers. When the reactive psychoses were finally admitted in ICD-8, those psychiatric schools that applied this concept for a great part of all psychoses were, of course, very happy. Their satisfaction, however, dwindled when it turned out that their Anglo-Saxon colleagues refrained from using this class. The comments to the ICD-8 stressed that this class should be used exceptionally and the glossary to ICD-9 expressly stated that the class "should be restricted to the small group of psychotic conditions that are largely or entirely attributable to a recent life experience." Thus in many countries few cases entered this class, whereas in some other countries it made up a large part of all psychoses. This situation, of course, drastically limited international comparisons.

There is no reason to believe that the mental disorders known as reactive or psychogenic psychoses in the Nordic countries and many other regions should be less frequent in the countries that do not use the term. The question is, Where are they classified in such countries? There is no doubt that many of them, especially in the United States, have been labeled schizophrenic reactions or schizophrenic episodes, acute schizophrenia, and so on. This is understandable with regard to psychoses of a mainly delusional type. But what about the greater part of the psychogenic psychoses, which are of the depressive type? They have probably been grouped among nonpsychotic disorders in spite of the fact that they fulfill all criteria attached to the concept of psychoses. Furthermore, the third group – reactive psychoses with disorders of consciousness – may be labeled hysteria, situational reaction, and so on.

To be fair, Nordic psychiatrists may occasionally use the diagnosis reactive psychosis too extensively. When you are treating a young psychotic, and you are not quite certain what the diagnosis should be, you will be inclined to use the diagnosis psychogenic psychosis, although at the bottom of your heart you may feel that it is probably a case of schizophrenia. Of course, this emotional mechanism in the diagnostician has implications for many other kinds of diagnoses, the decision being colored by the emotional attitude of the psychiatrist. Recent studies in Denmark have demonstrated that only a few of those psychotics who later turn out to be unquestionably schizophrenic do receive this diagnosis during their first admission, in spite of the fact that, in retrospect, the diagnosis was already certain at that time. The average interval between the time when the diagnosis could have been made and the time when it is really stated is about two years.

As for the problem of the classification of those psychoses that in Nordic countries are labeled reactive psychoses (ICD-8 no. 298), some of them will no doubt be placed in the class 308, acute reaction to stress. The glossary to ICD-9 says that these reactions are "very transient disorders of any severity and nature which occur in individuals without any apparent mental disorder in response to exceptional physical or mental stress . . . and which usually subside within hours or days." It is obvious that if these disorders can have "any severity and nature," some of them could naturally be placed under reactive psychoses, and that is what happens in Nordic countries and not in Anglo-Saxon countries.

In this connection, I should mention a concept that has been used widely in Denmark, especially in forensic psychiatry: the so-called abnormal singular reactions. The concept was created by the late Prof. Hjalmar Helweg in Copenhagen, who was a leading figure in Danish forensic psychiatry, and it arose as a result of his interest in a special communication problem between psychiatrists and lawyers. Serious crimes were sometimes committed by persons who were in an obviously psychotic state, which, however, lasted for only a few hours. It was difficult to convince judges that such persons had been suffering from a "disease" with a duration of only a few hours, since it did not comply with the popular concept of disease. It turned out that the term "abnormal singular reaction" was much more acceptable to them, and that, when this diagnosis was made, they would place the patient in the same legal box as ordinary psychotics, which of course was what Professor Helweg had intended.

The term "crisis" has become quite popular in the Nordic countries, as in many other countries. This rather vague term can be applied to many acute reactions to stress. It has become especially popular among those nonmedical professionals who come into contact with mentally deviant persons and feel that the treatment of these persons is their natural task and not that of psychiatrists. In many cases, this attitude is well founded. Such crises are so frequent and so short lasting that only a minority of them will ever come to the attention of psychiatrists. Johan Cullberg in Stockholm, who has for a number of years been the leader of the famous Nacka community psychiatric project, and who has written the best-known books about crisis therapy, has recently stated that when persons in such crises do come to the mental-health centers, most of them disappear quite soon. It is obvious that they do not feel that psychiatric therapy on dynamic lines, which is often applied to them, is really of any use for them. The conclusion may be that "crisis" is probably not a concept that should have a place in psychiatric classification. The word appears neither in ICD-9 nor in DSM-III.

The term "schizophreniform psychosis" was probably first used by Langfeldt (1939) in Norway. Shortly after the introduction of shock therapies, it became clear that, although some psychoses with schizophrenialike symptomatology responded well to these treatments, others did not. Langfeldt chose the term "schizophreniform" to distinguish the first group from the more malignant cases of true schizophrenias or process schizophrenias. Since then there has been a slightly different trend in terminology: Many psychiatrists use the term "schizophreniform" just to indicate that a given psychosis has a symptomatology similar to that of schizophrenia but may nevertheless be of a different nature. Schizophrenias are of course schizophreniform, but so also, at least in some stages, are psychoses following Huntington's chorea, different intoxications (especially by amphetamine), some psychogenic psychoses, and even some cases of manic-depressive disorder. Taken in this sense, schizophreniform is just a symptomatological concept. Unfortunately, outside Scandinavia "schizophreniform" is widely mistaken for a synonym of "psychogenic psychosis."

The term "schizoaffective" has become popular in Nordic countries, but not in a uniform way. Some psychiatrists use it often; others, not at all. Even among those who would like to use the term for purely descriptive purposes, it is a serious obstacle that in ICD-9 schizoaffective psychoses are classified just as a subgroup of schizophrenias. Those who feel that schizoaffective psychosis may be a subgroup of manic-depressive disorder, or perhaps a disease entity in itself, will not like to throw these cases into the schizophrenic basket.

Another term that has gained increasing attention in the Nordic countries during the 1980s is "cycloid psychosis." Carlo Perris (1974) at Umeå University, who is mainly responsible for this increased attention, adopted the term from Karl Leonhard (1957) in Berlin. Leonhard, like his teacher Karl Kleist, had been interested in atypical psychoses, in the sense that such psychoses were different from schizophrenia and manic-depressive disorder with regard to etiology, symptomatology, and course, often displaying a symptomatology that seemed to be a mixture of schizophrenic and manic-depressive symptoms. But in some cases it also displayed special symptoms that did not belong to either schizophrenia or manic-depressive disorder. Among these psychoses Leonhard singled out a group called cycloid psychoses, which were by definition characterized by a cycloid course in the sense that, as in manic-depressive disorder, there would be swings from one extreme to the other, with symptoms in one phase being exactly opposite to symptoms in the other phase. There were three subgroups: "anxiety-happiness psychosis," with panic at one extreme and ecstasy at the other; "motility psychosis," shifting between hyperkinesia and hypokinesia; and "excited-inhibited confusion psychosis," in which the dominant symptom was incoherence of thought, and in which it was more difficult to conceptualize the opposite state. Leonhard claimed that all these cycloid psychoses had a benign prognosis in the long run, and that further family investigations had shown homologous heredity.

In 1974 Perris published his monograph on the cycloid psychoses. In it he extended the concept to cases in which there were no swings between opposite phases and the main feature was polymorphic symptomatology. Perris felt that cycloid psychoses are something like a disease and that many of these cases have been falsely diagnosed as reactive psychoses, schizoaffective psychoses, atypical manic-depressive psychoses, and the like.

The interest in these cycloid psychoses has varied in the Nordic countries.

Whereas a new textbook of psychiatry published in 1983 in Gothenburg by Jan-Otto Ottosson regards cycloid psychoses as an obvious entity alongside schizophrenia and manic-depressive psychosis, this group is not even mentioned in the latest editions of other leading textbooks in Norway and Denmark; nor is it referred to in ICD-9 or in DSM-III. A number of psychiatrists in the Nordic countries will undoubtedly demand that cycloid psychoses be included as a class in ICD-10. On the other hand, if this class is introduced, the majority of Nordic psychiatrists will probably never use it. This again illustrates the limitations of the validity of classifications.

I also want to mention a special conceptual and terminological system that has been used in one of the psychiatric schools in Sweden, namely, that of Henrik Sjöbring (1973), who was professor of psychiatry at the University of Lund during the 1930s and 1940s. The basis of Sjöbring's system was what he called "analysis of personality." He argued that human personality involves four main components, each of which shows normal biological variation. Thus, if a person was subjected to mental or physical stress or lesion, the resulting symptomatology and course of illness would be influenced by these different personality components. Sjöbring's system has not been easy to understand, in part because he was not a gifted writer. Fortunately, some of Sjöbring's followers have provided clearer accounts of his system. It is evident that those who worked with Sjöbring found his system useful for understanding and describing patients and also for treating them. As long as Sjöbring's successor Erik Essen-Möller held the chair of psychiatry in Lund, Sjöbring's system remained in use, and the results of intensive research within the Sjöbring school have supported the validity of Sjöbring's concepts. Nevertheless, Sjöbring's terminology has not been generally accepted even in Sweden, and it does not seem likely that Swedish psychiatrists will demand that attention be paid to Sjöbring's terminology in future international classifications.

With regard to the technical aspects of classifications, for several decades Nordic psychiatrists have shown great interest in multidimensional classifications. The first to move in this direction were Essen-Möller and Wohlfahrt (1947), who distinguished between descriptive and etiological classification. In 1952, the Danish Psychiatric Association officially introduced a bidimensional classification in Denmark; the dimensions were etiology and gross psychiatric syndrome. This classification was in use until 1966, when Denmark accepted ICD-8. Essen-Möller (1961, 1971, 1973) further elaborated his classificatory system, and his work served as the basis for a multidimensional classification suggested by Ottosson and Perris in 1973. They proposed four dimensions: symptomatology, severity, etiology, and course. This system was published in *Psychological Medicine*. I would like to draw special attention to this system, as I think it has been especially successful in its description of personality variations. The classification has a coding system that appears to be practical.

In Scandinavia it is generally believed that ICD-10 should be multiaxial. Some, however, appear to have accepted the WHO's preliminary suggestion that the ICD-10 core classification should be unidimensional, which can be supplied with different axes for special purposes, and which also can be condensed or expanded in special situations, for instance, in developing countries.

Although DSM-III has received much attention in Nordic psychiatry, where many trials have been made, DSM-III will probably never be applicable internationally, since it has to be tailored to American conditions. In contrast, the WHO is under obligation to create an international classification that can be used equally well in all countries of the world.

Nordic psychiatrists have been favorably impressed by certain features of DSM-III: the multiaxial principle, the attempts to give exact diagnostic criteria and clear definitions of all terms. It has also been greatly appreciated that a number of publications have illustrated the use of DSM-III. At the same time, there are some elements in DSM-III that are felt to be somewhat disturbing. First, with regard to the diagnostic criteria, it is felt to be unrealistic, crude, and "unclinical" that a diagnosis should often depend on the *number* rather than on the type of the relevant symptom. Thus some kind of *weighting* of symptoms is considered necessary.

In addition, many are amazed at the classification of nonorganic psychoses. Many Scandinavian psychiatrists agree that the concept of schizophrenia should be defined in the restricted way in which it is currently used in he United States. But the group of "schizophreniform disorders" (defined in a way that differs radically from the original definition by Langfeldt) is not easy to accept, especially with regard to the sharp temporal divisions used for differential diagnosis. It is difficult to understand why a schizophreniform disorder stops to be schizophreniform if it lasts less than two weeks; if so, it is called a "brief reactive psychosis," but only if it follows a psychosocial stressor. If not, it is labeled "atypical psychosis," a term that is used in other contexts for schizophrenic disorders arising after middle age.

For Scandinavian psychiatrists, perhaps the only place to classify reactive or psychogenic psychoses according to DSM-III is under "brief reactive psychosis," which is frustrating, since many of our psychogenic psychoses last more than two weeks. In complete contrast to the Nordic concept of psychogenic psychoses, DSM-III indicates that the pertinent psychosocial stressor should be of a nature that "would evoke significant symptoms of distress in almost anyone." Nordic psychiatrists are convinced that, on the contrary, the origin of psychogenic psychoses often is of a "catathymic" nature, caused by a stress that only gives rise to a psychosis because it hits an especially vulnerable point in the affected patient. Still another problem with the notion is the fact that "brief reactive psychoses" must have a schizophreniform symptomatology. So there is no natural place within DSM-III for psychogenic psychoses that have depressive symptomatology, even though they constitute the majority of these psychoses. Only for those who display disorders of consciousness, is there obvious room within "dissociative disorders," the description of which shows clearly that some of these cases are true psychoses, and also that they are psychogenic.

There are many problems connected with the placement of reactive psychoses, problems that could be solved if the criteria for all relevant classes in future classifications were formulated in a sufficiently clear way.

REFERENCES

American Psychiatric Association 1980. *Diagnostic and Statistical Manual of Mental Disorders.* 3rd ed. (DSM-III). Washington, D.C.

Essen-Möller, E. 1961. On classification of mental disorders. *Acta Psychiatrica Scandinavica* 37: 119–126.

Essen-Möller, E. 1971. Suggestions for further improvement of the international classification of mental disorders. *Psychological Medicine* 1: 308–311.

Essen-Möller, E. 1973. Standard lists for three-fold classification of mental disorders. *Acta Psychiatrica Scandinavica* 49: 198–212.

Essen-Möller, E., and Wohlfahrt, S. 1947. Suggestions for the amendment of the official Swedish classification of psychiatric disorders. *Acta Psychiatrica Scandinavica Supplement* 47: 551–555.

Jaspers, K. 1913. *Allgemeine Psychopathologie. Ein Leitfaden für Studierende, Ärzte und Psychologen.* Berlin: Springer. English ed. (1963). *General Psychopathology.* Manchester: Manchester University Press.

Langfeldt, G. 1939. *The Schizophreniform States. A Catamnestic Study Based on Individual Re-examinations with Special Reference to Diagnostic and Prognostic Clues, and with a View to Presenting a Standard Material for Comparison with the Remissions Effected by Shock Treatment.* Copenhagen: Munksgaard.

Leonhard, K. 1957. *Aufteilung der endogenen Psychosen. Berlin: Akademie-Verlag.* English ed. (1979). *The Classification of Endogenous Psychoses.* New York: Irvington.

Ottosson, J. O., and Perris, C. 1973. Multidimensional classification of mental disorders. *Psychological Medicine* 3: 238–243.

Perris, C. 1974. *A Study of Cycloid Psychoses.* Copenhagen: Munksgaard.

Sjöbring, H. 1973. *Personality Structure and Development. A Model and Its Application.* Copenhagen: Munksgaard.

Wimmer, A. 1916. Psykogene Sindssygdomsformer. In *St. Hans Hospital 1816–1915,* ed. A. Wimmer, pp. 85–216. Copenhagen: G. E. C. Gads Forlag.

World Health Organization. 1957. *Manual of the International Statistical Classification of Diseases, Injuries and Causes of Death.* 7th rev. ed. Geneva.

World Health Organization. 1967. *Manual of the International Classification of Diseases.* 8th rev. ed. Geneva.

World Health Organization. 1977. *Manual of the International Classification of Diseases.* 9th rev. ed. Geneva.

5 *The Egyptian diagnostic system (DMP-I)*

AHMED OKASHA (Egypt)

HISTORICAL AND INTERNATIONAL BACKGROUND OF THE EGYPTIAN CLASSIFICATION

Anthropologists, historians, and students of cross-cultural psychiatry have observed that every society has its own views of health and illness, as well as its own classification of diseases. Descriptions of various syndromes appear in ancient Egyptian, Greek, and Roman texts. The modern concept of disease and nosology did not emerge in Western Europe until the late eighteenth century. The so-called developing nations contain more than two-thirds of the world population. They are little industrialized, overpopulated, and predominantly rural. Their economy is limited, and mental health has a low priority, with one or two psychiatrists for a million people. For this reason, many of these countries are forced to use nonpsychiatric services for mental-health care.

The developing countries need a classification that is simple, bias-free, clinically useful, and relevant to their psychiatric experience. We in Egypt, a developing country, faced the obligation of constructing a classification for mental disorders with an appropriate sociocultural frame for the following reasons:

1. To satisfy the need for statistical evaluation
2. To formulate a common language within a country that has an Anglo-Saxon, French, and some Soviet psychiatric influence, mainly because of the diversity of schools and trends
3. To consider cultural variations and types of services

The concept of discrete disorders and the medical model applied to psychiatry come under considerable criticism in Egypt from both within and outside the profession. Five lines of criticism have been debated:

1. The challenge to the legitimacy of psychiatry as part of medicine. The antipsychiatry movement denounced the basic premise that mental disorders are true illnesses. They argued that in the absence of anatomic or physiologic evidence of abnormality, the application of the concept of illness to behavioral, emotional, and cognitive states served the need for social control of deviants rather than representing genuine medical practice.
2. Interrater reliability of psychiatric diagnosis is low.

55

3. Psychiatric diagnosis has adverse social and psychological consequences.
4. There are no sharp boundaries between the normal and the abnormal, and many of the phenomena considered in diagnosis are extensions of normal phenomena such as anxiety and depression.
5. Psychiatrists from developing countries and cultural anthropologists have criticized the conventional diagnostic system for being rooted in Western European culture and for being irrelevant or invalid in other cultures; they have also argued that various cultures have different concepts of mental illness.

During the past decade, a small group of neo-Kraepelinian psychiatrists has emerged across the world and posed a number of propositions:

1. Psychiatry is a branch of medicine.
2. Psychiatric practice should be based on the results of scientific knowledge derived from empirical studies.
3. A boundary exists between the normal and the sick, and this boundary can be delineated reliably.
4. Within the domain of sickness, mental illnesses exist; they are not myths.
5. Psychiatry should focus treatment attention on people requiring medical care for substantial mental illnesses and give lower priority to those needing assistance for problems of living and unhappiness.
6. Research and teaching should explicitly and intentionally emphasize diagnosis and classification.
7. Diagnostic criteria should be used for classification, and research should validate such criteria.
8. Departments of psychiatry in medical schools should teach these criteria, instead of undervaluing them, as has been the case for many years.
9. Research efforts directed at improving the reliability and validity of diagnosis and classification should use advanced quantitative research techniques.
10. Research in psychiatry should use modern scientific methodology, especially that borrowed from biology.

DSM-III incorporates a number of developments from recent clinical experience and research. It places psychiatry once again within the classical medical model, wherein operational criteria are based mainly on manifest descriptive psychopathology tested for reliability, and a multiaxial system is used.

The radical changes in DSM-III (American Psychiatric Association, 1980) have meant breaking ranks with the World Health Organization, for they commit American psychiatry, at least for the rest of this decade, to using classification very differently from the ICD-9 (World Health Organization, 1978), which is used in most other countries. This is obviously a matter for regret and has generated a certain amount of ill-feelings. It is, of course, true that one of the cardinal functions of classification is to facilitate communication, and the WHO devoted much time and energy to persuading individual governments and national associations to use the ICD-9 instead of their own nomenclatures.

The Egyptian classification DMP-1 (1979) is based mainly on the ICD-8 (World Health Organization, 1969), French classification (INSERM, 1969), DSM-I (American Psychiatric Association, 1952), DSM-II (American Psychiatric Association, 1968), and the traditional British, American, and Egyptian textbooks. It contains 16 categories subdivided into various subcategories. International nomenclature is preserved whenever possible, the coding system is independent, and the corresponding international code is cited wherever appropriate. (See Appendix A.)

The purpose of this chapter is to compare two well-known systems of classification of mental disorders (the ICD-9 and DSM-III) with the Egyptian national system (*Diagnostic Manual of Psychiatric Disorders*, DMP-1). This has been constructed for local or, at most, regional use on the assumption that it has fulfilled some cultural requirements. The chapter also touches on some of the proposals for the classification of mental disorders and psychosocial factors in ICD-10.

COMPARING THE EGYPTIAN CLASSIFICATION WITH ICD-9 AND DSM-III

The Egyptian system, like ICD-9 and DSM-II, employs the descriptive method. All three systems consider etiology to some extent in certain areas, for example, in the use of Axis III of DSM-III, the use of physical codes in ICD-9, and the presentation of aetiological differentiation in DMP-1. In contrast to ICD-9 (in which a number of terms were included without a definition or a description in the glossary of terms), DSM-III and DMP-1 provide better categorical definitions. The revision conference of ICD-9 considered the problems that developing countries would face in using ICD-9, since specialized psychiatrists are not always available. Some of the delegates favored the use of a simplified form of ICD-9 for these purposes, whereas others favored accepting reasonably simple systems that are already established.

The organic mental disorders are considered as one category in DSM-III, whereas they are subdivided into five organic psychotic conditions and one nonpsychotic mental condition in ICD-9, and one psychotic and another nonpsychotic condition in DMP-1. Thus, the psychotic-nonpsychotic distinction is preserved in both ICD-9 and DMP-1. Etiology is coded independently in both ICD-9 and DSM-III, whereas it is incorporated into the global classification in DMP-1. (See Appendix B for a comparative listing.)

Transient organic psychotic conditions that are present in ICD-9 are not accepted in either DSM-III or DMP-1. The primary degenerative dementia of DSM-III, senile onset, corresponds to senile dementia in ICD-9 and DMP-1 (simple, depressed, paranoid, with acute confusional states, and other and unspecified). No further subtypes are presented in DMP-1. In DSM-III the same types apply for presenile dementia and multi-infarct dementia, whereas in ICD-9 there are no subtypes. The same applies in DMP-1 for the presenile dementia. But in the latter system, arteriosclerotic psychosis is classified into (1) psychosis with cerebral arteriosclerosis and (2) psychosis with other cerebrovascular disturbances.

In ICD-9 "non-psychotic mental disorders following organic brain damage" is unique, being represented in DSM-III only by "organic personality syndrome," and in DMP-1 by aetiological entities.

In DSM-III drug-intake disorders, whether abuse or dependence, are gathered under a "substance use disorders" category, whereas in ICD-9 they were separated into "alcohol dependence," "drug dependence," and "nondependent abuse of drugs." In both systems, the individual substance was a criterion for further differentiation. In ICD-9, alcoholic and drug psychoses are placed in different major categories, but they are placed together under substance-induced organic mental disorders in DSM-III. In DMP-1, all are grouped under the category of drug dependence, alcoholism, and alcoholic psychosis. In ICD-9, additional categories (alcoholic jealousy, other and unspecified) are present. On the same merits, two additional categories are observed in DMP-1 (alcoholic paranoid state and other alcoholic disorders).

Pathological drug intoxication is presented in ICD-9 but has no corresponding item in DSM-III. It is not present in DMP-1 either.

DMP-1 has not differentiated between abuse and dependence as ICD-9 did, although it has graded dependence into simple habituation and addiction. In DMP-1, alcohol pathological use is differentiated into

1. Simple chronic alcoholism, which corresponds to nondependent use in ICD-9
2. Intermittent alcoholic indulgence (dipsomania), which is not considered in DSM-III and is included in ICD-9 within the alcohol-dependence syndrome
3. Alcohol addiction, which is equivalent to dependence in the other two systems

There are also conceptual differences in certain terms used in the three systems. In DSM-III "substance abuse" means a pattern of pathological use causing impairment in social or occupational functioning for at least one month, whereas in ICD-9 it means that the maladaptive effect of a drug one has taken on one's own initiative is not detrimental to one's health or social functioning. This term is not used in DMP-1. The evidence for substance dependence is usually the development of tolerance or the presence of withdrawal symptoms. In ICD-9, it is considered a state of psychic and sometimes physical dependence evidenced by the presence of a compulsion, whether continuous or periodic, to take the drug, to experience its psychic effects, and sometimes to avoid discomfort from its absence; tolerance may not be present. In DSM-III a fifth digit was offered to differentiate the course. In DMP-1, "dependence" is replaced by the term "addiction," which is defined as being a state of chronic mild intoxication with a compulsion and a tendency to increase the dose, and withdrawal symptoms leading to personality deterioration. This is in contrast to the term "habituation," which means the desire for chronic repeated consumption of the drug to satisfy the desire, with no withdrawal symptoms.

DSM-III has 5 types of schizophrenic disorders, ICD-9 has 10 types, and DMP-1 has 10 types that are similar to the ICD-9 categories.

For the diagnosis of schizophrenic disorders in DSM-III, the following criteria must be fulfilled:

1. Deterioration from a previous level of functioning
2. Onset before the age of 45
3. Continuous symptoms for at least six months
4. Characteristic symptoms involving multiple psychological processes
5. Depressive or manic symptoms, if present, developed after psychotic symptoms
6. Not due to an organic mental disorder or mental retardation

In ICD-9 and DMP-1 only the first criterion is accepted, while others are not necessary to make the diagnosis. Further subclassification of schizophrenic disorders with respect to duration and course is presented in DSM-III, but not in the other two systems. The term "subchronic" is used to describe an illness that lasts less than two years and the term "chronic" to describe illness that lasts more than two years. Additional schizophrenic categories not present in DSM-III have been described in ICD-9 (i.e., simple schizophrenia, latent schizophrenia, and acute schizophrenic episode). The last item is considered a schizophreniform disorder in DSM-III. In DMP-1 the term "acute undifferentiated episode" stands for the ICD-9 "acute schizophrenic episode," and the term "incipient schizophrenia" for "latent schizophrenia" of ICD-9.

The concept of paranoid states does not differ in the three systems, but only four subcategories are observed in DSM-III, in comparison with six in ICD-9 and eight in DMP-1. In DMP–1, the absence of personality disorganization is a diagnostic criterion, and hallucinations are accepted in DMP-1 and ICD-9 but not in DSM-III. Of the four subtypes in DSM-III (paranoia, shared paranoid disorder, acute paranoid disorder, and atypical paranoid disorder), which are all used in ICD-9 under other terms, only three are considered in the DMP-1, excluding shared paranoid disorder. Other subtypes considered in DMP-1 are chronic delusional paranoid state, chronic hallucinatory paranoid state, chronic imaginative paranoid state, involutional paranoid state, and late paranoid state. ICD-9 includes simple paranoid state, paranoid, paraphrenia, shared paranoid disorder, and other and unspecified paranoid states. DSM-III has used the term "shared paranoid disorder" to replace "induced psychosis." It has introduced "acute paranoid disorder," which may fit in other or unspecified categories of ICD-9.

The term "psychotic disorders" not classified elsewhere in DSM-III is replaced to a large extent by other nonorganic psychoses in ICD-9 and by other functional psychoses in DMP-1. In DSM-III, four subtypes of this broad category are considered, whereas there are seven in ICD-9 and five in DMP-1. Schizophreniform disorder in DSM-III may be coded under undifferentiated schizophrenia, or acute schizophrenic episode in ICD-9, and under acute undifferentiated episode in DMP-1.

Brief reactive psychosis of DSM-III is coded under other and unspecified reactive psychosis in ICD-9, and under other functional psychosis in DMP-1.

Atypical psychosis in DSM-III roughly corresponds to forms of unspecified psychosis in DMP-1.

Regarding affective disorders, the salient features of DSM-III involve the grouping of all such disorders, encompassing both psychotic and neurotic conditions, and their subdivision into major affective disorders, other specific affective disorders, and atypical affective disorders. DMP-1 retains the term "manic depressive illnesses" for affective psychoses.

Neurosis, as a category, is accepted in both ICD-9 and DMP-1. In contrast, DSM-III does not use this as a major classificatory concept, but as categories in different symptom areas, that is, affective disorders, anxiety disorders, somatoform disorders, and dissociative disorders. Again, neurasthenia, although accepted in ICD-9 and DMP-1, is not present in DSM-III.

Psychosexual disorders are more elaborate in DSM-III than in either ICD-9 or DMP-1, and they include (1) gender identity disorders, (2) paraphilias, and (3) psychosexual disfunction. In ICD-9, sexual deviations and disorders account for 10 entities, whereas in DMP-1 they are considered as one entity under personality and character disorders and are divided into

1. Sexual stimulus disorders
2. Sexual expression disorders
3. Instinctual object disorders (the main criteria of which involve sexual behaviors contrary to accepted cultural norms, where sexual gratification is not obtained mainly or exclusively through penile-vaginal intercourse)

Factitious disorders are one of the new categories of DSM-III. It denotes a group of disorders involving voluntary control over produced mental and physical symptoms but not over their underlying motivation or mechanisms. The patient's aim is to assume the sick role.

Disorders of impulse control not classified elsewhere in DSM-III overlap to some extent with disturbances of conduct in ICD-9. Characteristically, in DSM-III the gratification during the act may or may not be followed by guilt; and the disorder involves symptoms related to impulse control. In DMP-1, these disorders are variants of personality disorders.

The term "somatoform disorders" introduced by DSM-III encompasses five subtypes. The corresponding syndromes in ICD-9 come from different areas: neurotic disorders and special symptoms or syndromes not elsewhere classified, for example, psychalgia. The corresponding syndromes in DMP-1 also pertain to different areas, such as special symptoms not elsewhere classified, isolated symptoms, hysterical neurosis of conversive type, hypochondriacal neurosis. Depersonalization disorder is placed in dissociative disorders in DSM-III, under neurotic disorders in ICD-9, and under special symptoms not elsewhere classified in DMP-1.

All reactions to stress are gathered into one broad category in DSM-III, and they are divided into acute and chronic reactions in ICD-9 and DMP-1.

Physiological malfunctions arising from mental factors and a group of psychic factors associated with disorders classified elsewhere in ICD-9 are included within the group of psychological factors affecting physical condition in DSM-III. Axis III is used in DSM-III to determine the physical system affected.

Again, some of the physiological malfunctions are placed in DSM-III under somatoform and psychosexual disorders.

With respect to personality disorders, DSM-III does not include here the concept of "explosive personality," which has been transferred to "impulse control disorder." Likewise, the "affective personality" has been transferred to cyclothymic and dysthymic disorders in DSM-III. This affective condition is termed "cyclothymic personality" in DMP-1. The "asthenic personality" of ICD-9 seems to correspond to "dependent personality" in DSM-III, and "passive-dependent personality" in DMP-1. The concept of sociopathic personality is termed "antisocial" in DSM- III, and "dyssocial character" in DMP-1. DMP-1 also includes immature personalities, characterized by childish behavior and lack of sense of responsibility, and character trait disorder, which involve marked exaggeration of specific behaviors without overall changes in personality structure.

The classification of mental retardation is quite similar across systems.

DMP-1 identifies psychiatric disorders related to epilepsy under a specific category, in contrast to DSM-III and ICD-9.

In DSM-III and ICD-9 conduct disorder of childhood has been classified as a separate entity with many different subcategories. In DMP-1, it has not been used as a diagnostic category, but variations of this disorder are grouped under other categories as "personality character trait disorder" (explosive, dyssocial, kleptomanic, pyromanic) and behavior disorder of childhood and adolescence (unsocialized aggressive reaction and group delinquent reaction).

In DSM-III the emotional disorders of childhood are classified into anxiety disorders and other disorders, whereas in ICD-9 they are considered one broad category with five specific types. In DMP-1 the emotional disorders are not presented under a special category, but the subtypes are included under behavior disorders. In DSM-III the anxiety disorders have three subtypes: separation anxiety, avoidant disorder, and overanxious disorder. In ICD-9 disturbances of emotions have the following subtypes: with anxiety; with misery; with sensitivity, shyness, and social withdrawal; with relationship problems; other or mixed and unspecified. DMP-1 defined the corresponding reactions as overanxious, withdrawing, runaway, adolescent turmoil, and other reactions of childhood. Thus, DSM-III is particular with regard to separation anxiety; ICD-9, with regard to the misery type and relationship problems; and DMP-1, with regard to the runaway, adolescent turmoil, and other reactions. DSM-III presents five types of eating disorders: anorexia nervosa, bulimia, pica, rumination, and atypical eating disorders. All of these are included under one category in DMP-1. DSM-III has subclassified stereotyped movement disorders into five types. In ICD-9 they are included either under physiological malfunction arising from mental factors, musculoskeletal factors (e.g., psychogenic torticollis), or special symptoms or syndromes not classified elsewhere – such as tics. In contrast, DMP-1 included these disorders under one undifferentiated category, that is, special symptoms not classified elsewhere, tics and other psychomotor disorders. Other disorders in childhood with physical manifestations were subdivided into five types in DSM-III: stuttering, functional enuresis, functional encopresis, sleepwalking, and sleep terror. In ICD-9 and DMP-1 they were included under special symptoms or syndromes not classified elsewhere.

Criteria for stuttering, enuresis, and encopresis are described in both DSM-III and ICD-9. Criteria for sleepwalking and night terror are not defined in ICD-9 and are not mentioned at all in DMP-1. Specific developmental disorders in DSM-III correspond to specific delays in development of ICD-9, and speech and learning disturbances in DMP-1. In DSM-III there are six subtypes of these disorders: reading, arithmetic, language, articulation, mixed, and atypical. In ICD-9 there are eight subtypes: reading, arithmetic, learning, speech or language, motor, mixed, other, and unspecified. In DMP-1, only speech and learning disturbances are mentioned, and no diagnostic criteria are presented.

Developmental disorders have been classified in DSM-III into pervasive disorders and specific developmental disorders. The pervasive disorders in this system have three subtypes: infantile autism, childhood-onset pervasive disorder, and atypical pervasive disorders. They correspond to psychosis with origin specific to childhood in ICD-9, and to miscellaneous (other) behavior disorder of childhood in DMP-1.

COMMENTS ON NOSOLOGICAL PROSPECTS

Looking to the future, it would seem worthwhile to attempt to make ICD-10 and DSM-IV uniform in order to arrive at one International Classification of Psychiatric Disorders. This would reduce the diversity of opinion and increase reliability among psychiatrists, as well as improve public opinion on the solidity of psychiatry.

Some observations on the basis of our participation in the WHO informal consultation on proposals for the classification of mental disorders and psychosocial factors in ICD-10, which took place in Geneva in April 1984, seem to be in order here. Compared with ICD-9, the main changes and innovations planned for ICD-10 appear to be the following: The broad rubrics of psychosis and neurosis are abandoned, although in various places on the classification the terms themselves are retained for use in a purely descriptive sense. All the mental disorders attributable to demonstrable organic causes, with the exception of those due to substance use, are grouped together regardless of whether their predominant manifestations are psychotic or nonpsychotic. Problems related to alcohol and other psychoactive drugs are brought together in a single group. The classification of schizophrenic disorders, and disorders possibly related to the schizophrenic spectrum of disease, would be expanded. Paranoid schizophrenia and residual schizophrenia would be identified at the three-digit level. A new category is introduced for acute, short-lived psychoses that are not obviously related to either schizophrenic or affective disorders. These disorders appear to be common in many developing countries but also occur in developed ones. All affective (mood) disorders, whether of psychotic intensity or not, are brought together into a single group. A major block of three-digit codes would be reserved for the neurotic disorders (adding the term "emotional" as a preferred synonym). The classification of emotional disorders presenting with somatic symptoms is revised and the various categories grouped together. The classification of personality disorders is simplified, and at the same time new categories are introduced for personality traits that do not warrant the designation disorder but are, nonetheless, of psychiatric significance. These conditions have been grouped together with personality change secondary to catastrophic experience or to psychiatric illness. The classification of disorders with an onset in childhood or adolescence is substantially expanded. The classification of psychosexual disorders is being thoroughly revised, and sexual deviations and disorders are being split into two subgroups.

The so-called cultural bound syndromes would appear either as inclusion terms or in a special index. The current list of such local syndromes is fairly extensive. It includes many reactive psychotic conditions such as Amoc and Lata, and many varieties such as spirit possession syndromes in Africa, Asia, and Latin America. Among neurotic conditions, one may note the acute panic reaction associated with a fear of shrinking of the genitals (the Koro syndrome of Malaysia), anxiety exhaustion related to studies (the Brain Fog syndrome of Africa), multiple physical and mental symptoms attributed to loss of semen (the Dahat of India), spirit possession (Al-zar in Egypt and Sudan), and many other conditions that are too poorly described to be understood. These may be included under subcategories in many standard classifications.

COMPARATIVE CONCLUSIONS

1. DMP-1 is based on DSM-II, ICD-8, and the French system.
2. DMP-1 is simpler than those systems.
3. DMP-1 follows certain cultural tendencies, such as gathering alcohol and other drugs together when considering the problem of substance abuse.
4. DMP-1 requires certain changes to make it more sophisticated but for the time being is satisfactory in view of the shortage of qualified specialists.
5. At present DMP-1 is only applied in university clinics, and enough time must be allowed for it to be applied in other centers before we can comment on its general usability.
6. The main difficulties noted from experience can be summarized as follows:
   a. In the absence of a multiaxial scheme, differentiation of diagnostic categories is incomplete.
   b. Intermingling of the clinical syndromes and their etiological bases adds to the difficulties of the clinician.
   c. The base amount of patient-care work required from clinicians leads them to use only the main categories and not go farther into subcategories.
   d. The DMP-1 classification of disorders of infancy and childhood is primitive and simple and needs more elaboration in order to take into consideration subcategories in ICD-9 and DSM-III, and the proposals for ICD-10.

APPENDIXES

A: The Egyptian Classification of Psychiatric Disorders (DMP-I)

01 *Mental retardation*
.0 Borderline mental retardation
.1 Mild mental retardation
.2 Moderate mental retardation
.3 Severe mental retardation
.4 Profound mental retardation
.5 Unspecified mental retardation
  0 Following infection and intoxication
  1 Following trauma or a physical agent
  2 With disorders of metabolism, endocrines or nutrition
  3 Associated with gross brain disease (postnatal)
  4 Associated with prenatal or cerebral anomalies
  5 With chromosomal abnormality
  6 Associated with prematurity
  7 Following major psychiatric disorder
  8 With psychosocial (environmental) deprivation
  9 With other and unspecified conditions
02 *Psychoses associated with organic brain syndromes*
.0 Senile and presenile dementia
.1 Psychosis associated with intracranial infection
.2 Psychosis associated with other cerebral condition
.3 Psychosis associated with general systemic condition
.9 Psychosis with other and unspecified conditions
03 *Non-psychotic conditions associated with organic brain syndromes*
04 *Psychiatric disorders of epilepsy*
05 *Drug dependence, alcoholism and alcoholic psychoses*
.0 Drug dependence
  .00 Simple habituation
  .01 Addiction
.1 Alcoholism
  .10 Simple chronic alcoholism
  .11 Intermittent alcoholic indulgence (dipsomania)
  .12 Alcohol addiction
.2 Alcoholic psychoses
  .20 Delirium tremens
  .21 Korsakov's psychosis
  .22 Alcoholic hallucinosis
  .23 Alcohol paranoid state
.8 Other conditions associated with drug dependence
.9 Other alcoholic disorders
06 *Manic and depressive illnesses*
.0 Manic-depressive illness, depressive type
.1 Manic-depressive illness, manic type

.2 Manic-depressive illness, circular type
.3 Manic-depressive illness, mixed type
.4 Involutional melancholia
.5 Depressive illness not elsewhere specified
.6 Manic illness not elsewhere specified
.9 Others

07 *Schizophrenia*
.0 Acute undifferentiated episode
.1 Incipient
.2 Schizo-affective
.3 Paranoid
.4 Catatonic
.5 Hebephrenic
.6 Simple
.7 Chronic undifferentiated
.8 Residual
.9 Other types

08 *Paranoid states*
.0 Acute or subacute paranoid episode
.1 Chronic delusional paranoid state
.2 Chronic hallucinatory paranoid state
.3 Chronic imaginative (fantastic) paranoid state
.4 Involutional paranoid state
.5 Late paranoid state
.6 Paranoia
.9 Other paranoid states

09 *Other functional psychoses*
.0 Acute undifferentiated psychosis
.1 Acute confusional psychosis
.2 Acute reactive and situational psychosis
.3 Chronic reactive and situational psychosis
.9 Others

10 *Neuroses*
.0 Anxiety neurosis
.1 Hysterical neurosis
   .10 Conversion type
   .11 Dissociative type
.2 Phobic neurosis
.3 Obsessive compulsive neurosis
.4 Depressive neurosis
.5 Neurasthenic neurosis
.6 Hypochondriacal neurosis
.7 Reactive and situational neurosis
.9 Others

11 *Personality and character disorders*
.0 Personality pattern disorder
   .00 Schizoid personality
   .01 Paranoid personality
   .02 Cyclothymic personality
   .03 Obsessive personality

.04 Antisocial personality
.1 Character trait disorder
    .10 Explosive personality
    .11 Kleptomanic character
    .12 Pyromanic character
    .13 Dyssocial character
    .14 Hypochondriacal character
    .15 Malingering
.2 Immature personalities
    .20 Passive dependent personality
    .21 Hysterical personality
    .22 Inadequate personality
    .23 Emotionally unstable personality
.3 Sexual deviation
    .30 Sexual stimulus
    .31 Sexual expression
    .32 Instinctual object
.9 Others

12 Psychophysiologic disorders
.0 Psychophysiologic skin disorder
.1 Psychophysiologic musculo-skeletal disorder
.2 Psychophysiologic respiratory disorder
.3 Psychophysiologic cardio-vascular disorder
.4 Psychophysiologic gastro-intestinal disorder
.5 Psychophysiologic genito-urinary disorder
.6 Psychophysiologic endocrine disorder
.7 Psychophysiologic disorder of organ of special sense
.9 Psychophysiologic disorders of other types

13 Behaviour disorders of childhood and adolescence
.0 Hyperkinetic reaction of childhood (or adolescence)
.1 Withdrawing reaction of childhood (or adolescence)
.2 Over-anxious reaction of childhood (or adolescence)
.3 Runaway reaction of childhood (or adolescence)
.4 Unsocialized aggressive reaction of childhood (or adolescence)
.5 Group delinquent reaction of childhood (or adolescence)
.6 Adolescent turmoil state
.9 Others

14 Special symptoms not elsewhere classified
.0 Speech and learning disturbance
.1 Tic and other psychomotor disturbance
.2 Disorder of sleep
.3 Feeding disturbance
.4 Disorders of sphincteric control
.5 Cephalalgia
.6 Impotence
.7 Frigidity
.8 Depersonalization
.9 Others

15 Conditions not classifiable under any of the previous categories
16 No psychiatric disorder

B: Comparative Listing of ICD-9, DMP-I, DSM-III and Proposed ICD-10

ICD-9	DMP-I	DSM-III	Proposed ICD-10 (1987)
ORG. PSYCH. COND.	01 Ment. retard.	• Dis. 1st evid. in infan., child. & adol.	F0 Org. & symp. dis.
290 Sen. & presen. org. psych. cond.	02 Psych. assoc. with OBS.	• Org. ment. dis.	F1 Psychoact. subs. dis.
291 Alc. psych.	03 Non-psych. cond. assoc. with OBS.	• Subs. use dis.	F2 Schiz. & other psych.
292 Drug psych.	04 Psychiat. dis. of epilep.	• Schiz. dis.	F3 Affect. (mood) dis.
293 Trans. org. psych. cond.	05 Drug depend., alcoholism & alc. psych.	• Paranoid dis.	F4 Neurotic, stress & somatoform dis.
294 Other org. psych. cond.	06 Manic & dep. illnesses	• Psych. dis. not else. class.	F5 Physiol. dysfunct. assoc. with ment. facts.
OTHER PSYCHOSES	07 Schizophrenia	• Affective dis.	F6 Abnorm. of adult pers. & behaviour
295 Schiz. psych.	08 Paranoid state	• Anxiety dis.	F7 Ment. retard.
296 Affect. psych.	09 Other funct. psych.	• Dissociative dis.	F8 Develop. dis.
297 Paranoid state	10 Neuroses	• Somatoform dis.	F9 Behav. & emot. dis. usually starting in child. or adult.
298 Other psychotic cond.	11 Pers. & charac. dis.	• Psychosex. dis.	
299 Psych. with origin spec. to child.	12 Psycho-physiol. dis.	• Factitious dis.	
NEUROTIC, PERS. & OTHER NON-PSYCH. MENT. DIS.	13 Behav. dis. of child. & adol.	• Dis. of impulse control not else. class.	
300 Neurotic dis.	14 Special symp. not else. classified	• Adjust. dis.	
301 Personality dis.	15 Cond. not classif. under any previous categ.	• Psychol. factors affecting physic. cond.	
302 Sex. dev. dis.	16 No psychiat. dis.	• Person. dis.	
303 Alc. dep. synd.		• V codes for cond. not attrib. to ment. dis. that are focus of attent. or treatment	
304 Drug depend.		• Additional codes	
305 Non-depend. abuse drugs			
306 Physiol. malfunc. from ment. factors			
307 Spec. symp. or synd. not else. cl.			
308 Acute reac. to stress			
309 Adjust. reaction			
310 Spec. non-psych. ment. dis. follow. OB damage			
311 Dep. dis. not else. cl.			
312 Dist. cond. not else. cl.			
313 Dist. emot. spec. to child. & adol.			
314 Hyperkin. synd. of child.			
315 Spec. delay of develop.			
316 Psychic fact. assoc. with diseas. class. else.			
317 Mild ment. retard.			
318 Other spec. ment. retard.			
319 Unspec. ment. retard.			

REFERENCES

American Psychiatric Association 1952. *Diagnostic and Statistical Manual of Mental Disorders* (DSM). Washington, D.C.

American Psychiatric Association 1968. *Diagnostic and Statistical Manual of Mental Disorders* (DSM-II). Washington, D.C.

American Psychiatric Association 1980. *Diagnostic and Statistical Manual of Mental Disorders*. 3rd ed. (DSM-III). Washington, D.C.

Egyptian Psychiatric Association 1979. *Diagnostic Manual of Psychiatric Disorders* (DMP-1). Cairo.

Institut de la Santé et de la Recherche Medicale (INSERM). Section Psychiatrie. 1969. *Classification français des troubles mentaux. Bulletin de l'Institut National de la Santé et de la Recherche Medicale.* vol. 24, supplement no. 2.

Spitzer, R., Williams, J., and Skodol, A. 1983. *International Perspectives of DSM-III.* Washington, D.C.: American Psychiatric Press.

World Health Organization 1969. *Manual of the International Statistical Classification of Diseases, Injuries and Causes of Death.* 8th rev. ed. (ICD-8). Geneva.

World Health Organization 1978. *Manual of the Ninth Revision of the International Classification of Diseases* (ICD-9). Geneva.

6   *Diagnosis and classification of mental disorders and alcohol- and drug-related problems in Nigeria*

AYO BINITIE (Nigeria)

Some of the more important goals of diagnosis and classification in the developing countries of Africa are to promote the understanding of African culture as it relates to Europeans, to enhance communication between the African and European psychiatric communities, and ultimately to develop a common language. When, for example, we talk of the peculiarities of depression in Africans, we imply

1. That the syndrome exists in the African setting
2. That in some ways depression in Africans is different from depression in Europeans
3. That it is possible to distinguish depression in Africans from depressions in Europeans

These inferences raise the question of what combination of genes and environment in an African setting contributes to the clinical picture hitherto regarded as classical. The example that we have given represents an exercise in appraising African culture by using a European yardstick. The converse experience of appraising European culture by means of an African yardstick has rarely occurred. Lest this statement become too theoretical, a practical example should clarify the point. What kind of Europeans are plagued by the syndrome of *Ogbanje* in Ibo or *Abiky* in Yoruba? Which Europeans are troubled by a malignant ancestor? Who among Europeans is plagued by *Olokun*, the goddess of fertility and wealth? At a more prosaic level, which Europeans are harmed by the machinations of witches and wizards? These afflictions are a matter of everyday occurrence in African countries and have persisted through generations. Are these syndromes simply absent in the European population? Or do they have cultural equivalents there?

The present position of psychiatric classification in Nigeria must be viewed from a historical perspective. The majority of Nigerian psychiatrists have been trained in the United Kingdom. The early pioneers, such as Thomas Lambo, exerted a dominant influence on the practice of psychiatry both in Nigeria and in London. The classification system that Lambo learned in the United Kingdom was in turn passed on to medical students, doctors, and teachers of medicine in Nigeria. This tradition has been further reinforced by his successor in office,

65

T. Asuni, and the younger generation of psychiatrists who also received their training either in London or Edinburgh (sometimes in both). The influence of Kraepelin on the classification of psychiatric disorders, as well as the modifications made by Eugene Bleuler, are still evident in Nigerian psychiatry. In actual day-to-day practice, however, many psychiatrists have found that pathoplastic factors influence psychiatric diagnosis, so that many classically described syndromes show much variation when applied to live patients in the Nigerian setting (Binitie, 1977). In order to understand such divergence from the classical syndromes it is necessary to examine in some detail the classification system currently being used by Nigerian psychiatrists.

CLASSIFICATION OF PSYCHIATRIC DISORDERS

Nigerian psychiatrists consider psychiatric disorders to be either functional or organic. Under the rubric of "organic psychoses" they include both acute and chronic brain syndromes. This category encompasses such conditions as the senile and presenile dementias, arteriosclerotic and senile psychoses, and epilepsy. In general, the organic psychoses present few diagnostic difficulties, since these disorders follow a typical medical model, and tests are frequently available to confirm the diagnoses.

However, the functional disorders require further comment. Nigerian psychiatrists recognize two broad categories of functional disorder: "psychosis" and "neurosis." Differentiation between these two categories is based partly on the intensity of the symptomatology presented and partly on the presence or absence of insight; thus, such severe symptomatology as hallucinations and delusions, disorders of thinking, gross abnormalities of behavior, and severe mannerisms frequently result in a diagnosis of psychosis, whereas milder symptoms – such as palpitations, heat in the body, fear, shaking of hands and legs, dryness of the mouth, frequent stooling and diarrhea – lead to a diagnosis of neurosis.

Thus, the bases for the neurotic classification are frequently stated to be both the presence of insight and an absence of the constellation of symptoms that psychiatrists regard as psychotic. Although borderline states are considered, it is clear that Nigerian psychiatrists generally apply recognizable criteria for arriving at the diagnosis of the various syndromes.

SCHIZOPHRENIA

In actual practice, most Nigerian psychiatrists make a diagnosis of schizophrenia whenever auditory hallucinations are present. The content of the hallucinations is important. The more bizarre the content, the more likely the psychiatrist is to diagnose schizophrenia. Thus, voices that abuse, command, or direct the patient tend to suggest a diagnosis of schizophrenia. Another diagnostic criterion considered indicative of schizophrenia is the presence of thought disorder, for example, thought insertion, broadcasting, and blocking. In the presence of such symptoms, there is no hesitation whatsoever in formulating a diagnosis of schizophrenia. Similarly, the presence of catatonic features, even in the absence of other symptoms, will be sufficient for the psychiatrist to arrive at a diagnosis of schizophrenia. In contrast, the presence of delusions, although useful, contributes only modestly to the making of such a diagnosis. In addition to hallucinatory and delusional symptoms, the presence of affective flattening, incongruous affect, and a history of personality change are considered suggestive of a schizophrenic syndrome.

Concerning the subcategories of schizophrenia, the classic categories are recognized by Nigeria psychiatrists, namely, simple, hebephrenic, paranoid, and catatonic. The African experience suggests that simple schizophrenia is infrequently present. The few patients so diagnosed have usually been referred to psychiatric departments by law enforcement agencies. Hebephrenic schizophrenia is more frequently diagnosed and includes those patients with more florid types of symptomatology. Catatonic symptomatology is infrequent; however, when present, it usually leads to a diagnosis of catatonic schizophrenia. The presence of systematized paranoid ideas – often in addition to auditory hallucinations – will culminate in a diagnosis of paranoid schizophrenia.

So far, no mention has been made of the pathoplastic effects of culture and the manner in which such disorders present themselves in the typical Nigerian community. Such effects occur, however, and they are readily recognizable for what they are. Thus, instead of the X-rays and gases beamed at the patient in a Western culture, witches and wizards trouble him or her in a typical Nigerian setting, particularly in the rural and less sophisticated areas. The more schooled the Nigerian, the more likely he or she is to leave witches and wizards in the countryside and assume the most technological symptoms of a European patient.

AFFECTIVE STATES

For a long time it was believed that depression did not occur in the traditional African population. Sufficient evidence has now been accumulated to show that this is not true. Lambo (1956, 1960), Buchan (1961), Collomb and Zwingelstein (1961), Field (1958), and Binitie (1981a,b, 1983) have demonstrated that this condition is common. Difficulty in the diagnosis of depression in the African setting results from the pathoplastic effect of the culture-modifying symptoms, so that it is difficult to recognize the condition to be the same as that of the classical European affective syndrome. Instead, the African patient frequently exhibits with many bodily complaints, such as heat in the head or body, worms crawling all over the body, worms in the head, tightness of the head, or gas in the stomach. Such somatic complaints may so dominate the picture that the true nature and significance of the symptoms are lost.

Guilt and suicidal ideation or acts are symptom patterns common to depression in European countries. Although not absent in African cultures, such features are rare in Nigeria. Thus, these cardinal symptoms which are highly suggestive of "depression" in European cultures are almost completely masked when an affective disorder occurs in an African population. It is the experience of Nigerian psychiatrists that the African equivalent of European "guilt" is the projection of hostile ideas onto social agencies within the culture or onto other aspects of the environment; such depressed patients often complain of witches and wizards scheming against them. In addition to somatic complaints, other important features of affective disorder, as it presents in African cultures, include the presence of depressive dreams (when the patient sees dead people) and loss of libido. Males may experience impotence. Hallucinations, when they occur, focus on themes of death and killing.

In summary, while the depressed African patient exhibits many somatic or bodily complaints, a sense of European guilt is absent or rare. Instead, witches and wizards plague the patient. There is, in addition, a loss of energy, interest and drive comparable to that found in European patients. The condition is chronic if untreated.

A variety of factors must be taken into consideration when differentiating reactive from endogenous types of depression. Family history may provide important diagnostic clues. Severity – as well as the presence or absence of precipitating factors – also plays an important role. However, variability of mood has not been found very useful in making judgments as to whether a patient is suffering from reactive or endogenous depression, and the sleep pattern is only marginally helpful.

Depression is quite prevalent in the Nigerian population and constitutes the third most common diagnostic condition (after anxiety and schizophrenic disorders) in most clinics. A few specialty centers – in particular, the teaching hospitals – record more depressed patients than schizophrenics (according to hospital statistics).

Involutional melancholia

Although Nigerian psychiatrists recognize that involutional melancholia is not a separate syndrome from depression, many retain this diagnostic category because of the distinct form this disorder takes in the afflicted persons and also because of such patients' rapid response to ECT.

Mania

This condition presents no special diagnostic difficulties for the African psychiatrist. The happy, jocular aspect of the manic patient, his elation and overactivity – together with his or her bombastic, boastful behavior – help to identify the syndrome. Additional features that may be present, such as grandiose delusions and paranoid ideas, help to clinch the diagnosis.

MANIC-DEPRESSIVE CIRCULAR OR CYCLOID PSYCHOSIS

In this condition, depression may alternate with mania in rapid succession, or there may be several episodes of depression followed by a single attack of mania. The criteria for the elements of this diagnosis are identical to those for mania and depression.

EXCITEMENT STATES

This condition is especially important and interesting since nothing comparable has been described in the European literature. Nigerian psychiatrists themselves are in fact not in agreement about the existence of this syndrome. A paper presented at an annual conference of a psychiatric association concerning the existence of this syndrome attracted a lively debate and a great deal of controversy as to whether the patients so diagnosed were in fact not cases of hypomania or mania, or – alternatively – catatonic schizophrenia; other psychiatrists have suggested that there is a hysterical component in this syndrome. It is clear that this kind of condition ought to be the subject of intensive research.

The condition is in some ways similar to amok, in that a sense of acute excitement is present. Such patients tend toward overactivity and are characterized by an outpouring of verbiage and an excessive output of energy. In contrast to the patient with hypomania whose speech is flighty, the verbal production of a patient in an excitement state is relatively circumscribed. For example, in the section of Benin where I practice, one suffering from an excitement state may make speeches to deities who are worshiped by the local inhabitants. Thus, others in the community may explain the condition by saying that the patient is possessed by a particular god or goddess and prescribe a suitable sacrifice to correct the situation.

The syndrome is episodic, often with long intervals between attacks. Characteristically, such attacks will come on suddenly, produce intense and profound activity, and lead to both a disruption of family life and a frenzy of religious activity. An episode frequently lasts one or two weeks but rarely longer. When it remits, the patient is restored to complete normalcy. No trace of the syndrome can be found. It is clear that such a clinical picture cannot be adequately classified by traditional diagnostic frameworks.

Spirit possession is found in shrines and more recently in new types of religious circles. In these instances, there is a total sense of control in an organized setting. Some follow-up studies suggest that some of those cases initially diagnosed as suffering from excitement state were eventually classified as schizophrenic or depressed. In most cases, however, the diagnosis continued to be that of an excitement state not fitting any diagnostic category currently in use.

NEUROSES

Neurotic conditions recognized in African psychiatry include anxiety states, depression, hysteria, obsessional neurosis, compensation neurosis, hypochondriasis, and neurasthenia.

Anxiety states

The syndrome "anxiety" encompasses phobias of various types. In addition, other features of this syndrome include psychic anxiety, somatic symptoms and autonomic symptoms (e.g., fear, palpitations, tremor of the fingers), and autonomic symptoms referable to the cardiovascular or respiratory system. Such clear-cut criteria generally lead to a consensus on the presence of this neurosis.

Depression

Criteria for making this diagnosis in general were discussed in the section on affective states. It is a common notion in African psychiatry that the presence of auditory hallucinations excludes a patient from this category. The term "neurotic depression" tends to be reserved for the milder variety of depression in which social factors, such as isolation and work stress, appear to precipitate the condition.

Hysteria

The key feature of this diagnostic category is the presence of abnormal bodily symptoms that are not in keeping with any known anatomical or physiological malfunction. Any part of the body may be affected.

Obsessional neurosis

This type of neurosis is not common in Africa, but it does occur. Obsessional thoughts and compulsions are the key criteria for arriving at this diagnosis.

Compensation neurosis

This condition – which is becoming more common in the larger urban centers – is really a form of hysteria in which the major source of conflict is the need for compensation.

Hypochondriasis

Although some Nigerian psychiatrists still employ the diagnosis of hypochondriasis, the majority of them recognize the condition as a form of depression. The cardinal symptoms of hypochondriasis are a preoccupation with bowel functions and other somatic complaints.

Neurasthenia

This condition is reserved by some Nigerian psychiatrists for patients in which the dominant picture is a lack of energy, accompanied by some anxiety symptoms. It is likely that the majority of these cases may be diagnosable with a depressive condition, while a few may meet anxiety state criteria.

ALCOHOLISM

The use of alcohol is rapidly expanding in the developing countries. A number of factors are involved in this expansion: greater affluence and a growing middle class that can afford drinking, as well as a heavy media campaign advertising alcohol. Young persons may use alcohol to feel manly or to forget the week's drudgeries. Furthermore, the frustrating effects of dislocation – common in many African countries – can lead to alcoholism. Weekend drunkenness is now a feature of life in many of the developing countries. In spite of this tremendous and widespread abuse of alcohol in Africa, few alcoholics seek psychiatric treatment. The vast majority remain in the community, coping as best they can with their disability. Surveys among both illiterate and literate citizens have shown that alcohol abuse is not regarded as an illness (e.g., Binite & Uku, 1982). Only when a major complication occurs, such as delirium, hallucinosis, or a paranoid reaction, is the psychiatrist consulted.

PERSONALITY DISORDERS

Personality disorder diagnoses do not yet represent a major preoccupation of psychiatrists in the developing countries. Such disorders become a problem only in relation to forensic psychiatry, that is, when crimes have been committed and the mental state of the accused is called into question. The most common of these diagnoses is psychopathic personality. This type of personality disorder is characterized by emotional immaturity coupled with a lack of forethought and frequently leads to seriously irresponsible conduct; it is a common adjunct to the diagnosis of toxic psychosis among Indian hemp smokers.

PSYCHOSIS FOLLOWING INGESTION OF HEMP

In no diagnostic area is there so much disagreement between psychiatrists practicing in Africa and those in Europe as in the sphere of the use of hemp, cannabis, or marijuana and its effect on mental health. The majority of psychiatrists working in Africa hold the view that the use of cannabis can produce a psychosis (Asuni, 1964; Lambo, 1965; Boroffka, 1966). In addition, marijuana is believed to precipitate latent psychoses with schizophrenic or depressive pictures. Binitie (1972), reporting on two cases of psychosis in children following ingestion of hemp, wrote that "the clinical picture suggests an organic rather than a functional psychosis" and that the features include redness of the eyes, disturbed, restless behavior and an inability to do simple calculations, together with a minor to moderate degree of clouding of consciousness. This clinical picture is a common occurrence in the wards of many psychiatric hospitals in Africa, as well as in other developing countries.

REFERENCES

Asuni, T. 1964. Sociopsychiatric problems of cannabis. *Bulletin on Narcotics*, 16: 17–28.

Binitie, A. 1972. Psychosis following the ingestion of hemp in children. *Psychopharmacologia* 44: 301–302.

Binitie, A. 1977. Psychological basis of certain culturally held beliefs. *Internal J. Social Psychiat* 23: 204–208.

Binitie, A. 1981a. Psychiatric disorders in rural practice in the Bendel State of Nigeria. *Acta Psychiat. Scand.* 64: 273–280.

Binitie, A. 1981b. The clinical manifestation of depression in Africans. In *The Prevention and Treatment of Depression*, ed. T. A. Ban, R. Gonzales, A. S. Jablensky, N. A. Sartorius, and F. E. Vartanian. Baltimore: Johns Hopkins University Press.

Binitie, A. 1983. The depressed and anxious patient care and treatment in Africa. *Int. J. Mental Health* 12: 44–57.

Binitie, A., and Uku, R. 1982. Attitude of illiterate Nigerians to mental illness. In *Mental Health in Africa*, ed. O. A. Erinosho and N. W. Bell. Ibadan: University Press Publishing House.

Boroffka, A. 1966. Mental illness and Indian hemp in Lagos, Nigeria. *East African Med. J.* 43: 377–384.

Buchan, T. 1961. Depression in African patients. *South African Medical Journal* 4: 1055–1058.

Collomb, H., and Zwingelstein, T. 1961. Les états depressifs en milieu Africaine, ed. T. A. Lambo. *Report of the First Pan African Psychiatric Conference*. Ibadan: Ibadan Government Press.

Field, M. G. 1958. Mental disorders in rural Ghana. *Journal of Mental Science* 104: 1043–1051.

Lambo, T. A. 1956. Neuropsychiatric observations in the Western Region of Nigeria. *Brit. Med. J.* 2: 1388–1394.

Lambo, T. A. 1960. Further neuropsychiatric observations in Nigeria. *Brit. Med. J.* 2: 1696–1704.

Lambo, T. A. 1965. Medical and social aspects of drug addiction in West Africa with special emphasis on psychiatric aspects. *Bulletin on Narcotics*, 17: 1–3.

7 Principles of the Chinese Classification of Mental Disorders (CCMD)

SHEN YU-CUN AND CHEN CHANGHUI (People's Republic of China)

On three different occasions since 1978 the Chinese Medical Association of Neurology and Psychiatry outlined a national classification of mental disorders following detailed discussions at a National Academic Conference (Chinese Neuropsychiatric Association, 1982). The current Chinese Classification of Mental Disorders (CCMD) was last revised at the National Professional Conference of Psychiatry held in October 1984. (See the appendix to this chapter.)

The current revision of the CCMD is based not only on broad principles of clinical practice among Chinese psychiatric professionals but also on the results of international academic communications. Since 1980, those classifications relevant to mental disorders in ICD-8 (World Health Organization, 1967) and ICD-9 (World Health Organization, 1978) – as well as the classification and diagnostic criteria for mental disorders in DSM-III (American Psychiatric Association, 1980) – have been translated and widely disseminated among Chinese professionals in the psychiatric field. In addition, a number of pilot tests and comparison studies have been completed. They include important data that were also considered during the current revisions of the CCMD (Chen Changhui and Shen Yu-cun, in press).

The following points were taken into consideration in the revision of the CCMD:

1. A classification must reflect advancements and updated knowledge from related scientific fields.
2. A classification must also demonstrate adequate stability and rational continuity with earlier systems; without such characteristics, diagnostic confusion would ensue in both medical practice and research activity, particularly in a country as vast as China.
3. A classification system must both be advantageous to Chinese performance in mental health and contribute to international academic activities.

The specific principles adopted during the formulation of the current CCMD-3 at the National Professional Conference of Psychiatry were as follows:

1. In our classification system, a nosological approach has been maintained. If an etiological factor or factors have been ascertained for a given mental disorder, then that disorder is categorized as a separate entity in the classification.

73

For example, the category "organic psychotic conditions" includes subcategories representing those disorders associated with intracranial infections, intracranial injury, cerebrovascular disorder, intracranial neoplasms, and epileptic psychosis; similarly, the category "psychoses associated with physical illness" includes subcategories for those psychoses associated with infectious disease, as well as various visceral, endocrine, and metabolic diseases; the category "toxic psychoses and drug and alcoholic dependence" includes subcategories for psychosis induced by drugs, drug dependence, alcohol dependence, toxic psychosis of carbon monoxide, and psychosis induced by pesticide.

In CCMD-3, both manic-depressive psychosis and involutional melancholia are subsumed under the category of affective psychoses, an approach similar to that of ICD-9 (World Health Organization, 1978). However, reactive psychosis and its subgroup, reactive depression, are treated as independent entities. Furthermore, depressive neurosis has been categorized as a subgroup of the neuroses. This was suggested by recent studies that show endogenous depression and involutional melancholia to be biologically different from reactive depression and neurotic depression. According to one study that examined the role of central neurotransmitter metabolism and neuroendocrine activities in various depressive disorders, involutional and manic-depressive patients showed much higher Dexamethasone Suppression Test (DST) escape rates (66.7 percent and 52.0 percent, respectively) than did neurotic and reactive depressives (both 7.7 percent only) (Zhou Dongfeng et al., 1984).

2. Consistent with ICD-9, neurasthenia is listed in CCMD-3 as a subgroup under "neuroses." Although neurasthenia had appeared in the classification system of DSM-II (American Psychiatric Association, 1968), it was deleted in DSM-III (American Psychiatric Association, 1980). The retention of neurasthenia in CCMD is based not only on long-term psychiatric practice in China but also on a pilot study completed in 1983. In this study, 50 outpatients being treated at the Clinical Department of the Institute of Mental Health, Beijing Medical College (now renamed Beijing Medical University), for a diagnosis of neurosis were interviewed with a 30-item schedule developed by psychiatrists of the institute. The instrument was based on the first few sections of the Present State Examination (Wing, Cooper, & Sartorius, 1974), as slightly modified by Xu Youxin et al. (1985). The schedule included 12 items (1–12) representing the symptoms of neurasthenia, 3 items (13–15) for anxiety, 4 items (16–19) for hypochondriasis, and 11 items (20–30) for depressive neurosis. The purpose of the schedule was to facilitate the process of arriving at a potential diagnosis. The four raters, who interviewed outpatients, fully agreed on the diagnoses in 42 cases of the 50 examined. After being evaluated according to the criteria for neuroses designed by the Clinical Psychiatric Research Unit of the Institute (Xu Youxin et al., 1983), the 42 with concordant diagnoses were found to consist of 25 cases with neurasthenia (59.5 percent), 4 with anxiety (9.5 percent), 5 with hypochondriasis (11.9 percent), 7 with depressive neurosis (16.7 percent), and 1 with some other diagnosis (2.4 percent). These results indicate clearly

that neurasthenia exists as a separate disease entity, at least in the Chinese population.

3. In order to avoid overdiagnosis of schizophrenic disorders, schizoaffective psychosis has been separated from schizophrenia and listed under the category for psychotic disorders not classified elsewhere, as in DSM-III (290.70). Owing to the uncertainty inherent in such a classification, it is suggested that operational diagnostic criteria – for example, for inclusion, exclusion, course, and duration – be adopted before the diagnosis of schizoaffective disorder is applied in clinical practice.

4. Owing to the potential for change in disease trends among the Chinese population and the need to facilitate international academic exchange in the psychiatric profession, drug dependence and alcoholic dependence have been regarded as independent subentities and retained in a category separate from intoxication with psychoses.

5. It is generally accepted that our current knowledge is limited in scope and insufficient to handle all diagnostic situations. Thus, in order to provide the psychiatrist with the space and flexibility to cope with the complexity and variety of real-life diagnostic needs, a residual category – described as "other" – has been retained at the end of each major item.

Although the design of the CCMD-3 system has been completed, any comment or suggestion from either home or abroad is welcome. The CCMD-3 will surely benefit both professional practice in mental health and also clinical and research activities throughout our country. Despite such anticipated improvements, certain points in CCMD-3 have generated some debate. It is hoped that those now practicing the profession will gain new knowledge by applying the system and that, on the basis of these further insights, CCMD-3 will be revised when the time is ripe.

APPENDIX 1: CLASSIFICATION OF MENTAL DISEASES AUTHORIZED BY THE CHINESE MEDICAL ASSOCIATION, NEUROPSYCHIATRIC BRANCH (NOVEMBER 1984)

1. Organic mental disorders. This category refers to any psychosis induced by various types of brain impairment but excludes those psychoses induced by physical disorders or intoxication. (Note: Numbers within parentheses after the diagnostic terms correspond to ICD-9 codes.)

1.1 Psychotic disorder associated with intracranial infectious disease (293, 310.8)
1.2 Psychotic disorders associated with impairment of brain
1.2.1 Psychosis induced by brain trauma (293)
1.2.2 Personality disorder following brain trauma (310.1)
1.2.3 Syndrome following brain trauma (310.2)
1.3 Psychoses associated with cerebrovascular disease

1.3.1 Arteriosclerotic psychosis (290.4, 310)
1.3.2 Psychosis following other cerebrovascular diseases (310)
1.4   Psychosis associated with intracranial neoplasm (294, 310)
1.5   Psychoses induced by cerebral degeneration (290, 294, 310)
1.5.1 Presenile dementia (290.1)
1.5.2 Senile dementia (290.0, 290.2, 290.3)
1.5.3 Other (290.8)
1.6   Epileptic psychoses
1.6.1 Epileptic consciousness disturbance (293.0)
1.6.2 Epileptic psychosis (294.8)
1.6.3 Epileptic dementia (294.1)
1.6.4 Epileptic personality disorder
1.6.5 Other
1.7   Other organic psychotic conditions (294)

2. Psychotic conditions associated with physical illness. This category includes conditions resulting from various systemic physical diseases; brain diseases and intoxication are excluded.

2.1 Psychosis associated with infectious disease (293)
2.2 Psychosis associated with visceral disease (293)
2.3 Psychosis associated with endocrine disorder (293)
2.4 Psychosis associated with metabolic disorder (293)
2.5 Other (293.8)

3. Toxic psychoses and drug and alcohol dependence. This category refers to psychotic conditions induced by the intake of substances, including drugs, alcohol, and other noxious substances.

3.1 Psychosis induced by drug (292.1)
3.2 Drug dependence (304)
3.3 Alcoholic psychotic disorder (291)
3.4 Alcoholic dependence (303)
3.5 Psychotic condition induced by carbon monoxide
3.6 Toxic psychosis induced by pesticide
3.7 Psychotic condition induced by the toxic effect of other substances

4. Schizophrenia (295). Without clear causal factors, schizophrenia is a common psychosis, with the first episode usually occurring in adolescence. Disturbances of thinking, emotion, perception, and behavior are characteristic of this condition and usually lead to discordance in mental activity. Although this type of disorder tends to persist over a long period of time, it is likely to have no conscious or intellectual disturbance associated with its course.

4.1 Schizophrenia, simple type (295.0)
4.2 Schizophrenia, hebephrenic type (295.1)
4.3 Schizophrenia, catatonic type (295.2)

4.4 Schizophrenia, paranoid type (295.3)
4.5 Schizophrenia, residual type (295.6)
4.6 Schizophrenia, deteriorative type
4.7 Schizophrenia, unspecified type
4.8 Other

5. Affective psychotic disorders. Although the causal factors are unknown, the affective disorders are all predominantly characterized by a disturbance of mood – either excitement or hypothymia – with corresponding changes in thinking and behavior. Usually, this group of disorders does not lead to personality defect. The milder forms may not develop to the degree of severity required for classification as a psychosis.

5.1 Manic-depressive psychoses (296.0)
5.1.1 Manic-depressive psychosis, manic type (296.0)
5.1.2 Manic-depressive psychosis, depressive type (296.1)
5.1.3 Manic-depressive psychosis, bipolar type (296.2, 296.3, 296.4)
5.1.4 Manic-depressive psychosis, other and unspecified (296.6)

6. Paranoid psychoses (297). With no known causal factors, these psychoses are characterized primarily by delusional symptoms, often persecutory or jealous in nature. These delusions tend to be systemic, but do not lead to personality defect.

6.1 Paranoia (297.1)
6.2 Paranoid state (297.0)
6.3 Induced psychosis (297.3)
6.4 Other (297.8)

7. Reactive psychoses (298). This small group of psychotic conditions should be restricted to those that are largely or entirely attributable to obviously stressful psychosocial factors; in such cases, the onset, development, and content of the psychotic symptoms are closely related.

7.1 Reactive confusion (298.2, 308.1)
7.2 Reactive excitement (298.1, 308.2)
7.3 Reactive depression (298.0, 309.0, 309.1)
7.4 Reactive paranoid state (298.3, 298.4)
7.5 Other

8. Other unclassified psychosis. This category includes those psychoses unclassifiable at present, such as schizoaffective psychosis, schizoid psychosis, atypical psychosis, and periodic psychosis.

9. Neuroses (300). Neuroses have the following common features: (1) These disorders are usually caused by the combined effects of predisposition and psychosocial factors; (2) such patients may complain of both psychological and physical disturbances, with no demonstrable relevant pathological basis found upon examination; and (3) except for some with hysteria, neurotic patients often have clear consciousness, considerable insight, and no serious behavioral disturbance. The course of these disorders tends to be rather long, but the patients are willing to accept treatment.

> 9.1 Anxiety (300.0)
> 9.2 Hysteria (300.1)
> 9.3 Phobia (300.2)
> 9.4 Obsessive-compulsive disorder (300.3)
> 9.5 Neurotic depression (300.4)
> 9.6 Neurasthenia (300.5)
> 9.7 Hypochondriasis (300.7)
> 9.8 Other neurotic disorders (300.8, 306, 307)

10. Physiological malfunction arising from psychological factors (306). These disorders are mainly characterized by various symptoms of physiological malfunction with no demonstrable pathomorphological basis and with no global disturbance in mental activity. Psychosomatic disorders are excluded.

> 10.1 Sexual functional disturbance
> 10.2 Sleep disorder (307.4)
> 10.3 Eating disorders (307.5)
> 10.4 Functional disorders of visceral organs
> 10.5 Other

11. Personality disorders (301). Persistent maladaptive and impaired patterns of behavior characterize individuals with this type of disorder; their interpersonal relationships are disturbed. Such individuals are generally recognizable by the time of adolescence or earlier, but the disorder may become less obvious in middle age.

> 11.1 Paranoid personality disorder (301.0)
> 11.2 Affective personality disorder (301.1)
> 11.3 Schizoid personality disorder (301.2)
> 11.4 Explosive personality disorder (301.3)
> 11.5 Anankastic personality disorder (301.4)
> 11.6 Hysterical personality disorder (301.5)
> 11.7 Asocial personality disorder (301.7)
> 11.8 Other

12. Sexual psychological disorders (302). These disorders include those abnormal behaviors characterized by the individual's achieving sexual pleasure and gratification through abnormal acts (partly or entirely) rather than normal sexual behaviors. Usually this type of disorder appears with no other psychotic manifestations.

12.1 Homosexuality (302.0)
12.2 Transvestism (302.3)
12.3 Exhibitionism (302.4)
12.4 Fetishism (302.8)
12.5 Voyeurism (302.8)
12.6 Other (302.8)

13. Mental retardation (317–319). This condition refers to arrested or incomplete mental development caused by congenital factors or childhood disorders and leading to subaverage intellectual functioning and maladaptive social behaviors. As the causal factors are not easy to identify in most cases, the clinical classification is usually based on severity of impairment.

13.1 Mild mental retardation (317)
13.2 Moderate mental retardation (318.0)
13.3 Severe mental retardation (318.1)
13.4 Profound mental retardation (318.2)
13.5 Unspecified

14. Child mental disorders (313–315). This category includes all mental disorders of children that could not properly be included in the preceding entries and that are characterized by features relevant to age and various stages of development.

14.1 Psychoses specific to childhood (299)
14.1.1 Infantile autism (299.0)
14.1.2 Infantile dementia (299.1)
14.1.3 Other (299.8)
14.2 Disturbance of emotions specific to childhood (313)
14.2.1 Anxiety reaction (313.0)
14.2.2 Panic reaction (313.0)
14.2.3 Depressive reaction (313.1)
14.2.4 Other (313.8)
14.3 Hyperkinetic syndrome of childhood (314)
14.4 Conduct disorders
14.5 Special delays in development (315)
14.5.1 Developmental reading difficulties (315.0)
14.5.2 Developmental arithmetic difficulties (315.1)
14.5.3 Developmental speech or language difficulties (315.3)
14.5.4 Other (315.8)
14.6 Special symptoms or syndromes not elsewhere classified (307)
14.6.1 Stammering and stuttering (307.0)
14.6.2 Tics (307.2)
14.6.3 Night terrors (307.4)
14.6.4 Functional enuresis (307.6)
14.6.5 Other and unspecified (307.9)
14.7 Other

REFERENCES

American Psychiatric Association. 1968. *Diagnostic and Statistical Manual of Mental Disorders*. 2nd ed. (DSM-II). Washington, D.C..

American Psychiatric Association. 1980. *Diagnostic and Statistical Manual of Mental Disorders*. 3rd ed. (DSM-III). Washington, D.C..

Chen Changhui, and Shen Yu-cun. In press. Study on the diagnostic criteria for schizophrenia. *Chinese J. Neurol. Psychiatry*.

Chinese Neuropsychiatric Association. 1982. Classification of mental disorders. Chinese Medical Association, 1981. *Chinese J. Neurol. Psychiatry* 15: 3–4.

Wing, J. K., Cooper, J. E., and Sartorius, N. 1974. *Description and Classification of Psychiatric Symptoms*. Cambridge: Cambridge University Press.

World Health Organization. 1967. *Manual of the Eighth Revision of the International Statistical Classification of Diseases, Injuries and Causes of Death (ICD–8)*. Geneva.

World Health Organization. 1978. *Manual of the Ninth Revision of the International Classification of Diseases, Injuries, and Causes of Death, (ICD–9)*. Geneva.

Xu Youxin et al. 1983. Some recommendations with regard to the diagnostic criteria for several types of neurosis. *Chinese J. Neurol. Psychiatry* 16: 236–238.

Xu Youxin et al. 1985. A preliminary report of a clinical study of four types of neuroses. WPA Transcultural Psychiatry Section Symposium, "Sociocultural aspects of mental health – East and West." Beijing, August 18–28.

Zhou Dongfeng et al. 1984. DST, urinary MHPG, SO_4 excretion, and platelet MAO activity in depression. National Symposium, "Affective disorders." Chinese Neuropsychiatric Association, Huangshan, September 28–October 4.

8 Basic principles in the development of DSM-III

ROBERT L. SPITZER AND JANET B. W. WILLIAMS
(USA)

The first official classification of mental disorders in the United States in 1840, had but one category: idiocy. Since that time, our classification systems have become increasingly complex and controversial, although many would say such is the price of progress. Our ultimate hope, of course, is that science will eventually reveal underlying similarities between some of the categories and that these will help to simplify the ways in which we classify mental disorders. In the face of this increasing complexity, it is useful to understand the process that guided the development of DSM-III, the basic goals adopted by the American Psychiatric Association's Task Force on Nomenclature and Statistics as it did its work, and the basic concepts that guided the development of DSM-III (Spitzer and Williams, 1985).

THE PROCESS

The process of developing DSM-III was guided by the Task Force on Nomenclature and Statistics, a supervisory steering committee that ultimately consisted of 19 distinguished psychiatrists and psychologists with broad expertise in the various diagnostic areas. This committee oversaw the proceedings of 14 advisory committees that did the actual detailed work of developing and revising successive drafts of the DSM-III text and criteria. These advisory committees, each comprising 4–18 individuals, included members of the task force in their special areas of interest and other individuals with special expertise in each specific area. In addition to these groups, there were liaison committees with many of the components of the American Psychiatric Association, as well as with other professional organizations such as the American Psychological Association, the American Psychoanalytic Association, and the Academy of Psychiatry and the Law.

An important part of the process was the conduct of national field trials in which several hundred clinicians from more than a hundred different clinical facilities, and some in private practice, evaluated more than twelve thousand patients with drafts of DSM-III. When a final draft was available, these clinicians participated in a formal reliability study that demonstrated a generally much

81

higher level of diagnostic reliability than had previously been obtained in non-research settings (Spitzer, Forman & Nee, 1979).

Throughout the six years of development of DSM-III, many public presentations were made of drafts of the classification and criteria, and several drafts of the text and criteria were made available to potential consumers before final publication. This process encouraged feedback from clinicians and researchers not directly involved in the development of DSM-III, of which much resulted in extensive changes in the proposed manual.

BASIC GOALS

Throughout their work, members of the task force and advisory committees were guided by a shared commitment to certain basic goals. The primary goal was that DSM-III be clinically useful. Although this may seem to be an obvious goal, it is worth enunciating because of the increased reliance that was placed on input from researchers as opposed to previous DSMs. It was important to reassure our clinical colleagues that we recognized that DSM-III was not going to be used only or primarily for research purposes, but that it must above all be useful to frontline clinicians for making treatment and management decisions in a variety of clinical settings.

A tremendous emphasis was placed on the importance of the reliability of DSM-III categories – that is, the degree to which clinicians can agree on the diagnoses they assign. Since DSM-III is widely used in the selection of research subjects, it was also important for research investigators to be able to use the same terms to describe the same kinds of subjects. This emphasis on reliability stems from a basic tenet that progress in psychiatry, perhaps even more than in the rest of medicine, will be hampered unless there is basic agreement on how patients are assigned to various diagnostic categories. It was also recognized that since DSM-III represented a fundamental change from DSM-II, increased reliability was necessary for its acceptability.

Whenever possible, changes in the classification were based on the results of research studies of the validity of the various categories. Unlike our predecessors who developed DSM-I and DSM-II, we were in the fortunate position of having available a much larger body of empirical studies. But it was not always easy to agree on the interpretation of the results of studies that were available, and a large part of our work with the advisory committees consisted of reaching a consensus about each point that could then be reflected in the diagnostic criteria.

Finally, the task force was aware of the need to maintain compatibility with ICD-9. As work began on DSM-III in 1974, we had the opportunity to inspect the proposed ICD-9, since it was available several years before it went into effect in 1979. It was felt that there had been significant advances in our field, primarily in the areas of specified diagnostic criteria and the multiaxial system, that had not been incorporated into ICD-9, and this justified our maintaining a system of classification that was somewhat independent. However, to the extent possible, we maintained compatibility with ICD-9 by incorporating changes proposed for DSM-III into the Mental Disorders chapter of the U.S. Clinical Modification of ICD-9: ICD-9-CM.

BASIC CONCEPTS

One of the basic concepts that the task force had to struggle with was the definition of a mental disorder. To be certain, the problem has not been solved in psychiatry, but neither has it been solved in the rest of medicine, for which there is no widely accepted definition of physical disorder. We found it useful to present, in the introduction to DSM-III, a simple, brief statement that describes the basic notion of what we mean by a mental disorder. This statement reads as follows:

A clinically significant behavioral or psychological syndrome or pattern that occurs in an individual and that is typically associated with either a painful symptom (distress) or impairment in one or more important areas of functioning (disability). In addition, there is an inference that there is a behavioral, psychological, or biological dysfunction, and that the disturbance is not only in the relationship between the individual and society.

Consider, first, why we say "clinically significant." We recognize that, strictly speaking, some pathological disturbances may be so mild that they do not justify being included in a clinically oriented classification of mental disorders. Next, we refer to a "behavioral or psychological syndrome or pattern" because, in the case of mental disorders, the presentation is primarily through psychological or behavioral symptoms. These symptoms, we say, are "typically associated with either distress or impairment in functioning." We do recognize that there may be milder forms of disorders that have not yet expressed themselves to the extent of causing distress or disability, but most mental disorders typically do.

The first part of the last sentence in our statement refers to our belief that there must be an inference that something within the organism represents a behavioral, psychological, or biological disturbance. The last part of the sentence touches on a complex subject involving sociocultural value judgments. We clearly want to indicate that conflict between an individual and society is not a sufficient basis for a judgment of mental disorder.

Another basic concept embodied in DSM-III is that there are often no sharp boundaries between these various disorders, although we refer to "mental disorders" and classify them as if they were all discrete entities. We often have to draw a somewhat arbitrary, although useful and necessary, boundary between one disorder and another, and between a disorder and normality. We do emphasize that what is being classified is disorders and not individuals. Some antipsychiatry rhetoric has accused DSM-III of classifying individuals, but this is quite incorrect. DSM-III classifies disorders that individuals may or may not have.

DSM-III takes an atheoretical approach with regard to etiology. In the 1950s, after Stengel conducted a survey to determine why the international classification system was so little used by various national groups, he concluded that clinicians did not like to use a classification system that bound them to a theory of etiology with which they did not agree (Stengel, 1959).

The DSM-III task force believed that, given our present state of ignorance about etiology, we should avoid including etiological assumptions in the definitions of the various mental disorders, so that people who have different theories about etiology can at least agree on the features of the various disorders without having to agree on how those disorders came about. An example of this is the category "neuroses." A psychoanalyst, a behaviorally oriented clinician, and a biologically oriented clinician have very different notions about how someone develops a phobia or perhaps about what we refer to as panic disorder with agoraphobia. However, we have found that these three clinicians can agree on the diagnosis, provided that the diagnosis is made on the basis of descriptive features and not on the basis of any particular etiologic theory.

The major exception to the atheoretical stance taken in DSM-III is found in the Organic Mental Disorders, where organic factors necessary for the development of the disorders have been identified or are presumed, and, therefore, are included in the defining criteria. Of course, we hope that, as our relative ignorance about the etiologies of the mental disorders is resolved, we will be able to move closer toward an etiologic classification.

DSM-III, like most classification systems, is based on the assumption that some disorders are more pervasive in their symptomatology and, therefore, can account for other syndromes with more strictly limited symptomatology. The classification, therefore, has a hierarchical structure. For example, affective disorders are said to take hierarchic precedence over anxiety disorders (although this notion has been called into question by recent research data). Thus, if a patient with a major depressive episode also has anxiety symptoms such as panic attacks, according to DSM-III only the affective disorder diagnosis would be given. But since recent research has demonstrated that individuals with both types of syndromes have different family histories than individuals with only either one of these syndromes, this particular hierarchy will probably be changed in the revision of DSM-III (Leckman et al., 1983).

Undoubtedly the most significant innovation in DSM-III is the use of specified diagnostic criteria, in contrast to the brief glossaries of DSM-I, DSM-II, ICD-8, and ICD-9, which merely included simple descriptions of the most common features of each disorder, without specifying which features are required for the diagnoses. These criteria represent clear statements of what features need to be present in order to make each diagnosis. Obviously, a major way to improve diagnostic reliability is to include specified diagnostic criteria.

Diagnostic criteria can have various formats. One type is based on a monothetic model in which several criteria are listed and each needs to be present in order to make the diagnosis. An alternative model is a polythetic one in which, for example, 10 features may be listed but only 4 are required in order to make the diagnosis (Widiger and Frances, 1985). When the criteria are based on a polythetic model, different patients may have different clinical features.

Some of the diagnostic criteria in DSM-III follow a monothetic model, some a polythetic model, and some a mixed model.

The diagnostic criteria in DSM-III are based in part on previous works, such as the Research Diagnostic Criteria (RDC) (Spitzer, Endicott & Robins, 1978) which in turn were elaborations of the Feighner criteria developed in St. Louis, Missouri (Feighner et al., 1972). Since these previous sets of diagnostic criteria covered only a small number of disorders (16–20), we had to work with experts in many areas to devise totally new criteria for DSM-III and had to test them and revise them – a lengthy process.

Recognizing that a psychiatric diagnosis, by itself, is certainly not adequate for treatment planning and needs to be supplemented by other sources of information, the task force incorporated into DSM-III a multiaxial system for patient evaluation. The DSM-III multiaxial system represents a bio-psycho-social approach to evaluation in that Axes I and II include all of the mental disorders, Axis III is for physical disorders, Axis IV for severity of psychosocial stressors, and Axis V is for rating the individual's highest level of adaptive functioning during the past year (Williams, 1985a,b).

Finally, the fundamental concept embodied by DSM-III is that the manual represents merely one cross-sectional cut in the ongoing process of developing a reliable and valid classification of mental disorders. Given our present state of ignorance, when deciding whether or not to add a new category to DSM-III, we did not so much ask, "Do we know that this category is valid and reliable?" since the answer to that question is rarely a firm yes, but "Will adding this category advance the field in some way? Is this a useful clinical distinction that needs to be made?"

Although at times we had to say to clinicians who proposed a particular category for DSM-III, "After working with you and trying to understand your concept, we do not think you have been able to clarify it yet so that it is reliable enough to study." We were also often able to say, "This is now at a stage where it can at least be tested." Most of the new categories in DSM-III, we think, have withstood such tests. The best example is the category of panic disorder (controversial at the time because we had removed it from the general concept of anxiety neurosis). Panic disorder has been found to have widespread clinical utility and has been supported by research both in the United States and abroad (Klein & Rabkin, 1981).

CONCLUSION

It now seems widely agreed that DSM-III represents a major step forward in our efforts to classify mental disorders accurately and is having a significant effect on diagnostic practice. DSM-III has also made major impact on psychiatric education (Williams, Spitzer & Skodol, 1985). But it is important to remember that DSM-III is only one step in a process in which we try to rely, as much as possible, on empirical data to derive diagnostic criteria that allow the field to test hypotheses after diagnoses, so that further revisions in our classifications can be empirically based.

REFERENCES

Feighner, J. P., Robins, E., Guze, S. B., Woodruff, R. A., Winokur, G., Muñoz, R. 1972. Diagnostic criteria for use in psychiatric research. *Archives of General Psychiatry* 26: 57–63.

Klein D. F., and Rabkin, J. G. 1981. *Anxiety: New Research and Changing Concepts.* New York: Raven Press.

Leckman, J. F., Weissman, M. M., Merikangas, K. R., Pauls, D. L., and Prusoff, B. A. 1983. Panic disorder increases risk of depression, alcoholism, panic and phobic disorders in families of depressed probands. *Archives of General Psychiatry* 40: 1055–1060.

Spitzer, R. L., Endicott, J., and Robins, E. 1978. The psychiatric status schedule and technique for evaluating psychopathology and impairment in role funtioning. *Archives of General Psychiatry* 23: 41–55.

Spitzer, R. L., Forman, J. B. W., and Nee, J. 1979. DSM-III field trials: I. Initial interrater diagnostic reliability. *American Journal of Psychiatry* 136: 815–817.

Spitzer, R. L., and Williams, J. B. W. 1985. Classification of mental disorders. In *Comprehensive Textbook of Psychiatry.* 4th ed. vol. 1., ed. H. Kaplan and B. Sadock, pp. 591–613. Baltimore, Md.: Williams and Wilkins.

Stengel, E. 1959. Classification of mental disorders. *Bulletin of the World Health Organization* 21: 601–663.

Widiger, T. A., and Frances, A. 1985. The DSM-III personality disorders: perspectives from psychology. *Archives of General Psychiatry* 42: 615–623.

Williams, J. B. W. 1985a. The multiaxial system of DSM-III: Where did it come from and where should it go? I. Its origins and critiques. *Archives of General Psychiatry* 42: 175–180.

Williams, J. B. W. 1985b. The multiaxial system of DSM-III: Where did it come from and where should it go? II. Empirical studies, innovations, and recommendations. *Archives of General Psychiatry* 42: 181–186.

Williams, J. B. W., Spitzer, R. L., and Skodol, A. E. 1985. DSM-III in residency training: results of a national survey. *American Journal of Psychiatry* 142: 755–758.

PART II

International views on specific syndromes

9 International perspectives on schizophrenic and related psychotic disorders

PETER BERNER AND WILLIAM KIEFFER (Austria)

At the beginning of the nineteenth century, Sydenham's (1922) model of medicine as the science of pathological "species" became firmly established in psychiatry. It stimulated efforts to identify distinct entities of mental illnesses. As early as 1850, the French psychiatrist Bayle (1826) had guided this search into two promising directions. Bayle's research on general paralysis suggested, on the one hand, that the diagnostic value of cross-sectional psychopathology might be questioned in view of changes in psychic symptomatology that may occur during the evolution of illness. On the other hand, Bayle's pathological-anatomical observations stressed the importance of searching for organic findings in order to establish an etiological classification. Unfortunately, research in this direction led only to the identification of some organic brain disorders, whereas the origin of the majority of psychopathological conditions remained unknown. It followed that the classification of those disturbances still had to be based on clinical data, among which those relating to course of illness came to acquire special weight after Baillarger (1854) and Falret (1850–1), having continued to explore mental disorders along Bayle's line, described the *maladie à double forme* (the manic-depressive illness).

Near the turn of the century, Kraepelin (1896) integrated the work of French and German predecessors and established his nosology, for which course and outcome served as the most important guidelines. In this system, dementia praecox, encompassing Hecker's hebephrenia, Kahlbaum's catatonia, and dementia paranoides, appears as a morbid condition that passes through a great variety of clinical pictures to arrive at a deficiency state in which emotion and volition are particularly impaired. At the beginning of the twentieth century, E. Bleuler (1911) initiated efforts to identify symptoms allowing a cross-sectional diagnosis among the clinical features occurring during the course of this illness, for which he coined the name "schizophrenia." Whereas Bleuler focused on symptoms directly related to a hypothetical illness process, K. Schneider (1939) searched for a cross-sectional diagnosis, having in mind a purely pragmatic and atheoretic classification.

89

PRINCIPLES UNDERLYING SCHIZOPHRENIC AND RELATED PSYCHOTIC CONCEPTS

All attempts to define schizophrenia ultimately refer either to Kraepelin, Bleuler, or Schneider. The divergencies with regard to the delimitation of schizophrenic from other "functional disorders" cannot, however, simply be explained by the adherence to one of these three diagnostic approaches. A more careful analysis reveals that even classifications claiming to be based solely on observation or pragmatic considerations also take various theoretical assumptions into account. Consequently, if one wants to see how schizophrenia and related psychotic disorders are viewed by different schools, the hypothetical principles underlying the different conceptions must be understood. At least seven theoretical assumptions have guided different schools in the selection of clinical features for the definition of schizophrenia:

1. Moebius's endogeny hypothesis (1893) stipulates that schizophrenia is genetically determined.

2. Kraepelin's nosological hypothesis (1913) states that dementia praecox leads to mental invalidity owing to a peculiar destruction of the psychic personality's inner integrity.

3. E. Bleuler's pathogenetic basic disturbance hypothesis (1911) conceives of schizophrenia as a group of disorders, not necessarily of the same etiology but having in common a hypothesized primary organic disturbance, possibly of endogenous nature, leading to clinically ascertainable features that he calls "basic symptoms." The most important aspect of the disturbance is the dissociation of psychic functions.

4. Jaspers's hierarchical principle (1913) assumes that neurotic symptoms or personality disorders correspond to the most superficial "levels" of psychic dysfunctioning, whereas affective, schizophrenic, and organic symptoms correspond to deeper "levels." When several symptoms that belong to various "levels" occur simultaneously or consecutively, diagnosis is determined by the deepest "level" reached.

5. Janzarik's concept of structural-dynamic coherency (1959) postulates that "dynamic instability" may lead to first-rank symptoms and partly to Bleuler's basic symptoms (for instance, ambivalence, inappropriate affect, depersonalization, or derealization). For Janzarik, "dynamic" is a fundamental realm embracing affectivity and drive, which he contrasts to the "psychic structure" containing behavior patterns and cognitive notions. Some parts of this structure become "dynamically invested," meaning that they are connected with positive, negative, or ambivalent feelings. Dynamics are only partly tied to structural elements; the rest constitute a reservoir of free-floating drive and emotion, which may undergo morbid changes manifesting as depletion on the one hand and derailments on the other. The latter may be either stable, as in expansion into a maniform state and restriction into a depressive state, or unstable. The instability is characterized by rapid fluctuations or "swings" between expansion and restriction, which Mentzos (1967) called *Mischbilder* (unstable mixed states),

with corresponding changes in the actualization of positively, negatively, and ambivalently invested parts of the structure. Higher levels of instability lead to an impairment of reality testing in the form of delusional impressions and perceptions, illusions, and hallucinations. The rapid swings in drive, emotional resonance, and affectivity overpower the patient so that feelings of will-deprivation, alien influence, depersonalization, derealization, and ambivalence may arise. Derailments, according to Janzarik, are devoid of nosological specificity. They may occur in affective, organic, or schizophrenic psychoses, and even perhaps in psychogenic psychoses. Depletion, by contrast, seems to take place only in schizophrenic and organic disorders.

6. The biorhythmic disturbance hypothesis for affective psychoses (Jung, 1952) assumes that changes in biorhythms are "fundamental" disturbances of the major affective disorders.

7. The dichotomy concept of endogenous psychoses depicts them in terms of either schizophrenia or manic-depressive illness. E. Bleuler (1911) and K. Schneider (1939) adopted this point of view in the course of their work. The concept received reinforcement through Mayer's (1921) and Kolle's (1931) catamnestic studies. These authors came to the conclusion that, because the course of some paraphrenic and paranoic illness ended up in deficiency states, these disorders belonged to schizophrenia.

VARIOUS EUROPEAN APPROACHES TO SCHIZOPHRENIA DEFINITION

Divergencies in the definition of schizophrenia seen in the various schools depend upon how they take the aforementioned hypotheses into consideration: Kraepelin's nosological hypothesis includes the endogeny concept and makes use of the hierarchical principle explicitly formulated later by Jaspers. In later editions of his textbook, Kraepelin also adopted the dichotomy concept. E. Bleuler clearly followed the hierarchical principle and the concept of dichotomy, as did K. Schneider, who also embraced the endogeny hypothesis. Follow-up studies carried out by the Bleulerian and Schneiderian schools (M. Bleuler, 1972; Müller, 1981; Huber, Gross & Schüttler, 1979) showed that the outcome of some of the patients diagnosed as schizophrenics by their cross-sectional criteria was favorable, and so they abandoned the poor prognosis hypothesis of Kraepelin. Psychiatrists adhering to one of these two schools and accepting the implied theoretical background will not conceive of endogenous psychoses as being other than schizophrenia or manic-depressive illness and will not combine the two into an independent schizoaffective illness entity. At best, schizoaffective psychoses are considered a subgroup of schizophrenia, as classified in ICD-9. Because of the impreciseness of some of Bleuler's and Schneider's criteria, the paucity of operational rules for diagnostic assignment (for example, one does not know what weight to give to accessory or second-rank symptoms), and the adherence to Jaspers's principles, followers of these schools have come to adopt a broad concept of schizophrenia, to the detriment of major affective disorder, on the one hand, and various psychogenic psychoses, on the other. The latter are therefore virtually restricted to some rare cases of paranoic developments.

The Scandinavian schools, by contrast, gravitated toward Kraepelin and considered "true" schizophrenia a poor outcome disorder that may be distinguished from psychogenic "schizophreniform" disorders by means of prognosis indicators that can be empirically established. In addition to symptomatological criteria, nonsymptomatological prognosis indicators such as onset, presence or absence of precipitating factors, childhood conditions, and marital status were taken into consideration. The Scandinavian approach narrows the concept of schizophrenia once again by removing from it the "reactive" or "psychogenic psychoses." It does not, however, really abandon Jaspers's principle: Manic-depressive traits are considered to indicate good prognosis and patients exhibiting them may be considered to be suffering from a "schizophreniform" disorder (Langfeldt, 1956).

French psychiatry also sides with Kraepelin in that it considers schizophrenia to be a disorder that manifests itself early (before the age of 40) and whose course leads to a permanent deficit (corresponding to the concept *démence précoce*). On the other hand, the French school has never accepted the dichotomy concept, insisting that there are independent functional delusional psychoses in addition to schizophrenia and manic-depressive illness. These can be distinguished from schizophrenia by means of the aforementioned illness course criteria and Bleulerian basic symptoms (Pull & Pull, 1981). Schneiderian criteria carry no diagnostic weight for schizophrenia; indeed, one finds the brunt of them part of the *syndrome d'automatisme mental de Clérambault*. In studies carried out between 1920 and 1926, Clérambault discovered that such symptoms manifest as an initial stage of the independent functional psychosis – the *psychose hallucinatoire chronique*. Yet, the syndrome has an autonomous character not necessarily leading to this psychosis (Clérambault, 1942). French authors nevertheless follow Jaspers's principle in disregarding affective features as indicative of a manic-depressive illness when coinciding with Bleulerian and Kraepelinian criteria for schizophrenia or with signs of other delusional psychoses (among which Schneiderian first- and second-rank symptoms also figure). Accordingly, schizoaffective psychoses are not found in French nosology. As for the endogeny hypothesis, the French school takes a subtle position: An endogenous predisposition is assumed for schizophrenia and some delusional psychoses (especially the *psychose hallucinatoire chronique*), which, when submitted to environmental influences, leads to morbid manifestation; other delusional entities are considered to be of psychogenic origin. On the basis of this prudent point of view concerning hypotheses and the aforementioned orientation on Bleulerian symptoms plus illness course for the diagnosis of schizophrenia, neither Bleulerian nor Schneiderian criteria serve to demarcate this illness from psychogenic disorders.

Points of view diverging from the aforementioned schools of thought, such as the attempt of some German authors (for instance Leonhard, 1968, 1957) to discard the dichotomy concept in favor of one accepting several endogenous psychoses, had no appreciable influence on diagnostic habits for schizophrenia at the international level until the beginning of the 1970s. Since then, a decisive transformation having two closely associated sources has been set in motion: On the one hand, Jaspers's principle concerning the separation between affective and schizophrenic psychoses is falling into disrepute; on the other, operational research criteria have been developed.

In English-speaking countries, the Bleulerian criteria for schizophrenia traditionally predominated. In the last 15 years these have been supplemented or replaced by the Schneiderian ones, which at the time appeared superior in fulfilling the growing need for easily comprehensible operational diagnostic criteria. Interest in long-term follow-up studies was also growing, and soon made it obvious that many cases attributed to schizophrenia cross-sectionally, especially according to Schneiderian standards, were really manic-depressive. During phases characterized by "schizophrenic" symptoms, such patients had also manifested affective features, but owing to Jaspers's principle these had been neglected. Consequently, many American authors simply reversed the hierarchical relationship between the two disorders.

DIAGNOSTIC CRITERIA FOR SCHIZOPHRENIA AND OTHER FUNCTIONAL PSYCHOSES

The clear methodical support elicited by this volte-face enhanced the development of operationally defined criteria for diagnostic inclusion and exclusion of schizophrenia. The search for inclusion criteria for schizophrenia led researchers to begin by choosing first-rank symptoms and those basic symptoms considered to be adequately well defined. On the other hand, the observation that some cases initially taken to be schizophrenic showed modifications of symptomatology in the direction of affective psychoses lent renewed and stronger support to Kraepelin's concept. As a result, symptomatological and nonsymptomatological prognosis indicators, especially those worked out empirically by the Scandinavian school, and illness course were chosen for inclusion and exclusion criteria. Thus, the overall goal was to establish a clear demarcation between "true" schizophrenia and psychogenic and affective psychoses. Demarcation from affective psychoses was especially supported by the declaration contained in many diagnostic systems that affective states corresponding to operational criteria for mania or depression exclude the diagnosis of schizophrenia.

These criteria for major affective disorders frequently contain elements chosen with reference to the biorhythmic-disturbance hypothesis (e.g., diurnal variations of mood and drive as well as sleep disturbances). Again, virtually no room will be found for schizoaffective disorder whenever this reversal of Jaspers's rule of level is applied. In DSM-III, for instance, this category is only retained "for those instances in which the clinician is unable to make a diagnosis with any degree of certainty between Affective Disorder and either Schizophreniform

Table 9.1. *Endogenomorphic-schizophrenic axial syndrome*

A. Incoherence
   Without marked pressure or retardation of thinking or marked autonomous
   anxiety; at least one of the following symptoms is required:
   1. Blocking. Sudden cessation in the train of thought; after a gap the previous
      thought may be taken up again or may be replaced by a different thought
   2. Derailment. Gradual or sudden deviation from the train of thought without gap
   3. Pathologically "muddled speech." Fluent speech, for the most part syntactically
      correct, but the elements of different thoughts (which, for the patient, may
      belong to a common idea) get muddled together
B. Cryptic neologisms
   The patient does not explain their private meaning spontaneously.
C. Affective blunting
   Without evidence of marked depression, tiredness, or drug effect. This term
   includes flatness of affect, emotional indifference, and apathy; essentially, the
   symptom involves a diminution of emotional response.

Note: Definitive, A and/or B present; probable, only C present.

Disorder or Schizophrenia" (American Psychiatric Association 1980, p. 202).
Functional psychoses unaffiliated to schizophrenic or manic-depressive disorders, such as paranoid disorder or paranoia in DSM-III, will only be considered
when neither schizophrenia nor manic-depressive disorder can be diagnosed.
How often such other psychoses will be diagnosed in different systems depends
upon the breadth of the diagnostic criteria used for schizophrenia and the
affective psychoses.

Many of the operational criteria currently in use for schizophrenia contain
more or less complicated combinations of elements chosen with reference to the
aforementioned theoretical assumptions. Since such algorithms allow a choice
of elements stemming from different theories, it is not possible to test the
theoretical assumptions each one of them represents, for instance, whether
Schneider's criteria are more prone to select more homogenous groups of patients
than Bleuler's or vice versa. Furthermore, inclusion into the algorithm of non-
symptomatical standards for the evaluation of the various hypotheses reduces
the possibility of testing them. Thus, the DSM-III requirement for diagnostic
assignment of an illness lasting 6 months precludes, to a certain extent, testing
the assumption that schizophrenia is a chronic disorder. The same observation
applies to the use of genetic data as an inclusion criterion, as contained, for
instance, in Feighner's St. Louis Criteria (Feighner, Robins, Guze, Woodruff
& Winokur, 1972).

The Vienna Research Criteria (1983) were conceived to avoid these pitfalls
(Berner, 1969). Table 9.1 shows that the Vienna Criteria for schizophrenia
represent a strictly theory-oriented approach. They are founded on the endogeny
hypothesis and the schizophrenia concept of E. Bleuler. They modify the latter

Table 9.2. *Endogenomorphic-cyclothymic axial syndrome*

A. Appearance of *biorythmic disturbances* (1 and 2 are necessary)
   1. Diurnal variations in affectivity or drive
   2. Sleep disturbance (early awakening or prolonged sleep or interrupted sleep)
B. Appearance of a marked *change in affectivity* following a period of habitual functioning (euphoric/manic or depressive or dysphoric [= irritable] or anxious)
C. Appearance of a marked *change in emotional resonance* following a period of habitual functioning
D. Appearance of a marked *change in drive* (reduced or increased) following a period of habitual functioning

Note: A and (B or C or D) are necessary.

Table 9.3. *Number of patients diagnosed as schizophrenic according to 11 different diagnostic formulations among 200 first admissions for functional psychosis to 2 mental hospitals in Vienna*

Schneider	
(at least one first-rank symptom)	121
ICD-9	97
Bleuler	
(at least one basic symptom)	91
DSM-III	
Schizophrenic and schizophreniform	80
Research diagnostic criteria	67
ICD-9	
Without schizoaffective psychosis	64
Bleuler	
(at least two "A"s)	53
DSM-III	
Schizophrenic	49
St. Louis Criteria	44
Vienna	
Endogenomorphic schizophrenic axial syndrome	36
Bleuler	
(at least three "A"s)	22

according to Janzarik's structural coherency model in that they exclude those basic symptoms considered to represent dynamic instability, since they are as devoid of diagnostic specificity as first-rank symptoms.

The Vienna concept for schizophrenia leaves room for any kind of dynamic derailment, but, in contrast to the derailments in manic-depressive illness, they are not thought to be accompanied by biorhythmical changes. Consequently, Jaspers's principle is not taken into consideration: In the presence of a clinical

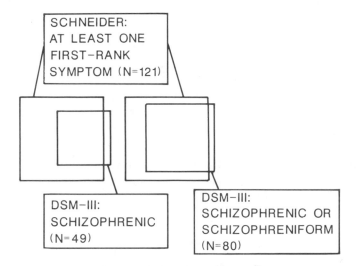

Figure 9.1. Above and opposite: Overlap between Schneiderian, Bleulerian, and Viennese criteria for schizophrenia and corresponding DSM-III criteria on a sample of functional psychosis patients

picture in which both the schizophrenic and the cyclothymic axial syndromes (see Tables 9.1 and 9.2, respectively) manifest together, a schizoaffective disorder will be diagnosed. According to a follow-up study in Vienna (Berner, Katschnig & Lenz, 1983), this seldom occurs (in only 4 out of 200 patients suffering from functional psychoses). Our concept for schizophrenia is narrower than many others, even those that incorporate manic and depressive syndromes as exclusion criteria, for we take unstable mixed states into account as well.

The Viennese outlook disregards the dichotomy hypothesis. The presence of our criteria for any one of our axial syndromes for affective disorder does not imply that they obligatorily represent a nosological entity. It is possible that derailments accompanied by biorhythmical changes are common to several distinct categories of affective disorders, such as bipolar, unipolar, or other "cycloid" psychoses. Psychoses falling outside the bounds of the schizophrenic and affective axial syndromes are diagnosed on a purely syndromatological level. Follow-up studies have shown that some of them later develop typical schizophrenic or affective symptoms, whereas others continue to escape nosological attribution. Future research may show them to be autochthonous nosological entities, such as the *psychose hallucinatoire chronique* or psychogenic psychoses.

Patient sampling is influenced by the diagnostic system used. Figure 9.1 and Table 9.3 illustrate this point and also indicate how narrow the Vienna concept is in relation to others. Figure 9.1 shows the overlap between the diagnostic formulations of Bleuler, Schneider, and the Viennese Criteria on the one hand and the DSM-III diagnosis of schizophrenia on the other. Table 9.3 compares the number of patients diagnosed as schizophrenic according to seven diagnostic formulations. For example, Berner, Katschnig and Lenz (1983) use the poly-

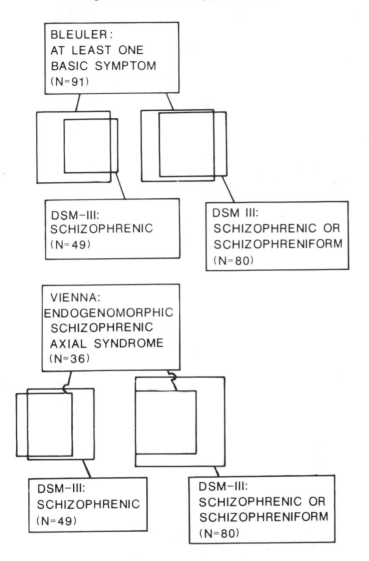

diagnostic approach. In the light of the previous considerations, additional future research directed toward a simultaneous application of many diagnostic criteria to the same patient population may prove to be a valuable heuristic instrument that may reveal differences between schools and cultures.

REFERENCES

American Psychiatric Association. 1980. *Diagnostic and Statistical Manual of Mental Disorders*, 3rd ed. (DSM-III). Washington, D.C.

Baillarger, J. 1854. De la folie à double forme. *Ann. Med. Psychol.* 6: 369–384.

Bayle, A. L. J. 1826. *Nouvelle doctrine des maladies mentales*. Paris: Gabon.

Berner, P. 1969. Der Lebensabend der Paranoiker. *Wien. Z. Nervenheilk* 27: 115–161.

Berner, P., Katschnig, H., and Lenz, G. 1983. DSM-III in German-speaking countries. In *International perspectives on DSM-III*, ed. R. L. Spitzer, J. B. W. Williams, and A. E. Skodol. Washington, D.C.: American Psychiatric Press.

Bleuler, E. 1911. *Dementia praecox oder Gruppe der Schizophrenien*. Leipzig: Deuticke. Reprint 1978. München: Minerva. English edition: *Dementia Praecox or the Group of Schizophrenias*. Trans. J. Zinkin. New York: International University Press, 1950.

Bleuler, M. 1972. *Die schizophrenen Geistesstörungen im Lichte langjähriger Kranken- und Familiengeschichten*. Stuttgart: Thieme.

Clérambault, G. de. 1942. *Ouevre psychiatrique*. Paris: PUF.

Falret, J. P. 1850–1. Leçons à l'hospice de la Sâlpetrière. *Gaz. des Hôp. 23 et 24 année*: 258.

Feighner, J. P., Robins, E., Guze, S. B., Woodruff, R. A., and Winokur, G. 1972. Diagnostic criteria for use in psychiatric research. *Arch. Gen. Psychiat.* 26: 57–63.

Huber, G., Gross, G., and Schüttler, R. 1979 *Schizophrenie*. Berlin: Springer.

Janzarik, W. 1959. *Dynamische Grundkonstellationen in endogenen Psychosen*. Berlin: Springer.

Jaspers, K. 1913. *Allgemeine Psychopathologie*. Berlin: Springer 8th ed. 1946. Berlin: Springer.

Jung, R. 1952. Zur Klinik und Pathogenese der Depression. *Zbl. ges. Neurol. Psychiat.* 119: 163.

Kolle, K. 1931. *Die primäre Verrücktheit*. Leipzig: Thieme.

Kraepelin, E. 1896. *Psychiatrie*. 5th ed. Leipzig: Barth. 6. Aufl., 1904. 7. Aufl., 1909–1915. 8. Aufl. 1899. English edition: *Dementia Praecox and Paraphrenia*. Trans. R. M. Barclay from 8th edition of *Psychiatry*. Edinburgh: Livingstone. 1921.

Kraepelin, E. 1913. *General Paresis*. Monograph series no. 14. New York: Nervous and Mental Disease Pub. Co.

Langfeldt, G. 1956. *The Prognosis in Schizophrenia*. Copenhagen: Munksgaard.

Leonhard, K. 1957. *Aufteilung der endogenen Psychosen*. Berlin (DDR): Akademie-Verlag. English edition: New York: Irvington Publishers, 1979.

Leonhard, K. 1968. Über monopolare und bipolare endogene Psychosen. *Nervenarzt 39*: 104–106.

Mayer, W. 1921. Über paraphrene Psychosen. *Z. Neurol.* 71: 187–206.

Mentzos, S. 1967. *Mischzustände und mischbildhafte phasische Psychosen*. Stuttgart: Enke.

Moebius, P. J. 1893. *Abriss der Lehre von den Nervenkrankheiten*. Leipzig: A. Abel.

Müller, C. 1981. *Psychische Erkrankungen und ihr Verlauf sowie ihre Beeinflussung durch das Alter*. Bern: Hans Huber.

Pull, C. B., and Pull, M. C. 1981. Des critères cliniques pour le diagnostic de schizophrénie. In *Actualités de la schizophrénie*, ed. P. Pichot. Paris: PUF.

Schneider, K. 1939. *Klinische Psychopathologie*. Leipzig: Thieme. 1980. 12, gegenüber der 8 unveränderten Aufl. Stuttgart: Thieme. English edition: *Clinical psychopathology*. Trans. M. W. Hamilton and E. W. Anderson from 3rd edition. New York: Grune and Stratton, 1959.

Sydenham, T. 1922. *Selected Works of Thomas Sydenham*. London: J. Bale, Sons and Danielson.

10 *The diagnosis and classification of autism*

Empirical studies relevant to nosology

DONALD J. COHEN, RHEA PAUL, AND FRED R. VOLKMAR (USA)

Most problems in the classification of autism have stemmed from the difficulties facing all diagnosis in childhood, including the developmental changes in the expression of childhood disorders and the lack of overarching theoretical perspectives. In addition, there have been specific problems related to the nosology for the most severe disorders. These include continuities among various early-onset conditions, relations between behavioral features and intellectual level, and controversies about the nature of etiology in relation to diagnosis. During the past decade, a consensus about the validity and nosology of various psychiatric disorders of childhood onset has begun to emerge as a result of greater diagnostic precision, the use of multiaxial classification schemes (Rutter, Shaffer & Shepherd, 1975; Cohen, 1976), and the availability of longitudinal data. The appearance of the American Psychiatric Association's 1980 *Diagnostic and Statistical Manual* (DSM-III), with its use of specific behavioral criteria for diagnosis, represents an advance in the diagnosis of childhood disorders and the search for methods for reliable and valid assessement.

DSM-III presented two innovations in relation to childhood disorders. First, it used a multiaxial approach that provided for the fuller description of autistic and other children by requiring information about medical conditions, psycho-social environmental stresses, and level of adaptation. Second, DSM-III emphasized the importance of phenomenological features rather than etiological or theoretical viewpoints in diagnosis, thus making it possible for professionals from various backgrounds to attempt to find common ground for clinical discussion and research. In relation to autism, the introduction of the concept of Pervasive Developmental Disorders (PDD) emphasized that these children and adults suffer from a range of disturbances affecting the emergence of basic psychological competences, including social development and language.

Soon after the appearance of DSM-III, researchers found problems in several areas, such as the suitability of the category Childhood Onset PDD as distinct from autism. These observations, and the emergence of new information about autism and other PDDs, have provided a basis for revising DSM-III and have increased our understanding of the central features of autism.

This chapter focuses on empirical studies conducted during the past several years by the Child Study Center research group relevant to the phenomenology of autism and issues in classification. The specific issues concerning autism and PDD are used to illustrate general features in childhood diagnosis and the relation between advances in nosology and empirical research.

DSM III: VALIDITY OF CRITERIA

To assess the validity of the major DSM-III criteria for autism, parents of 50 clearly autistic individuals completed a detailed structured questionnaire concerning the children's developmental history (Volkmar, Cohen & Paul, 1986). The autistic individuals ranged from 28 months to 33 years in age (mean 16.9 years) and had IQ's ranging from 6 to 90 (mean 33); all had received multidisciplinary evaluations in our center, where many have been followed for many years. From their data base, 62 specific items concerning the course of illness were abstracted and used to operationalize DSM-III criteria. Information obtained when the children were older agreed quite well with data obtained during early childhood, in contrast to the frequently encountered problems with retrospective data in relation to normal children.

The clinical information was subjected to principal components factor analysis. Three major factors emerged: social relatedness; responsivity and environmental reactivity (motor and affective symptoms and responses to the environment); and deviant language patterns. A fourth factor concerned developmental changes. Thus, the factor analysis provided supportive evidence for the emphases of DSM-III criteria concerning social relations and language. All patients satisfied DSM-III criteria for disturbed language development, but 18 failed to satisfy fully DSM-III's requirement that autistic individuals have a *pervasive* lack of social relations. These 18 patients exhibited some degree of attachment to their parents and siblings, and their social behavior was odd and deviant, although not utterly absent. Several higher-functioning individuals had thought problems, as revealed in their speech, which suggested delusional thinking, a behavior specifically excluded by DSM-III for the diagnosis of autism. Whether lower-functioning or mute children might also have thought problems cannot be determined.

Autism appears during the first years of life with either a period of relatively normal development before the onset or a deviant path of development from the very first days of life. Kolvin (1971) distinguished two major groups of "psychotic" children, those with an onset after five years and those with generally much younger age of onset. On the basis of his observations of early- and late-onset psychosis, DSM-III chose an age criterion of 30 months for autism and postulated a new disorder (similar in nature to autism) with an onset after that point; for no apparent reason, the age criterion was different from Kolvin's. The previously noted study and subsequent work has cast doubt on DSM-III's requirement that autism appear before age 30 months. In this group, six subjects by report of parents failed this criterion.

In a subsequent study, we examined the age of onset of 116 cases of children studied by us who were phenomenologically autistic (Volkmar, Cohen & Stier,

1985). All but 5 had an onset during the first 30 months; among those with later onset, emergent major physical problems or serious parental denial of earlier difficulties were prominent. For autism, age of onset is more properly characterized as "age of recognition," since the earliest signs may be subtle and the pathological process almost invariably can be traced in its origins to the very early periods of development.

Age of onset was further examined in our center during the past decade by a detailed review of the entire experience with 250 psychotic children, including those with early and late onset. A bimodal distribution was found: Almost all of the early-onset, autistic children were recognized before 48 months; the later-onset schizophrenic children were generally recognized after age 10.

On the basis of this and further work, described later in the chapter, we believe that the diagnosis of autism should be based on natural history and phenomenological features, and that any child satisfying the criteria should receive the diagnosis, regardless of age of onset. Using our large set of data concerning age of onset, a cutoff point of 36 months would include the vast majority of autistic children and one of 48 months virtually all.

The concepts "delusions" and "hallucinations" are so firmly part of the portrayal of schizophrenia that the framers of DSM-III sought to exclude children with these difficulties from the diagnosis of autism in order to differentiate autism from schizophrenia. However, drawing a line between the unusual thoughts and preoccupations of autistic individuals and the delusions of schizophrenic adults may be difficult, as revealed by clinical experiences and self-descriptions of brighter, older autistic people such as Tony, a young man whose autobiography we have presented (Volkmar & Cohen, 1985). Rather than serving as an exclusionary criterion, the unusual, repetitive, stereotypical, and odd thoughts of autistic children can provide interesting avenues into an understanding of their inner world.

In summary, DSM-III's criteria for autism have proven relatively robust. However, they are in need of revision for four reasons: (1) Autistic children are socially related; (2) they have an onset after 30 months, in some cases; (3) there is no sharp distinction between autism and childhood onset PDD; and (4) autistic children may have odd thoughts and experiences that cannot be differentiated from those found in older psychotic individuals. These themes are elaborated further in the following sections.

COMMUNICATION

DSM-III's description of autism focused on disturbances in language, rather than communication. The primary function of language, however, is to mediate social interaction, and language is the primary vehicle by which social interaction takes place among humans. The question of the primacy of linguistic deficits in autism has often been discussed. Although at one time language deficits were thought to cause autistic social-withdrawal, evidence such as the fact that young normal children communicate effectively nonverbally before the acquisition of language argues against this position. It is possible that autism stems from dysfunctions in particular cognitive and information-processing functions relating to social cognition, as suggested by the work of Sigman with young autistic children (Sigman et al., 1986), but other investigators have emphasized that the social deficits are related to disorders of neurological organization that are relatively independent of cognitive functioning (Fein et al., 1986). It would appear to us that the language and communicative deficits in autism arise from the more fundamental disorders of human relating. (See Paul, 1986, for a detailed discussion.)

In normal development, joint attentional routines between children and parents (Bruner, 1975) evolve into protodeclarative acts of preverbal communication (Bates, 1976) or precursors to first sentences that serve the function of making a comment on a shared topic. Autistic children are unable to form joint attentional routines, either on the basis of cognitive, perceptual, or more specific social deficits, and their failure to express intentions related to joint reference might thus be a reflection of the basic dysfunction in joint attention. With no desire or means for achieving or stably maintaining joint attention, autistic children would have no desire or capacity to learn language; they may satisfy their needs for protesting and requesting through nonverbal gestures and non-specific utterances. Even in higher-functioning autistic individuals, with good syntactic abilities, the fundamental disturbance in joint attention may be seen in more subtle disturbances in shared topicality and cognitive inference. These verbal autistic children and adults may master the syntactic and phonological systems of language but fail to integrate these language features with their semantic and pragmatic counterparts. This is possible since syntactical abilities may arise from relatively specific language-learning strategies distinct from semantic ones (Curtis, 1981).

In studies of verbal autistic children and adults, we have investigated the autistic person's ability to gauge another person's mental or cognitive state, and have shown that even brighter autistic people have difficulties in assessing what their conversational partner considers the topic of conversation, knows about the world, has been able to gather from the discourse that has already taken place, has foregrounded for the purpose of the conversation, and the like. Since so much conversational exchange is predicated on the shared ability of both speakers to go beyond the literal meaning of the message and to infer something about implicit intentions and cognitive states, such a deficit can result in pervasive disturbances in dyadic conversation. In one study (Paul & Cohen, 1984b), we examined autistic individuals' abilities to respond to contingent queries or request for clarification of three types (Gallagher, 1981): requests for confirmation (*Child*: I watched "Dynasty" on TV last night; *Interviewer*: You watched "Dynasty"?); neutral requests for repetition (*Interviewer* asks with a rising tone, "What?"); and requests for specific constituent repetition (*Child*: I left the book in the bedroom; *Interviewer*: You left what in the bedroom?). Compared with retarded children, the autistic children had more problems in language development relative to their mental age, including reduced sentence length and paucity of conversation, as well as poor imitation. Contrary to the general description of autistic children as withholding or negativistic (about which more will be said later), the children responded to queries 93 percent of the time, as often as retarded children. Although they tried to comply with the requests, they did not do as well as retarded individuals in one specific area: They were less likely to provide the specific constituent item requested. They had trouble particularly in understanding what the interviewer really wanted to know, or more generally, in the social cognitive ability to take the place of the other in the conversation.

In a related study, we (Paul & Cohen, 1985) examined how an autistic individual responds to an indirect request. Indirect requests are those sentences in which the illocutionary intent of the utterance does not match the surface form. For example, the sentence "Can you pass the salt?" is on the surface a question that can be answered either yes or no. It is obvious to normal people, in most situations, that this is not a question but a request. Paul and Feldman (personal communication) found that autistic individuals tend to respond literally to such questions. In our formal study, autistic children were asked a series of questions, based on the work of Carrell (1981), of the form: "Can you color the circle blue?"; "The circle really needs to be colored blue"; "I'd be very happy if you make the circle blue"; and so on. When the requests were made in a highly structured fashion, autistic children did as well as retarded children, and both groups were able to function like normal 4- to 6-year-olds and comply with the request. When the situation was unstructured, however, the autistic individuals did worse than the retarded, especially in relation to sentences that required greater semantic processing. Like Tager-Flusberg (1981), we found syntactic processing to be commensurate with developmental level, whereas semantic and pragmatic processing was more impaired and emerged most clearly in unstructured situations.

From a clinical and educational point of view, the most impressive feature of autistic language dysfunction is that the majority of individuals are mute or have relatively little language. Studies of higher-functioning individuals with language may shed some light on the most profoundly impaired, since there appears to be a spectrum of severity with no sharp cutoff point. Even people capable of normal syntax and phonology have persistent disturbances in communication and have difficulty extracting implicit or implied information about the other person's cognitive state and intentions and using this knowledge to aid in language processing and in formulating an appropriate response. Thus, there appears to be a developmental continuity from the autistic infant's disturbance in social communication (eye contact, shared stimulus of interest, and the like) and the brighter autistic person's disturbance in social engagement. Social communication, rather than language, appears to be the primary or core deficit. (See also Wetherby & Prutting, 1984.)

The diagnostic centrality of social communication emerged, as well, from studies that we conducted on the natural history of childhood autism and children with severe language disturbances (Paul, Cohen & Caparulo, 1983; Paul

& Cohen, 1984a). We examined speech, language, performance intelligence, school placement, behavior, and other characteristics of autistic and language-disordered children over the course of many years. Children with serious language impairments who had markedly unusual social relatedness had very guarded prognoses. Over the course of years, they increasingly resembled children with autism. In fact, the outcome of such children may be worse than that of higher-functioning autistic children. Prognostically, relatively better receptive language abilities early in life are related to greatest improvement in social skills later, but language improvement, although it may be impressive in some children, is generally less clear than are gains in adaptive skills. DSM-III suggested that language disorders should not be diagnosed in the presence of mental retardation, but the majority of language-impaired children are retarded and may show greater impairments in language than in other areas of functioning. In summarizing this area of investigation, we now believe that (a) in children who have serious disturbances in both social relating and language impairment, the diagnosis of autism is more relevant to longer-term outcome and (b) the degree of intellectual retardation does not preclude making a specific diagnosis of language impairment.

BIOLOGICAL FACTORS

Given the early onset, lifelong duration, severity, and breadth of disturbance in autism, one would expect that biological deficits would easily be discovered and replicated. The opposite, however, has been the case. Although all autistic individuals deserve a thorough biomedical evaluation as part of their clinical care, for the majority no biological basis for their disorder can be found using current methods.

Studies of neurological functioning in autism, with appropriate control groups, including retarded and other developmentally and psychiatrically disturbed children, are limited. Chief among the biological observations has been the appearance of seizures during adolescence in a considerable minority of the more retarded, autistic population, but the basis of this is unknown. The only neurochemical finding that has been well replicated is that about 40 percent of autistic individuals have elevated levels of blood serotonin; however, no correlations between this finding and any clinical feature are known, nor is this specific since other retarded individuals also have elevated blood serotonin. (For a detailed review of neurochemical findings, see Anderson & Hoshino, 1986.) We and others have examined electroencephalograms (EEGs) and computed brain tomograms among autistic individuals. The several studies that have been done suggest that there is a subgroup of children with abnormalities in the EEG and computed brain tomograms, but there are no specific abnormalities, and most patients have normal examinations (Harcherik et al., 1985). Recent positron emission studies (PET scans) have not revealed consistent abnormalities either. In a study in our laboratory, we found that a high percentage of autistic children retain primitive snouting reflexes, consistent with the clinical observations of their frequent mouthing (Minderaa et al., 1985). More sophisticated electrophysiological studies using event-related potentials have suggested that there may be disturbances in processing information, but in general have failed to reveal "hard-wired" or neurological damage, as have gross autopsy findings. The autistic syndrome has been found to occur in the presence of various types of insults to the nervous system, including seizure disorders, rubella syndrome, inborn errors of metabolism, and the like, as well as in association with chromosomal abnormalities (such as the Fragile X chromosome syndrome). Genetic studies, including family and twin studies, have supported the concept that there is a genetic contribution to autism, at least in certain situations; however, most cases of autism remain sporadic, and there are no biological features currently known to distinguish the sporadic cases from those with a familial predisposition.

Mental retardation or deficiency is seen in up to 80 percent of all autistic children, and intellectual level (or IQ) is a relatively stable characteristic of autistic children over the span of decades. Although social relatedness tends to improve and behavior may be modified considerably by education, intellectual level does not tend to rise. Children with higher intellectual levels tend to have lower incidence of seizures and to do much better in later-life adaptation to education and work. As we note later, consideration of IQ is thus an important aspect of diagnosis and should be specifically measured and recorded in all autistic children. Questions about the validity of IQ measures have been raised because of the difficulties involved in testing autistic children, and in the past many were considered "untestable." Today investigators and clinicians feel that reliable and valid measurement is possible in almost all cases, given well-trained examiners and sufficient time. Poor performance tends to be an adequate reflection, then, of the child's abilities and cannot be ascribed to noncompliance or negativism.

Thus, in surveying the range of biological and medical conditions that have been found among autistic children, apparently none has yet emerged that can be used as a basis for diagnosis or subclassification. Clearly, the search for such markers and correlates is a high priority for all investigations related to autism. Such work can use increasingly complex and precise methods for studying neurobiological processes in patients; thoughtful application of these approaches and awareness of their methodological limitations and artifacts will be essential in advancing clinical understanding (Young, Leven & Cohen, 1985).

BEHAVIORAL STUDIES

Studies of the behavior of autistic individuals provide another avenue into the phenomenology of autism. In a reanalysis of previous experimental data, we suggested that the lack of compliance of autistic individuals with specific tasks could be understood as a reflection of competence rather than negativism; it appeared that autistic individuals performed tasks that they understood and could respond to (Volkmar & Cohen, 1982).

To follow up this line of inquiry, we examined the effects of treatment structure on the behavior of 19 autistic individuals (Volkmar, Hoder & Cohen, 1985). Three conditions of treatment structure were operationally defined by staff:child ratio and ranged from highly structured (1:1) activities, tasks with intermediate levels of structure (1:2), and tasks with relatively less structure (1:4). Subjects were observed in their usual residential treatment setting as they interacted with familiar staff members. Thus it was possible to minimize the effects of potentially confounding variables such as novelty of the situation. A time-sample procedure was used to collect data relating to the frequency of stereotypes, self-injurious behaviors, direction of the subject's gaze (at staff, task, or elsewhere), vocalization and echolalia, and response to requests. In the more structured situations, there was significantly less stereotypy or self-injury, and the autistic individuals directed their visual attention more appropriately. Moreover, subjects were generally compliant with requests made by caregivers. When they understood the request and could perform the task – for example when the request was nonverbal and the task was nonverbal – the autistic children and adolescents were compliant. These results suggest the importance both of high staff-to-child ratios for facilitating behavioral functioning and of observational setting in the assessment of behavioral characteristics. Subsequent studies have also shown that compliance of autistic individuals to demands is primarily a function of developmental level rather than intrinsic "negativism" or lack of cooperation.

To pursue the question of autistic negativism and gaze aversion experimentally, we studied how autistic individuals utilize information from faces (Volkmar, Sparrow, Rende & Cohen, personal communication). Autistic and normal individuals were compared in their ability to complete a series of puzzles depicting photographs of human faces. Puzzles varied along three dimensions: complexity (3, 6, or 9 pieces), familiarity (familiar person or unfamiliar face), and configuration (picture is normal or picture is scrambled with parts of face rearranged randomly). As expected, autistic individuals took longer to complete the puzzles than normals; both groups did best on the easiest puzzle. Most important, however, both the autistic individuals and the normals made use of the information provided by the normal facial arrangement. Rather than engaging in global gaze avoidance, autistic individuals appear to use facial information and to look at others in specific contexts; however, they fail to master fully the use of gaze in regulating dialogue, in intentionally avoiding or acutely focusing gaze to limit or enhance social contact.

These studies highlight the importance of viewing behavior of autistic individuals from a variety of perspectives; in particular, it is important to consider behavior within the context of other aspects of the individual's development and psychosocial environment.

ASSESSMENT METHODS

Kanner (1973), in his original description of the syndrome, suggested that autistic children are not retarded. We know now that this view is not correct. Although autistic individuals often exhibit variability in different aspects of the cognitive development, most autistic persons are mentally retarded. As for other children, IQ scores are predictive of later development. A variety of diagnostic checklists and rating scales have been developed for other aspects of autism, such as the Rimland E–2 checklist, the Behavior Rating Instrument for Autistic and Atypical Children (BRIAAC), and the Autism Behavior Checklist (ABC) (see Parks, 1983, for a review). Although these instruments may be useful for some purposes (e.g., for documenting current symptoms or obtaining historical information specifically relevant to aspects of disordered development), their utility is limited by problems of validity and reliability. Most of these instruments have been developed specifically for autistic persons and thus lack a normative basis. They tend to focus on symptoms that are thought to be specifically related to autism (such as gaze aversion or stereotypy) and may be more useful for arraying autistic individuals along dimensions of symptomatology than for diagnosis or comparison with normal populations. An exception is the BRIAAC, which is designed for codifying observations in a more clinical setting and which has been used with some small populations of normal and retarded children. The BRIAAC, however, is limited in several key features: For example, it does not make use of historical or parental information, it is closely related to level of development, and it is not useful after the preschool years (Cohen et al., 1978).

We have recently completed a study using a well-standardized, normative assessment instrument, the revised Vineland Adaptive Behavior Scales (Volkmar et al., personal communication), which is based on a detailed interview with a parent or primary caregiver. This instrument yields measures of adaptive behavior in three main domains: communication, daily living, and social skills, in comparison to the normal population. Scores can also be calculated for nine subdomains (receptive, expressive, and written language; personal, domestic, and community activities; and interpersonal, play, and coping skills), which constitute the three major domains. In our study of 57 individuals (35 autistic and 22 nonautistic developmentally impaired children and adults), the Vineland revealed significant differences between the groups that could be accounted for primarily in terms of interpersonal relationships and other social skills. The differences between groups could not be accounted for on the basis of mental age. A quotient was devised for assessing relative social disability based on the Vineland Score and mental age from a standardized IQ test; when this quotient was used, it became even clearer that the area of greatest disparity between the retarded and autistic individuals was that of social relatedness and interpersonal skills. A well-standardized instrument (such as the Vineland) offers the greatest potential for precision in describing and measuring the social deficits of autistic individuals. This possibility represents an important topic for future research.

DIAGNOSTIC FEATURES

Social development in autism is both *delayed*, as in retardation syndromes, and *deviant*. By emphasizing the deviant quality of autistic social dysfunction, clinicians and investigators mean that some aspects of autistic social behavior are not observed even in quite young normal infants and are not accounted for by limitations in cognitive abilities. Primarily, the autistic social deviance relates to the quality or tone of social relations: autistic persons' inability to appreciate the affective experiences and mental frame of others, to understand the emotional climate, and to express their own emotions in a meaningful fashion – their inability to know, in a basic sense, how their own mind functions and that others have minds of their own. The precise characterization of this deviance, which was central to Kanner's earliest descriptions, has, however, received less research emphasis than other aspects of the autistic syndrome, such as language.

To determine whether the autistic social dysfunction is present, clinicians assess various areas of functioning through observation, interviews with the parents, and formal assessment of the child's behavior and cognitive abilities. This evaluation reviews four major areas:

1. *Communicative acts*: the individual's verbal and nonverbal attempts at communication, through behavior (such as pointing or looking at objects, turning away, calling attention to oneself, using eye contact to guide conversational turn-taking, etc.) or speech (using words to truly communicate desires, protest, call attention, elaborate, inform, etc.)

2. *Attachment*: the child's physical proximity and use of others for comfort and security, and specific differences in his or her relations with primary caregivers and others

3. *Sociability*: the degree to which the child is interested in people rather than things, including his or her recognition of differences among people, attraction to people and their actions, and so on

4. *Understanding and expressing emotions*: the child's ability to understand the feelings of others (including the capacity for empathy) and to display a range of emotions that are suitable to the context

For the purpose of classification, *autistic social dysfunction* is a dichotomous variable. It is present or absent. Its presence is the cardinal criterion for the diagnosis of autism. However, in clinical and research work, it is very important to have a much more fine-grained assessment of areas of social and other adaptive functioning. DSM-III provides for this through the multiaxial system. Axis V, which is the highest level of adaptive functioning, is particularly relevant to autism, if it is elaborated appropriately. We propose that Axis V be completed for autistic children through the use of reliable and valid assessment methods for both adaptive functioning (such as the Vineland, described previously) and intellectual ability (such as the WISC, Stanford Binet, or other appropriate measures of intelligence). These two factors, which are essential for the diagnosis of mental retardation, are highly relevant for understanding any developmentally disabled child or adult. Using the Vineland and an IQ measure, it is possible to create a Social Quotient that can indicate the severity, relative to intellectual impairment, of a child's social adaptation. In the future, this may provide for phenomenological subclassification of autistic children and adults.

Age

The diagnostic criteria for autism, like clinical descriptions of autistic individuals, have focused on very young autistic children. This would be similar to a typology for congenital heart disease that described only its manifestations during the newborn period, but failed to provide for its natural history. It is all the more inappropriate now, as we are increasingly aware of the educational and vocational needs of autistic adolescents and adults.

The diagnosis of autism can be sustained throughout adulthood on the basis of the continued presence of the basic disturbance in social communication and, even for brighter adults, the inability to fully engage in the world of social intercourse. Even bright autistic adults may be unable to follow the story line of soap operas or enjoy normal humor. They may speak well but in a stilted monotone and may be unable to initiate or sustain friendships with peers. Basically, these autistic individuals continue to have major problems in registering, empathically understanding, or decoding implicit meanings and to use this information to regulate social behavior. For these autistic adults, the diagnosis of autism remains suitable. For the rare autistic person who no longer shows the autistic social dysfunction, another diagnosis, if appropriate, should be given (usually this is a personality diagnosis, such as schizoid personality). Autistic individuals may develop other psychiatric problems that require diagnosis, such as depression, generalized anxiety disorder, anorexia nervosa, and the like. The important point, diagnostically, is that autistic children generally develop into autistic adults, and the concept of "residual autism" fails to convey the developmental continuities in the underlying deficit. The concept "infantile" autism is not appropriate for the lifelong disorder.

High- and low-functioning autism

Clinicians have used various terms to differentiate two large subgroups of autistic individuals: (1) those who tend to be nonverbal, to have more behavioral problems (such as abuse and aggression), to have more neurological difficulties, and to be more retarded; and (2) those who have language skills, are more normal in appearance, seem to be drifting about in their own world or pulled into a shell, and have normal or near-normal intelligence. Obviously, there is much overlapping between groups, and one value of the multiaxial system is that it dissects the range of functioning in many different areas and does not simply group children in a single category. The terms "high" and "low" functioning have been used to distinguish the two major groups just portrayed, but these terms are unfortunate owing to their ambiguity and evaluative tone.

To preserve the intention of subclassification, we recommend, for the time being, the use of "intellectual functioning." For high functioning, we suggest the use of a nonverbal IQ of 70 or a global IQ of 55, and we designate these children as suffering from Kanner's autism; for the less fortunate children, whose intellectual level, as well as other areas of functioning, is grossly impaired, we suggest the term "autistic pervasive developmental disorder." The tremendous differences between the nonverbal, mute child with an IQ of 15 and a bright, eccentric and college-educated young man with an IQ of 115 deserve to be noted nosologically. More important, future work should help define norms that are sensitive to the clinical areas of impairment for both autistic children and adults; such norms will make it possible to place individuals in the perspective of a spectrum of dysfunctions that is more similar to the clinical point of view.

DIAGNOSTIC CRITERIA

On the basis of this approach we (Cohen, Volkmar & Paul, 1986a; Cohen, Paul & Volkmar, 1986) recommend that the diagnostic criteria for autism be based on disturbances in two areas of human development:

1. *Autistic social dysfunction*: gross and sustained impairments in socialization and reciprocal social relations, including dysfunctions involving communicative intentions, attachment, sociability, and the expression and understanding of emotions

2. *Gross deficits in social communication and language development*: including mutism or peculiar speech patterns and impairment in nonverbal (gesture, gaze, facial expression, etc.) and verbal communication (defining the shared topic, establishing rapport, maintaining dialogue, taking turns, understanding implicit messages)

Because of the developmental similarities in these two areas, it might be possible to consider them together as constituting a single, overarching diagnostic characterization – *autistic dysfunction of socialization and social communication* – which would be defined polythetically by the types of symptoms noted above.

In addition to these two major areas of dysfunction, autistic children and adults have a variety of intriguing and disturbing behaviors, which they may share with other developmentally disordered and retarded individuals. These include an impoverishment of imagination and play, obsessions and odd preoccupations, stereotypic and manneristic movements, insistence on preserving physical objects and routines in the same fashion, fascination with mechanical objects, and deviant (increased or diminished) responses to certain types of environmental stimuli. Although these characteristics are not diagnostic of autism, their presence is confirmatory or suggestive that the individual is autistic.

The revisions of DSM-III that are now under way are consistent with the emphases in this approach to diagnosis. The work group's recommendations, as synthesized by Dr. Lorna Wing, include three types of diagnostic criteria: social, communicative, and the range of associated features noted above.

If diagnostic criteria are used rigorously, there will be many children with early onset disorders who will not receive the diagnosis of autism. For these children, clinicians have used various terms, such as autisticlike, psychotic,

Asperger's syndrome, atypical development, atypical personality development, symbiotic psychosis, schizoaffective disorder, childhood schizophrenia, borderline, and other conditions. Under the conventions of DSM-III, many of these children would be categorized as having atypical pervasive developmental disorder. Other, nonautistic early-onset disorders are probably more frequent than autism and clearly deserve greater research to define a more specific nosology (Dahl, Cohen & Provence, in press). Many of the historical categories (e.g., atypical development) remain in need of rigorous study and are of more heuristic than scientific use.

For the present, we have utilized the concept "multiplex developmental disorders" to characterize one large, heterogeneous subgroup of children with early-onset, nonautistic disorders (Cohen, Volkmar & Paul, 1986b). These children suffer from profound and persistent problems in the regulation of anxiety (with fears and panic), social development (with attachments to others marked by mixtures of dependency and hostility, and rapid shifts in relations characterized by "splitting and ambivalence"), and cognitive problems (with distortions in reality testing, delusions, paranoid tendencies, magical thinking, and the like). The natural history of such children is sometimes toward frank childhood schizophrenia, but they may develop serious personality disorders as well. Clearly, future research will be required to develop adequate diagnostic criteria and establish the validity of these "atypical" pervasive developmental conditions.

In addition to diagnosing children with autistic and nonautistic "psychotic" conditions, clinicians must differentially diagnose children whose major problems lie in the sphere of language development. Meticulous study is needed to define the areas of both expressive and receptive competence. In childhood, pure receptive language disorder is rarely – if ever – seen, and both types of language disorders are commonly associated with mental retardation. Therefore, we define a language disorder using the convention of a ratio of language competence to mental age. An expressive or receptive language disorder is diagnosed if the ratio of expressive or receptive language ability to mental age is less than 70. Moreover, if a child has an autistic social dysfunction, and satisfies the criteria for autism, this diagnosis preempts the diagnosis of language disorder since autism includes language dysfunction as a primary diagnostic feature (Cohen, Volkmar & Paul, 1986a).

CONCLUSIONS

During the last several years, there has been a consensus among clinicians and investigators about the core psychological disturbances of childhood autism. The primacy of the social dysfunction, which so impressed Leo Kanner, has again emerged in the forefront of research in the area. Whether disturbances in this area lead to or "cause" the other dysfunctions cannot be known; most likely, increased understanding of the fundamental matrix out of which autism emerges will remain elusive until more is known about the biology of social relatedness, a field to which clinical research on autism may contribute. In child psychiatry, classification schemes reflect the state of knowledge and also show what remains to be learned. It is useful today that the diagnosis of autism is made without reference to theoretical viewpoints about etiology, beliefs about what treatment or treatments are most effective, and other factors that are, of course, of great clinical and theoretical importance.

Diagnostic emphasis on communicative functioning and socialization reflects what is known about autism, from infancy throughout adulthood, from individuals with profound mental retardation to those with normal intelligence.

Although we are firmly convinced that autism reflects a series of underlying disturbances in biological maturation of the central nervous system, the precise nature of these disturbances remains an open question. Thus, it would be premature to use biological findings available today for diagnosis or subclassification, although the presence of these findings (including inborn errors of metabolism, brain dysfunctions, chromosomal abnormalities, abnormal EEGs and computed tomograms, and the like) is of great interest and theoretical relevance. Furthermore, it is fundamental to the scientific method to be honest about how little is currently understood concerning the normal physiology of processes such as socialization, let alone how these processes may be disrupted in relation to autism and similar disorders.

During the next several years, research on classification and diagnosis may be facilitated in two ways:

1. The development of scales and measures more suitable for assessing autistic children's functioning and specific behavioral methods would assist in subclassifying children and better delineating areas of disturbance. The advances made with methods such as the Vineland scales, along with sensitive behavioral, naturalistic, and cognitive measures, are apparent. Research methodologies involving the assessment of mutuality, joint attention, and the like, along with methods for studying communication and language, will help define areas of specific impairment in autistic individuals in general and, more likely, relative impairment for different individuals.

2. Advances in biological research may provide us with more robust findings about the biological substrate of the disorder(s). Nothing would be more useful than the determination of specific genetic factors, physiological or neuroanatomical lesions, or biochemical abnormalities. The autistic syndrome most likely is etiologically quite heterogeneous, and further biological research will probably add to the multiple causes of the condition. The availability of behavioral measures and diagnoses will help in sorting out the various types of etiologies, the relation between genotype and behavioral expression, and the nature of various artifacts (Young, Leven & Cohen, 1985).

For too many decades, controversy about the etiology and treatment of autism has impeded progress in understanding autism and in sharing knowledge among professionals committed to the welfare of autistic children and adults. Today, it should be possible for investigators and clinicians from varying perspectives to share information about clinical characteristics, behavioral change, and relevant treatments, using generally accepted diagnostic conventions. Regardless of theoretical orientation, we are all united by the shared recognition of how little can be done, on the basis of current knowledge, to alter the prognosis for the great majority of autistic individuals. The application of scientific canons concerning evidence and conjecture or hypothesis will enable investigators from varying backgrounds to discuss openly what is known and what remains to be studied. Research on classification and diagnosis is aimed at synthesizing this knowledge and facilitating this type of open communication.

ACKNOWLEDGMENTS

We wish to thank the staff of Benhaven and Dr. Amy Lettick, its director, for collaborating in many of our studies. This research was supported by NICHD grant 03008, Mental Health Clinical Research Center grant MH 30929, the Childrens Clinical Research Center, the John Merck Fund, The MacArthur Foundation, and Leonard Berger.

REFERENCES

Anderson, G., and Hoshino, Y. 1986. Neurochemistry. In *Handbook of Autism and Pervasive Developmental Disorders*, ed. D. Cohen and A. Donnellan. New York: Wiley.

Bates, G. 1976. *Language in Context*. New York: Academic Press.

Bruner, J. 1975. The ontogenesis of speech acts. *Jour. Child Language* 2: 1–20.

Carrell, P. 1981. Children's understanding of indirect requests: comparing child and adult comprehension. *Jour. Child Language* 8: 329–345.

Cohen, D. 1976. The diagnostic process in child psychiatry. *Psych. Annals* 6: 404–416.

Cohen, D. 1978. Agreement in diagnosis: Clerical assessment and behavioral rating scales for pervasively disturbed children. *Jour. Amer. Acad. Child Psychiatry* 17: 589–603.

Cohen, D., Paul, R., and Volkmar, F. 1986. Issues in the classification of pervasive developmental disorders: provisional diagnostic axes and categorical criteria. *Jour. Amer. Acad. Child Psychiatry* 25: 213–220.

Cohen, D., Volkmar, F., and Paul, R. 1986a. Issues in the classification of pervasive developmental disorders: history and current status of nosology. *Jour. Amer. Acad. Child Psychiatry* 25: 158–161.

Cohen, D., Volkmar, F., and Paul, R. 1986b. Classification of pervasive developmental disorders and associated conditions. *Handbook of Autism and Pervasive Developmental Disorders*, ed. D. Cohen and A. Donnellan. New York: Wiley.

Curtis, S. 1981. Dissociations between language and cognition: cases and implications. *Jour. of Autism and Developmental Disorders* 11: 15–30.

Dahl, K., Cohen, D., and Provence, S. In press. Issues in the classification of developmental disorders of early onset. *Jour. Amer. Acad. Child Psychiatry*.

Fein, D., Pennington, B., Markowtix, P., Braverman, M., and Waterhouse, L. 1986. Towards a neuropsychological model of infantile autism: Are the social deficits primary? *Jour. Amer. Acad. Child Psychiatry* 25: 198–212.

Gallagher, T. 1981. Contingent query sequences within adult–child discourse. *Jour. Child Language* 8: 51–62.

Harcherik, D., Cohen, D., Paul, R., Ort, S., Shaywitz, B. A., Volkmar, F., Rothman,

S., and Leckman. J. 1985. Computed brain tomographic scanning in four neuro-psychiatric disorders of childhood. *Amer. Jour. Psychiatry* 142: 731–734.

Kanner, L. 1973. *Childhood Psychosis: Initial Studies and New Insights.* Washington, D.C.: V. H. Winston & Sons.

Kolvin, I. 1971. Studies in the childhood psychoses: I. Diagnostic criteria and classification. *British Jour. Psychiatry* 118: 381–384.

Minderaa, R., Volkmar, F., Hansen, C., Harcherik, D., Akkerhuis, G., and Cohen, D. 1985. Brief report: snout and visual rooting reflex in infantile autism. *Jour. Autism and Developmental Disorders* 15: 409–416.

Parks, S. 1983. The assessment of autistic children: a selective review of available instruments. *Jour. Autism and Developmental Disorders* 13: 255–267.

Paul, R. 1986. Communication. In *Handbook of Autism and Pervasive Developmental Disorders,* ed. D. Cohen and A. Donnellan. New York: Wiley.

Paul, R., and Cohen, D. 1984a. Outcomes of severe disorders of language acquisition. *Jour. Autism and Developmental Disorders* 144: 153–160.

Paul, R., and Cohen, D. 1984b. Responses to contingent queries in adults with mental retardation and pervasive developmental disorders. *Applied Psycholinguistics* 5: 349–357.

Paul, R., and Cohen, D. 1985. Comprehension of indirect requests in adults with mental retardation and pervasive developmental disorders. *Jour. Speech and Hearing Research* 28: 1–5.

Paul, R., Cohen, D., and Caparulo, B. 1983. A longitudinal study of patients with severe developmental disorders of language learning. *Jour. Amer. Acad. Child Psychiatry* 22: 525–534.

Rutter, M., Shaffer, D., and Shepherd, M. 1975. *A Multiaxial Classification of Child Psychiatric Disorders.* Geneva: World Health Organization.

Sigman, M., Ungerer, J., Mundy, P., and Shuman, T. 1986. Cognition. In *Handbook of Autism and Pervasive Developmental Disorders,* ed. D. Cohen and A. Donnellan. New York: Wiley.

Tager-Flusberg, H. 1981. On the nature of linguistic functioning in early infantile autism. *Jour. Autism and Developmental Disorders* 11: 45–56.

Volkmar, F., and Cohen, D. 1982. A hierarchical analysis of patterns of noncompliance in autistic and behavior-disturbed children. *Jour. Autism and Developmental Disorders* 12: 35–42.

Volkmar, F., and Cohen, D. 1985. The experience of infantile autism: a first person account by Tony W. *Jour. Autism and Developmental Disorders* 15: 47–54.

Volkmar, F., Cohen, D., and Paul, R. 1986. An evaluation of DSM-III criteria for infantile autism. *Jour. Amer. Acad. Child Psychiatry* 25: 190–197.

Volkmar, F., Hoder, L., and Cohen, D. 1985. Compliance, "negativism," and the effect of treatment structure on behavior in autism: a naturalistic study. *Jour. Child Psychology and Psychiatry* 26: 865–877.

Volkmar, F., Stier, D., and Cohen, D. 1985. Age of recognition of pervasive developmental disorder. *Amer. Jour. Psychiatry* 142: 1450–1452.

Wetherby, A., and Prutting, C. 1984. Profiles of communication and cognitive-social abilities in autistic children. *Jour. Speech and Hearing Research* 27: 364–377.

Young, J., Leven, L., and Cohen, D. 1985. Neurochemical strategies in clinical research. In *Psychiatry,* ed. R. Michels and J. Cavenar. Philadelphia: J. B. Lippincott.

11 *Acute and transient psychoses*

A view from the developing countries

NARENDRA N. WIG (Egypt) AND R. PARHEE (India)

During the past two or three decades, several reports from developing countries have described a class of psychotic disorders frequently termed "acute psychosis" or "transient psychosis." These psychoses are generally rapid in onset, have a short duration, and are followed by complete recovery. The patient tends to have florid psychotic symptoms established within a period of a few days, with delusions, hallucinations, and great emotional turmoil. Sometimes the symptoms seem to be precipitated by marked mental stress. It is difficult to classify these disorders within the conventional Western framework of psychiatric diagnostic systems.

HISTORICAL BACKGROUND

Scientific interest in the nosology of psychiatric disorders began to crystallize around the middle of the nineteenth century in Europe with detailed observations of psychiatric patients in terms of symptoms, causes, and outcomes. Kraepelin (1896) was the first to bring together diverse entities under the rubric of "dementia praecox," separating it from the other major psychotic disorder, namely, manic-depressive psychosis. Kraepelin focused primarily on outcome: deterioration versus nondeterioration. This was in contrast to a simple constellation of symptoms. Dementia praecox was characterized by slow deterioration, as well as hallucinations, delusions, stereotypies, and disordered affect. However, Kraepelin himself pointed out that about 13 percent of dementia praecox patients did not deteriorate and presumably recovered without major defect. Kraepelin's brilliant treatise was followed by Bleuler's (1911) conception of schizophrenia, or "split mindedness," which was based on a hierarchy of symptoms that he described as primary and secondary. Within this group of psychotic disorders, Kraepelin included three basic types of dementia praecox: catatonic, hebephrenic, and paranoid. A fourth type, simple schizophrenia, was described later. Over the years many other subtypes such as schizoaffective, pseudoneurotic, acute, and latent have been added to this list.

The occurrence of a nonorganic, nonaffective psychosis, acute in onset and transient in course, has always been a problem with traditional psychiatric classifications based on Kraepelin's dichotomy of dementia praecox and manic-

115

depressive psychosis. Probably most of these special cases do not go to mental hospitals and perhaps for this reason nineteenth-century psychiatrists did not pay enough attention to them. With the emergence of general hospital psychiatric units and community psychiatric centers, there is better recognition of these cases.

Although the conventional British and American psychiatric classification systems largely ignored these disorders until recently, other national classificatory systems seem to have recognized their presence. French psychiatrists, for example, have long recognized *bouffée délirante*, a rapid onset psychosis with good outcome, characterized by unsystematized and polymorphous delusions with some clouding of consciousness and affective disturbances (Pichot, 1985). In Germany, Leonhard described "cycloid psychosis," which differs from classical schizophrenia and affective psychosis (Cranach & Hippius, 1985). Some varieties of cycloid psychosis closely resemble the acute and transient disorders referred to above. The concept of psychogenic or reactive psychoses has been prominent in Scandinavian psychiatry since the beginning of the century when Wimmer (1916) published his famous monograph on "psychogenic psychoses." The psychogenic psychosis is thought to be caused by major mental trauma. These psychoses are considered benign, usually last only a few weeks, and are followed by complete recovery (Strömgren, 1985).

EXPERIENCE FROM DEVELOPING COUNTRIES

During the last 50 years, many reports from countries in Asia, Africa, and Latin America have confirmed the occurrence of acute and transient psychotic disorders (Wig, 1984; Wig et al., 1985; Varma & Savita, 1985). Only recently, however, have more organized clinical research studies with follow-up designs been reported.

In India, Wig and Singh (1967) drew attention to the occurrence of acute atypical psychosis cases that do not fit into the traditional categories of schizophrenia or affective psychosis. Wig and Narang (1969) described cases of acute short-lived psychoses with marked hysterical features, following some major life event, for which they suggested the name "hysterical psychosis." Many more reports of acute psychoses from India have appeared in recent years (Singh & Sachdev, 1980; Kapur & Pandurangi, 1979; Pandurangi & Kapur, 1980; Kuruvilla & Sitalakshmi, 1982).

Reports of cases of acute atypical psychosis on the African continent have appeared frequently (Carothers, 1953; Collomb, 1966; Jilek & Jilek-Aall, 1970; German, 1972). German (1972) has provided an excellent review of the condition as it exists in sub-Saharan Africa. His description is very similar to reports from India and other Asian countries. The onset of symptoms is acute, often precipitated by some important life event. The constellation of symptoms varies in different reports, but generally the condition consists of a state of excitement with disorganized behavior that includes mixed elements of confusion, affective changes, and thought disturbances. According to German (1972), the presence of "amorphous, easily precipitated and recurrent transient psychosis" is one of the main differences observed in clinical psychiatry in Africa in comparison with other parts of the world. This type of psychosis is more common in the economically underprivileged and socially deprived classes set within a background of poor physical health and in a social setting where such behavior under stress is culturally acceptable. The duration of such psychosis is usually brief, with or without antipsychotic drugs or electroconvulsion therapy.

A major multicentered study was recently conducted by the Indian Council of Medical Research (ICMR). More than three hundred cases of psychotic illness from four centers in India, with victims aged between 15 and 60 years and with an acute onset (i.e., full development of psychosis within a period of two weeks), were investigated in detail and followed up for one year. The most striking feature of this study was that more than 75 percent of the victims had fully recovered with no relapse of psychotic illness by the time of a one-year followup (Indian Council of Medical Research, 1985). In a similar study sponsored by the World Health Organization and conducted in New Delhi with cases of acute first-episode psychosis, Wig and Parhee (1984) reported that nearly 70 percent of the cases suffered from only a single episode of illness during the course of a one-year follow-up. The ICD-9 diagnosis at the time of initial assessment did not differentiate cases with good recovery from those with poor outcome in either the ICMR- or the WHO-sponsored studies. Irrespective of whether the cases were originally diagnosed as schizophrenia, manic-depressive psychosis, or nonorganic psychosis, more than 70 percent had completely recovered at the end of one year. Another striking feature of these studies was the difficulty in classifying acute psychotic cases into either schizophrenia or manic-depressive psychosis, the traditional categories of psychotic disorder. Only 49 percent of the sample in the WHO-sponsored study, and 60 percent in the ICMR study were given a diagnosis of schizophrenia or manic-depressive psychosis at initial assessment.

In view of the difficulty of assigning cases of acute psychosis to the existing ICD-9 diagnostic categories on the basis of the presenting clinical picture, an attempt was made in the ICMR study to develop a purely descriptive diagnostic classification. This categorization depended entirely on the predominent clinical manifestations of the patient at the time of the initial contact. Ten categories (types) were developed to cover the range of observed behavior in these cases, and each category was operationally defined. These were (1) predominantly excited, (2) predominantly withdrawn, (3) predominantly depressed, (4) predominantly elated, (5) predominantly paranoid, (6) predominantly confused, (7) predominantly hysterical, (8) predominantly spirit possession, (9) mixed, and (10) others. It was observed that more than 50 percent of the cases belonged to the two descriptive categories of predominantly excited and paranoid types. The next two common categories of acute psychosis were withdrawn and depressed types (25 percent). The remaining categories accounted for the remainder of the cases (25 percent).

SALIENT FEATURES OF ACUTE TRANSIENT PSYCHOSIS

The studies in developing countries mentioned earlier seem to have confirmed the following features of acute transient psychosis:

1. Cases of acute and transient psychosis are regularly and frequently seen in the psychiatric services of developing countries.
2. By and large, these are good outcome cases. More than two-thirds of the victims seem to recover fully by the end of the year without any relapse, and another 10–15 percent may have one relapse but are quite well by the end of the year.
3. Current knowledge suggests that acute transient psychosis is not a unitary concept but a mixture of heterogeneous disorders.
4. There is no uniform clinical picture. The symptomatology seems to be rapidly changing over time. The most common presentation seen in India is disorganized social behavior, with generalized excitement and persecutory delusions.
5. The initial diagnosis according to standard classifications (e.g. schizophrenia, manic-depressive psychosis) does not seem to be significantly correlated with the outcome, as most victims recover by the end of the year.
6. Major psychological or physiological stress at the beginning of acute psychosis is not universally present. It is seen in less than half of the cases.
7. According to the strict criteria, many of the cases of acute psychosis do not fit well with either ICD-9 or DSM-III classifications and have to be labeled "atypical psychosis" or "psychosis not otherwise specified."

THE CURRENT STATUS OF ACUTE TRANSIENT PSYCHOTIC DISORDERS IN INTERNATIONAL PSYCHIATRIC CLASSIFICATION

The WHO International Classification of Diseases (ICD-9) and the American Psychiatric Association's (1980) *Diagnostic and Statistical Manual* (third edition, DSM-III) are currently the two most widely accepted systems of classification of mental disorders. Unfortunately, neither of them seems to deal adequately with the problem of acute and transient psychosis, particularly as seen in developing countries, where the majority of the world population lives.

Unlike the DSM-III system, the current ICD-9 does not have explicit diagnostic criteria, but it does contain a glossary to help the user (World Health Organization, 1978). Unfortunately, this glossary does not clearly indicate where to classify the acute psychoses described above. For example, most psychiatrists from India, having been brought up in the Anglo-American tradition of psychiatry, tend to regard these cases as variants of either schizophrenia or manic-depressive psychosis, although the classical features of these conditions are missing. These cases are often listed under "acute schizophrenic episode" (295.4) although the description given in the ICD-9 glossary (e.g., dreamlike state with perplexity) is usually missing in most of the cases.

The other alternative in ICD-9 is to include these cases under code number 298, that is, "other nonorganic psychoses," provided the condition is "largely or entirely attributable to a recent life experience." This is a major limitation of ICD-9. As pointed out earlier, it has not been easy to demonstrate the presence of a significant life event in more than half of the cases. Furthermore, the subcategories of code 298 are not adequate. For example, states of simple excitement, withdrawal, or hysterical dissociation of psychotic type, as well as spirit possession syndromes seen in many parts of the world, are difficult to fit into the present ICD-9.

The DSM-III system seems to recognize these conditions better as it clearly separates them from schizophrenia and manic-depressive psychosis, and allocates them to a separate section entitled "psychotic disorders not elsewhere classified." This section contains four categories: schizophreniform disorder, brief reactive psychosis, schizoaffective disorder, and atypical psychosis. Unfortunately, a large number of cases of acute and transient psychosis, as discussed in this chapter, do not fit into the first three categories and again end up as "atypical" cases.

The diagnostic criteria for schizophreniform disorder in DSM-III involve the presence of all the criteria for schizophrenia, except that the duration of illness should be less than six months and more than two weeks. There are two problems with using this definition. First, recent studies have shown that a large number of cases of acute transient psychosis develop a full-blown picture in less than two weeks. Second, schizophrenia as conceptualized in DSM-III is a chronic disorder. It is not clinically sound to use the criteria of a chronic psychosis (e.g., thought broadcast, thought insertion, delusion of control, passivity, affective blunting, etc.) to describe an acute psychotic condition in which gross behavior disturbance, generalized excitement or withdrawal, changing content of delusions, and so on, are the main features.

The diagnosis of brief reactive psychosis in the DSM–III is limited to cases in which a recent life event appears as the causative factor. Unfortunately, the "duration-of-symptom" criterion again limits the usefulness of this diagnosis. The current description strongly suggests that such psychotic conditions must resolve in two weeks. But this does not appear to occur in many acute and transient psychotic cases. Revision of this section of DSM-III will no doubt improve its usefulness for developing countries.

CONCLUSION

Acute and transient psychiatric disorders are regularly and frequently seen in the mental health services of developing countries. Their recognition and management is of great public health concern, since most of them recover spontaneously. The available information does not justify classifying them as either schizophrenia or affective disorders. Both the current WHO international classification (ICD–9) and the American Psychiatric Association's classification (DSM-III) fail to provide a satisfactory system for describing these disorders.

Until more knowledge is obtained about acute and transient psychoses, it would be better to put them in a new category in international classifications.

REFERENCES

American Psychiatric Association 1980. *Diagnostic and Statistical Manual of Mental Disorders.* 3rd ed. (DSM-III) Washington, D.C.

Bleuler, E. 1911. Dementia praecox oder Gruppe der Schizophrenien. In *Handbuch der Psychiatrie,* ed. G. Aschaffenburg. Leipzig: Deuticke.

Carothers, J. C. 1953. *The African Mind in Health and Disease.* WHO Monograph Series no. 17. Geneva: World Health Organization.

Collomb, H. 1966. Aspects particuliers de la psychiatrie africaine. In *Cliniques Africaines.* Paris: Gauthior-Villars.

Cranach, M. von, & Hippius, H. 1985. State of diagnosis and classification in German speaking countries. In *Mental Disorders, Alcohol and Drug Related Problems, International Perspectives on Their Diagnosis and Classification.* Amsterdam: Excerpta Medica. International Congress Series 669.

German, G. A. 1972. Aspects of clinical psychiatry in sub-Saharan Africa. *British Journal of Psychiatry* 121: 461–479.

Indian Council of Medical Research 1985. Final report of the project: "The phenomenology and natural history of acute psychosis" (mimeographed copy available from Indian Council of Medical Research, New Delhi).

Jilek, N. G., and Jilek-Aall, L. 1970. Transient psychoses in Africans. *Psychiatrica Clinica* 3: 337–364.

Kapur, R. L., and Pandurangi, A. K. 1979. A comparative study of reactive psychosis and acute psychosis without precipitating stress. *British Journal of Psychiatry* 135: 544–550.

Kraepelin, E. 1896. *Psychiatrie.* Leipzig: Barth.

Kuruvilla, K., and Sitalakshmi, N. 1982. Hysterical psychosis. *Indian Journal of Psychiatry* 24: 352–359.

Pandurangi, A. K., and Kapur, R. L. 1980. Reactive psychosis – a prospective study. *Acta Psychiatrica Scandinavica* 61: 89–95.

Pichot, P. 1985. Psychiatric nosology in France and Francophone tradition. In *Mental Disorders, Alcohol and Drug Related Problems, International Perspectives on Their Diagnosis and Classification.* Amsterdam: Excerpta Medica. International Congress Series 669.

Singh, G., and Sachdev, J. S. 1980. A clinical and follow-up study of atypical psychoses. *Indian Journal of Psychiatry* 22: 167–172.

Strömgren, E. 1985. World-wide issues in psychiatric diagnosis and classification and the Scandinavian point of view. In *Mental Disorders, Alcohol and Drug Related Problems, International Perspectives on Their Diagnosis and Classification.* Amsterdam: Excerpta Medica. International Congress Series 669.

Varma, V. K., and Savita, M. 1985. Diagnosis and classification of acute psychotic disorders in the developing world. *Indian Journal of Social Psychiatry* 1: 11–21.

Wig, N. N. 1984. Diagnostic et classification en psychiatrie. Aspects transculturels. In *Confrontations Psychiatrique No. 24,* Edition et Administration. Paris: Specia.

Wig. N. N., Kusumanto, S. R., Shen Yu-Cun, and Sell, H. 1985. Problems of psychiatric diagnosis and classification in the Third World. In *Mental Disorders, Alcohol and Drug Related Problems, International Perspectives on Their Diagnosis and Classification.* Amsterdam: Excerpta Medica. International Congress Series 669.

Wig, N. N., and Narang, R. L. 1969. Hysterical psychosis. *Indian Journal of Psychiatry* 11:93.

Wig, N. N., and Parhee, R. 1984. Classification of acute psychotic states. Paper presented at the WHO/Asean Forum on the Status of Diagnosis and Classification of Mental Disorders, Alcohol and Drug Related Problems in the Third World. Jakarta, Indonesia, February. (Copies available from World Health Organization, Geneva.)

Wig, N. N., and Singh, G. 1967. A proposed classification of psychiatric disorders for use in India. *Indian Journal of Psychiatry* 9: 158–171.

Wimmer, A. 1916. Psykogene Sindssygdomsformer (Psychogenic varieties of mental diseases). In *St. Hans Hospital 1816–1915*, ed. A. Wimmer, pp. 85–216. Copenhagen: G. E. C. Gads Forlag.

World Health Organization 1978. *Mental Disorders: Glossary and Guide to Their Classification in Accordance with the Ninth Revision of the International Classification of Diseases.* Geneva.

12 Schizoaffective psychosis

An empirical comparison of diagnostic approaches

MICHAEL ZAUDIG, MICHAEL VON CRANACH,
HANS-ULRICH WITTCHEN, GERT SEMLER, AND
HERBERT STEINBÖCK (Federal Republic of Germany)

INTRODUCTION

The concept and classification of schizoaffective disorders are still controversial. A variety of terms are used, with shifting meanings, again and again disputing Kraepelin's principle of the two-disease entities. Nevertheless, most psychiatrists agree that the basic structure of the classification system Kraepelin originated is still dominant in psychiatry. One of his major organizing principles was that mental diseases could be grouped on the basis of their long-term course. In 1896 Kraepelin proposed that psychotic disorders be divided into dementia praecox and manic-depressive insanity. Dementia praecox (schizophrenia) was seen as being inevitably deteriorative, whereas manic-depressive insanity was seen as leading to recovery. But Kraepelin himself had to accept that 13 percent of his dementia praecox cases had a good prognosis and remained well without any defect. Some of these cases were classified as periodic dementia praecox, a kind of psychosis, in which affective and schizophrenic symptoms were present simultaneously, with a periodic course and full recovery of the patient not being unusual. The predominant reaction to this observation was the assumption that this variable prognosis refers to a third entity or a group characterized by schizophrenia with recurrent course and complete recovery (Kendell, 1983). Strong efforts were, therefore, made to distinguish a schizophrenia with a favorable prognosis from "true" schizophrenia with a chronic or deteriorating course. Langfeldt (1937) introduced the concepts of good- and poor-prognosis schizophrenias, defining the former as "schizophreniform psychosis" and the latter as "true" schizophrenia. Schizophreniform psychoses are "acute, precipitated by problems of living or by organic factors; recovery from episodes is usual; and there is some evidence of a relationship between schizophrenic illness and primary affective disorders" (Langfeldt, 1939). In Scandinavian countries the terms "reactive psychosis" (Astrup & Noreik, 1966; McCabe, 1975) and "psychogenic psychosis" (Faergerman, 1963) are widely used to describe a group of acute, good-prognosis schizophrenias.

Unrelated to Kraepelin's system of classification is the concept of "degeneration psychosis" that Wernicke (1900) introduced in Germany and that can be traced back to the French notion of *les dégénérés* (Legrain, 1886). The kind of psychosis was characterized by a sudden onset, a polymorphous symptomatology, and a recurrent course; Kleist (1921) and Schröder (1926) strongly defended the autonomy of the degeneration psychosis. In 1928 Kleist coined the term "cycloid psychosis" for a group of features consisting of "degeneration psychosis" and "delusional affective psychoses," a heterogeneous group of acute psychoses. Leonhard (1957) divided the cycloid psychoses into three subtypes: the motility psychosis, the confusion psychosis, and the anxiety-elation psychosis. Cycloid psychoses were assumed to have a recurrent and bipolar course with full recovery from each episode. This concept has been further developed by Perris's (Perris, 1974; Perris & Brockington, 1981) introduction of operational criteria.

Independently of this German cycloid concept, French psychiatrists developed a taxonomy that was not influenced by Kraepelin's dichotomy. Since Legrain (1886) and Magnan (1893), many acute psychoses have been designated *bouffée délirante*. Magnan regarded these short-lasting psychoses as an expression of a constitutional weakness (degeneration). According to Ey (1954), the disorder arises with dramatic suddenness, a polymorphous delusional state and various affective disturbances; the mood constantly changes from exaltation to terror, to perplexity, to anxiety and depersonalization. A single episode lasts no more than a few weeks, remission is complete, and relapse is usual. There are two variants: the classical *bouffée délirante* as described by Magnan and a reactive condition in which psychosocial precipitants are considered to be of etiological significance. In 1983, Pull, Pull, and Pichot introduced operational criteria.

In 1983 the term "schizoaffective" was coined by Kasanin. He described nine young adults who had become acutely psychotic with emotional turmoil, a blending of affective and schizophrenic symptoms, and "distortion of the outside world and presence of false sensory impression" (Table 12.1). Patients with this kind of psychosis recovered completely within a few weeks or months, although there was a marked tendency of the psychosis to recur later. Kasanin's "acute schizoaffective psychoses" resembles the concepts of schizophreniform mentioned earlier (reactive, degenerative, and cycloid psychosis), as well as *bouffée délirante* and Kraepelin's periodic dementia praecox. All these "traditional" acute psychoses have in common acute onset, polymorphous symptomatology such as schizophrenic symptoms, excitement, overactivity, "emotional turmoil," manic and/or depressive mood disturbance, short duration, full recovery, and a better outcome than typical schizophrenia.

In 1965 Vaillant described "the efforts of psychiatry to rename the recovered schizophrenic." He systematically compared the following features in 16 studies: acute onset, acute schizophrenic picture with symptoms of psychotic depression, confusion or disorientation, good premorbid adjustment, a clear precipitating event, and remission to the premorbid level of adjustment (see also Tsuang & Simpson, 1984).

Under the heading of "schizoaffective psychosis," Procci (1976) updated Vaillant's (1965) review, comparing in addition Vaillant's remitting schizo-

Table 12.1. *Criteria by J. Kasanin for schizoaffective psychosis*

1. A group of nine cases is presented in which there is a blending of schizophrenic and affective symptoms.
2. The psychosis is characterized by
   a. A very sudden onset
   b. A setting of marked emotional turmoil with a distortion of the outside world and presence of false sensory impressions in some cases.
3. The psychosis lasts a few weeks to a few months and is followed by recovery.
4. Patients are young people, in their 20s or 30s, in excellent physical health, in whom there is usually a history of a previous attack in late adolescence.
5. The prepsychotic personalities of the patients show the usual variation found in any group of people.
6. Some of the factors favoring recovery include good social and industrial adjustment, the presence of a definite and specific environmental stress, the interest in life and its opportunities, and the absence of any passivity or withdrawal.

phrenia (1965) as well as Stephens, Astrup, and Magrum's (1966) "recovered schizophrenics," the Fowler et al. (1972) "good prognosis schizophrenia," and McCabe's "reactive psychosis" (1975). To Vaillant's criteria he added family history of depression and psychomotor excitation. Procci concluded that all these psychoses – subordinated to Kasanin's original term "schizoaffective" – probably represent a "variant of affective disorder or an independent entity bearing a similarity to affective disorder." Consequently, Kasanin's original term "schizoaffective" was shifted to a synonym for acute psychoses with similarity to affective psychoses. Following Procci's conclusion, Pope and Lipinski (1978) argued in a critical review that schizoaffective disorder represents a form of affective disorder, primarily bipolar affective disorder.

With the introduction of operational criteria in psychiatry (Feighner et al., 1972), strictly defined operational criteria for schizoaffective disorder were presented by Welner, Croughan, and Robins (1974), Spitzer, Endicott, and Robins (1978), and Kendell (1979). In addition, a distinction between schizoaffective mania and schizoaffective depression was established. This "modern idea of concurrent schizoaffective psychosis" (Brockington & Meltzer, 1983) ignores the "psychological setting" (such as Kasanin's emotional turmoil or excitement, confusion, ecstasy, anxiety, and motility disturbances) and just focuses on clear-cut manic or depressive syndromes in combination with typical schizophrenic symptoms. This modern view of schizoaffective disorder is reflected in the definition of ICD-9 (World Health Organization, 1978) and the revision of DSM-III (American Psychiatric Association, 1987), specifying bipolar and depressive types. In DSM-III (American Psychiatric Association, 1980) "schizoaffective disorder survives only as a diagnostic category of last resort" (Tsuang & Simpson, 1984) and belongs to "psychotic disorders not elsewhere classified" without operational criteria.

At present two major concepts for schizoaffective psychosis are used:

1. The more traditional concepts such Kasanin's "schizoaffectives," *bouffée délirante*, cycloid psychosis, schizophreniform and reactive psychoses
2. The modern idea of "concurrent" schizoaffective psychosis such as Welner's, Spitzer's, and Kendell's criteria, and recently the criteria of DSM-III-R

In DSM-III and ICD-9 both aspects of traditional and modern definitions are included and therefore the definitions are equivocal.

As mentioned earlier, a variety of terms have been applied to schizoaffective psychoses, but confusion still exists regarding the nosological position of these psychoses. Are they a subgroup of schizophrenia as in ICD-9, a variant of affective disorders, or a third disease entity? In order to test the latter hypothesis one has to find a homogenous group of psychoses that could be empirically delineated from schizophrenia and affective disorder. For this purpose, the operational criteria for cycloid psychosis, *bouffée délirante* and Kendell's schizoaffective illness were examined.

DIAGNOSTIC CRITERIA

Perris introduced operational criteria for cycloid psychosis (Perris & Brockington, 1981) (Table 12.2). He did not accept the three Leonhard (1980) subtypes and asserted that "the clinical picture of cycloid psychosis is most frequently characterized by the occurrence of features belonging to any of the subtypes described by Leonhard." In Perris's account, the symptomatology includes confusion, mood-incongruent delusions, hallucinatory experiences, pan-anxiety, ecstasy, motility disturbances, mood swings, and polymorphic symptomatology. The onset is sudden and the psychotic picture is full blown. The disease follows a relapsing course without any obvious relation to events and with full recovery from each episode. Perris emphasizes three cardinal features: the presence of some confusion, polymorphic symptomatology, and acute onset in a "full blown psychotic condition" (Perris & Brockington, 1981).

The predictive validity of Perris's concept has been confirmed by Cutting, Clare, and Mann (1978) and Brockington and Leff (1979), who found that cycloid psychoses are not synonymous with the modern concepts of schizoaffective psychoses such as Welner's or the Research Diagnostic Criteria (Spitzer, Endicott & Robins, 1978). In previous investigations (Zaudig & Vogl, 1983; Vogl & Zaudig, 1985) we were able to distinguish cycloid psychosis from "concurrent schizoaffective psychoses" (Brockington & Meltzer, 1983).

Upon investigating schizoaffective psychosis in French psychiatry, Pull, Pull, and Pichot (1983) developed operational criteria for *bouffée délirante* (Table 12.3). They proposed operational diagnostic criteria that included the following: acute onset, short duration, delusions and/or hallucinations of any type, de-

Table 12.2. *Perris's criteria for cycloid psychoses*

A. An acute psychotic condition in patients ranging from 15 to 50 years of age.
B. The condition has a sudden onset (within few hours or at most a few days).
C. For a definite diagnosis, the occurrence of at least four of the following symptoms is required:
   1. Confusion of some degree, mostly expressed as perplexity or puzzlement
   2. Mood incongruent delusions of any kind, most often with a persecutory content
   3. Hallucinatory experiences of any kind, often related to themes of death
   4. An overwhelming, frightening, and pervasive experience of anxiety, not bound to particular situations or circumstances
   5. Deep feelings of happiness or ecstasy, most often with a religious coloring
   6. Motility disturbances of an akinetic or hyperkinetic type, which are mostly expressional
   7. A particular concern with death
   8. Mood swings in the background, not so pronounced as to justify a diagnosis of an affective disorder.
D. There is no fixed symptomatological constellation. On the contrary, the symptomatology may change frequently in the course of the same episode, often showing bipolar characteristics.

Table 12.3. *Diagnostic criteria for* bouffée délirante *(Pull et al.)*

A. Age at onset: approximately between 20 and 40 years
B. Onset: acute, without any prior psychiatric history (other than identical episodes)
C. No chronicity: active phases fade away completely in several weeks or months possibly recurring under the same form; the patient remaining devoid of all abnormality in the interval
D. Characteristic symptoms (all of the following):
   1. Delusions and/or hallucinations of any type
   2. Depersonalization/derealization and/or confusion
   3. Depression and/or elation
   4. Symptoms vary from day to day, even from hour to hour
E. Not due to any organic mental disorder, alcoholism, or drug abuse

personalization/derealization and/or confusion, and depression or elation, with symptoms varying daily or hourly.

It is our opinion that the two aforementioned concepts pertain to the same kind of psychosis, and that Perris's concept of cycloid psychosis is probably more comprehensive than *bouffée délirante*. Cycloid psychosis appears to correspond to ICD-9 schizoaffective psychosis, and *bouffée délirante* to ICD-9 acute paranoid reaction (298.3). However, the ICD-9 nomenclature and classification fails to convey these special concepts in full (Pichot, 1982).

Table 12.4. *Kendell's criteria for schizoaffective illness*

The patient must fulfill the criteria for schizophrenia *or* paranoid psychosis *and* depression *or* mania.

Criteria for schizophrenia
One nuclear symptom (thought insertion, thought withdrawal, thought broadcasting, thought echo, voices discussing patient, delusions of control or autochthonous delusions). In a patient too withdrawn, suspicious or thought-disordered to give a history, 2 fully rated objective signs from the following list of 11 (1 from any 2 groups):
Group 1: (Behavior) mannerisms, posturing, stereotypies, catatonic phenomena or behavior suggesting hallucinations
Group 2: (Affect) suspiciousness, perplexity, blunting incongruity
Group 3: (Speech) neologisms, incoherence, nonsocial speech

Criteria for paranoid psychosis
The patient must have a preoccupying delusion involving the external world. These may be delusions of influence (by paranormal phenomena, physical forces), persecution, reference, misinterpretation, assistance, infidelity, pregnancy, or a fantasy lover. They must be persistent and preoccupying and the patient must show conviction by defending them against argument or acting on them.

Criteria for depression
The patient must have 4 fully rated items from a list of 16 symptoms (sadness, hopelessness, suicidal intent, loss of interest, inferiority, pathological guilt, delusions of guilt, hypochondriacal delusions, nihilistic delusions, insomnia, loss of appetite, loss of libido, loss of emotions, muddled thoughts or poor concentration, morning depression) and 3 signs (observed sadness, agitation, retardation).

Criteria for mania
The patient must have 3 fully rated symptoms from the following list of 5 symptoms and 7 signs:
Symptoms: euphoria, racing thoughts, tirelessness, delusions of special powers, delusions of grandiose identity
Signs: overactivity, distractibility, irreverent behavior, embarrassing behavior, hypomanic affect, pressure of speech, flight of ideas.

Note: Two partly rated items count as one fully rated item. The symptoms and signs are defined as in the glossary of Wing's Present State Examination (Wing, Cooper & Sartorius, 1974).

We next describe a version of the modern idea of "concurrent schizoaffective psychosis," a term coined by Brockington and Meltzer (1983). Beside the criteria of Welner, Croughan, and Robins (1974) and Spitzer, Endicott, and Robins (1978), Kendell (in Brockington & Leff, 1979) introduced and operationalized a distinction between schizoaffective depression and schizoaffective mania. According to Kendell's criteria for schizoaffective psychosis (Table 12.4), the patient must fulfill the criteria for schizophrenia (1 nuclear symptom out of 7) or paranoid psychosis (1 out of 8 symptoms) as well as for depression (4 fully rated items out of 19 signs and symptoms) or mania (3 fully rated items out of 13 signs and symptoms). This deliberately broad concept is of interest because, as Brockington and Leff (1979) have pointed out, stricter criteria like those of Welner and the Research Diagnostic Criteria have already decided that many of Kendell's schizoaffectives belong to either the schizophrenic or the affective categories, thus resolving their nosological status arbitrarily.

AIMS

The present study examines the extent to which modern criteria for schizoaffective psychosis, such as Kendell's (1983), and traditional criteria, such as Perris's (1974) cycloid psychosis and Pull's (1983) *bouffée délirante*, represent a homogeneous group of schizoaffective psychosis patients. By using these diagnostic concepts it should be possible to separate them from affective and schizophrenic psychoses, thus stressing the hypothesis of an independent group of psychoses.

METHODS

This study is part of a research program on the comparability of diagnostic systems, an aspect of which is reported by Semler, Wittchen, and Zaudig (see Chapter 20 of this volume). One hundred two acute psychiatric inpatients were examined. Ninety of them received a diagnosis of psychosis according to ICD-9 (Figure 12.1). Of the 61 schizophrenic patients (ICD–9), 1 was classified as hebephrenic, 24 as paranoid, 21 as residual, and 15 as schizoaffective. Of the 27 patients with affective psychosis (ICD-9), 7 were classified as unipolar depression, 11 as bipolar manic, and 9 as bipolar depression. Two patients received the diagnosis of paranoid disorder. These ICD-9 project diagnoses were assigned in a weekly case conference by consensus of all psychiatrists working on the project.

All patients were examined with three instruments: (1) the CIDI, a fully standardized interview (Robins, Wing & Helzer, unpublished manuscript, 1985), (2) the Present State Examination (Wing, Cooper & Sartorius, 1974), and (3) the DSM-III checklist (Helzer et al., 1985). In order to allow a more detailed examination of schizoaffective psychoses from a descriptive point of view special attention was given to cross-sectional and longitudinal aspects by using checklists containing the criteria of Kendell, Perris, and Pull. They were applied to the three instruments mentioned above. A history of at least one previous episode followed by full recovery was required for the diagnosis of schizoaffective psychosis.

RESULTS

According to the ICD-9 project diagnosis, 15 patients received a definite diagnosis of schizoaffective psychosis. Of these, 13 (87 percent) fulfilled the

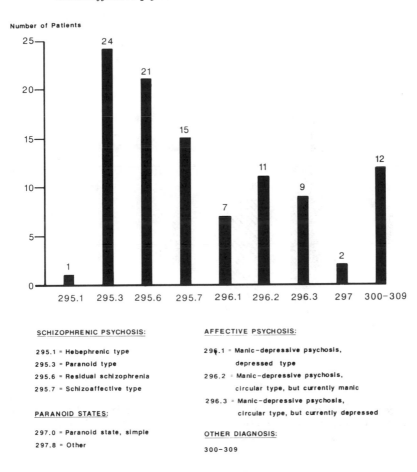

Figure 12.1. ICD-9 diagnosis of the "project sample" (N ≡ 102)

criteria of Kendell, 7 (47 percent) the criteria of cycloid psychosis (Perris's criteria) and 4 (27 percent) Pull's criteria for *bouffée délirante*. Table 12.5 presents the specificity and sensitivity of these three criterion sets vis-à-vis the ICD-9 diagnoses of psychotic disorders, and Table 12.6 exhibits the concordance (kappa and Yule y) between ICD-9 diagnoses and the three criterion sets.

Taking ICD-9 criteria for schizoaffective psychosis as a "yardstick," Kendell's criteria demonstrated a high sensitivity (87 percent), only medium specificity (53 percent), and low concordance with it ($k = .19, y = .46$), neither significantly above chance concordance. Perris's and Pull's criteria had a much higher specificity (98 percent in both cases) and less sensitivity (47 percent and 27 percent, respectively). Perris's criteria of cycloid psychosis revealed considerable concordance ($k = .53, y = .71$, both at $P < 0.01$), with ICD-9 schizoaffective

Number of patients

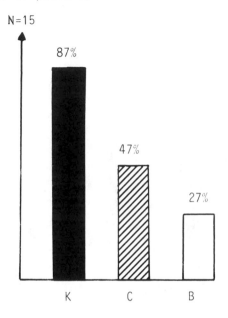

Figure 12.2. Concordance (sensitivity) of Kendell's criteria (K), Perris's criteria of cycloid psychosis (C), and Pull's criteria of *bouffée délirante* (B) with 15 cases of schizoaffective psychosis (ICD-9 295.7)

Table 12.5. *Comparison of the ICD-9 project diagnosis with Kendell's criteria (K) of schizoaffective psychosis, Perris's criteria of cycloid psychosis (C), and Pull's criteria of* boufée délirante *(B) in 87 of 102 cases*

ICD-9 project diagnosis	N	Specificity (%)			Sensitivity (%)		
		K	C	B	K	C	B
295.3	24	56	91	95	83	8	8
295.6	21	53	89	93	76	0	0
295.7	15	53	98	98	87	47	27
296.1	7	43	91	93	0	0	0
296.2	11	46	91	93	45	9	0
296.3	9	46	90	94	44	0	0

Table 12.6. *Concordance between the ICD-9 project diagnosis with Kendell's criteria (K) of schizoaffective psychosis, Perris's criteria of cycloid psychosis (C) and Pull's criteria of* bouffée délirante *(B) in 87 of 102 cases*

ICD-9 project diagnosis	N	Kappa			Yule's y		
		K	C	B	K	C	B
295.3	24	.27	−.00	.04	.43*	−.02	.12
295.6	21	.18	−.14	−.10	.31		
295.7	15	.19	.53**	.32	.46	.71**	.59*
296.1	7	−.13	−.08	−.06			
296.2	11	−.03	.00	−.08	−.08	.00	
296.3	9	−.02	−.09	−.07	−.09		

Note: ** $p < .01$. * $p < .05$.

Table 12.7. *Concordance (Cohen's kappa) between ICD-9 295.7, Kendell schizoaffective psychosis (K), cycloid psychosis (C), and* bouffée délirante *(B)*

Diagnostic definitions	Number of patients (N = 102)	Diagnostic definitions		
		K	C	B
ICD-9 295.7	15	.19	.53**	.32
Kendell (C)	54	—	.16	.11
Cycloid psychosis (C)	9	—	—	.79***
Bouffée délirante (B)	6			

Note: ** $p < .01$. *** $p < .001$.

psychosis, whereas Pull's criteria had a modest concordance ($k = .32$, $P > 0.05$; $y = .59$, $P < 0.05$).

Comparing Kappa coefficients between each pair of the three sets of criteria, we found (Table 12.7) a high concordance between the diagnostic criteria of Pull and those of Perris ($k = .79$, $p < 0.01$). In contrast, the concordance of these two sets of criteria with that of Kendell was below chance agreement. These results underline the distinction between traditional and modern criteria for schizoaffective psychosis.

On examining relationships with ICD-9 non-schizoaffective psychoses, Table 12.5 shows that of the 24 paranoid schizophrenic patients, 20 (83 percent) met Kendell's criteria, 2 (8 percent) met Perris's criteria, and 2 (8 percent) met

Pull's criteria. Of 21 patients with residual schizophrenia, 16 (76 percent) ful-filled Kendell's criteria, and none fulfilled the criteria of Perris or Pull. A similar result was obtained with the 11 bipolar manic patients: 5 (45 percent) fulfilled Kendell's criteria, 1 (9 percent) Perris's criteria, and none Pull's criteria. Of the 72 nonschizoaffective psychotics (1 hebephrenic and 2 paranoid psychotics excluded), 45 (62 percent) met Kendell's criteria. The minimal overlap of cycloid psychosis (4 percent, $n = 3$) and *bouffée délirante* (3, $n = 2$) with the 72 nonschizoaffective psychosis patients points out the exceptional position of these two sets of diagnostic criteria.

COMMENT

The concepts of *bouffée délirante* and cycloid psychosis appear to be quite similar ($k = .79$) and to form a rather homogeneous subgroup within the schizoaffective psychoses. They are quite different from the "modern idea of concurrent schizoaffective psychoses," such as Kendell's criteria, with which they have a low concordance. These results are in line with previous investi-gations (Zaudig & Vogl, 1983; Vogl & Zaudig, 1985) using different metho-dologies and different patient samples. When investigating the relationship of cycloid psychosis to ICD-9 schizoaffective psychosis, we found moderate con-cordance between them, medium sensitivity, and very high specificity. Regard-ing *bouffée délirante*, we could confirm Pichot's statement (1982) that the criteria of *bouffée délirante* have no adequate ICD-9 equivalent; both concordance and sensitivity were low. Cycloid psychoses and *bouffée délirante* could be easily distinguished from both affective and schizophrenic psychoses, and can be interpreted as forming a homogeneous group of psychoses. It has been argued (Pope & Lipinski, 1978) that the presence of affective symptoms and a relapsing course suggest that these patients are suffering from a variant of affective dis-order. The clinical picture, however, is quite different from affective psychosis. In contrast, Kendell's deliberately broad concept showed a high overall sensi-tivity to nonschizoaffective psychoses, that is, considerable overlapping with affective and schizophrenic psychoses, in addition to showing low concordance and modest specificity with ICD-9 schizoaffective psychosis. Kendell's criteria are, therefore, best to cover a broad spectrum of schizoaffective psychosis and are very useful as a "screening" approach in further research in this field. In conclusion, the results of the present study underline the exceptional position of traditional concepts of cycloid psychosis and *bouffée délirante* as conforming a rather homogeneous diagnostic group. They are not synonymous with modern or, in Brockington and Meltzer's (1983) terms, "concurrent" concepts of schizo-affective disorder. Furthermore, there is strong evidence that the traditional concepts of schizoaffective disorder, not its modern or concurrent concepts, can be delineated clearly from affective and schizophrenic disorders, thus suggesting a separate illness and challenging Kraepelin's dichotomy.

ACKNOWLEDGMENTS

We thank Tobias von Geiso, M.D., Toni Vogt, M.D., and the other interviewers for their careful assessments and clinical examinations. Werner Mombour, M.D., offered helpful comments.

REFERENCES

American Psychiatric Association. 1980. *Diagnostic and Statistical Manual of Mental Disorders*. 3rd ed. (DSM-III) Washington, D.C.
American Psychiatric Association. 1987. *Diagnostic and Statistical Manual of Mental Disorders*, 3rd ed., revised (DSM-III-R). Washington, D.C.
Astrup, C., and Noreik, K. 1966. *Functional Psychosis: Diagnostic and Prognostic Models*. Springfield, Ill.: Charles C. Thomas.
Brockington, J. F., and Leff, J. P. 1979. Schizoaffective psychosis: definitions and incidence. *Psychological Medicine* 9: 91–99.
Brockington, J. F., and Meltzer, H. Y. 1983. The nosology of schizoaffective psychosis. *Psychiatric Developments* 4: 317–338.
Cutting, J. C., Clare, A. W., and Mann, A. H. 1978. Cycloid psychosis: an investigation of the diagnostic concept. *Psychological Medicine* 8: 637–648.
Ey, H. 1954. *Etudes Psychiatriques*. Vol. 3. *Bouffées délirantes et psychoses hallucinatoires aigües*. Etude no. 23, p. 203. Paris: Desclee de Brouwen.
Faergerman, P. M. 1963. *Psychogenic Psychoses*. London: Butterworth.
Feighner, J. P., Robins, E., Guze, S. E., Woodruff, R. A., Winokur, G., and Muñoz, R. 1972. Diagnostic criteria for use in psychiatric research. *Archives of General Psychiatry* 26: 57–63.
Fowler, R. C., McCabe, M. S., Cadoret, R. J., and Winokur, G. 1972. The validity of good prognosis schizophrenia. *Archives of General Psychiatry* 26: 182–185.
Helzer, J. E., Robins, L. N., McEvoy L. T., Spitznagel, E. L., Stolzman, R. W., Farmer, A., and Brockington, J. F. 1985. A comparison of clinical and Diagnostic Interview Schedule diagnoses. Physician reexamination of long-interviewed cases in general population. *Archives of General Psychiatry* 42: 657–666.
Kasanin, J. 1983. The acute schizoaffective psychosis. *American Journal of Psychiatry* 13: 97–126.
Kendell, R. E. 1983. Schizophrenia. In *Companion to Psychiatric Studies*, 3rd ed., ed. R. E. Kendell and A. K. Zealley. Edinburgh: Churchill Livingstone.
Kendell, R. E., Brockington, J. F., and Leff, J. P. 1979. Prognostic implications of six alternative definitions of schizophrenia. *Archives of General Psychiatry* 36: 25–31.
Kleist, K. 1921. Autochthone Degenerationspsychosen. *Zeitschrift für die gesamte Neurologie und Psychiatrie* 69: 1–11.
Kraepelin, E. 1896. *Psychiatrie, ein Lehrbuch für Studierende und Ärzte*. 5th ed. Leipzig: Barth.
Langfeldt, G. 1937. *The Prognosis in Schizophrenia and the Factors Influencing the Course of Disease*. Copenhagen: Munksgaard.
Langfeldt, G. 1939. *The Schizophreniform States*. Copenhagen: Munksgaard.
Legrain, M. 1886. *Du Délire Chez les Dégénérés*. Paris: Librairie A. Deshaye et E. Lecrosnier.
Leonhard, K. 1957. The cycloid psychoses usually misdiagnosed as schizophrenias. *Psychiat. Neurol. Med. Psychol.* 9: 359–365.

Leonhard, K. 1980. *Aufteilung der Endogenen Psychosen*. Berlin: Akademie-Verlag.

McCabe, M. S. 1975. Reactive psychosis: a clinical and genetic investigation. *Acta Psychiatrica Scandinavica*. Supplement 259: 1–133.

Magnan, V. 1893. *Leçones Cliniques*. 2nd ed. Paris: Bataille.

Perris, C. 1974. Study of cycloid psychosis. *Acta Psychiatrica Scandinavica*, Supplement 253.

Perris, C., and Brockington, J. F. 1981. Cycloid psychosis and their relation to the major psychosis. In *Biological Psychiatry*, ed. C. Perris, G. Struew, and B. Jansson. Amsterdam: Elsevier/North Holland Biomedical Press.

Pichot, P. 1982. The diagnosis and classification of mental disorders in French-speaking countries: background, current views and comparison with other nomenclatures. *Psychological Medicine* 12: 475–492.

Pope, V. G., and Lipinski, J. F. 1978. Diagnosis in schizophrenia and manic-depressive illness. *Archives of General Psychiatry* 35: 811–828.

Procci, W. R. 1976. Schizo-affective psychosis: fact or fiction? *Archives of General Psychiatry* 33: 1167–1178.

Pull, C. B., Pull, M. C., and Pichot, P. 1983. Nosological position of schizoaffective psychoses in France. *Psychiatria Clinica* 16: 141–148.

Schröder, P. 1926. Über Degenerationspsychosen. *Zeitschrift für die gesamte Neurologie und Psychiatrie* 105: 539–547.

Spitzer, R. L., Endicott, J., and Robins, E. 1978. Research diagnostic criteria: rationale and reliability. *Archives of General Psychiatry* 35: 773–782.

Stephens, J. H., Astrup, C., and Mangrum, J. C. 1966. Prognostic factors in recovered and deteriorated schizophrenics. *American Journal of Psychiatry* 122: 1116–1121.

Tsuang, M. T., and Simpson, J. C. 1984. Schizoaffective disorder: concept and reality. *Schizophrenia Bulletin* 10: 14–25.

Vaillant, G. E. 1965. A historical review of the remitting schizophrenias. *Journal of Nervous and Mental Disease* 138: 48–56.

Vogl, G., and Zaudig, M. 1985. Investigation of operationalized diagnostic criteria in the diagnosis of schizoaffective and cycloid psychoses. *Comprehensive Psychiatry* 26: 1–10.

Welner, A., Croughan, J. L., and Robins, E. 1974. The group of schizoaffective and related psychosis: critique, record, follow-up and family studies. I. A persistent enigma. *Archives of General Psychiatry* 31: 628–631.

Wernicke, C. 1900. *Grundriss der Psychiatrie*. Leipzig: Thieme.

Wing, J. K., Cooper, J. E., and Sartorius, N. 1974. *Measurement and Classification of Pychiatric Symptoms*. (German translation edited by M. von Cranach, Beltz-Verlag, Weinheim and Basel , 1982). Cambridge: Cambridge University Press.

World Health Organization. 1978. *Mental Disorders: Glossary and Guide to Their Classification in Accordance with the Ninth Revision of the International Classification of Diseases*. Geneva.

Zaudig, M., and Vogl, G. 1983. Zur Frage der operationalisierten Diagnostik schizoaffectiver und zykloider Psychosen. *Archiv für Psychiatrie und Nervenkrankheiten* 233: 385–396.

13 Affective (mood) disorders and anxiety disorders

Considerations for developing ICD-10

GERALD L. KLERMAN (USA)

INTRODUCTION

Recent diagnostic classification systems have included separate categories for affective disorders (or mood disorders) and for anxiety disorders. This approach to classification represents a major departure from previous classification systems, which subsumed these disorders under psychotic or neurotic categories.

Principles of classifying nonorganic conditions

In modern medicine, classification systems are ideally based on etiology. In most classifications of psychiatric disorders, the etiologic approach is applied to disorders due to organic neurologic disease and disorders due to the effects of alcohol and psychiatric drugs. For classification of most nonorganic conditions, however, etiologic principles have been of only limited value.

The separation of nonorganic disorders into psychotic and neurotic groups has a descriptive basis – implied etiology and also treatment prescription. Psychotic states are usually presumed to be due to biological etiology (genetic, endogenous, metabolic, or degenerative), whereas neurotic disorders are usually related to psychosocial causes (including developmental problems, reactions to stress, and maladaptive personality patterns). The treatment prescriptions that follow from this presumptive etiology involve the use of drugs and somatic therapy for psychoses and the use of psychotherapies – whether psychodynamic, interpersonal, or behavioral – for neuroses.

In the 1960s and 1970s, the psychotic-neurotic separation proved scientifically inadequate and was criticized. Many neurotic conditions were shown to have genetic-familial associations, as in the research on panic and agoraphobia, as well as on many forms of depression. Drug treatment proved highly efficacious for phobias, anxiety states, so-called neurotic depressions, and stress reactions.

Once the psychotic-neurotic distinction as a basis for classifying nonorganic disorders is abandoned in the DSM-III and the draft of ICD-10, the most reasonable basis for classification is to group together disorders on the basis of their major presenting clinical manifestation. This classificatory principle was

135

adopted for DSM-III and appears in some aspects of the proposed ICD-10, as exemplified by the category of affective disorders (or mood disorders).

Emotions, mood, and affect

At times, emotion, mood, and affect are used interchangeably. But the semantic convention is that *emotion* refers to the broad overall concept within which *mood* and *affect* are distinguished from each other on the basis of temporal frame. *Affect* usually refers to the minute-to-minute or hour-to-hour fluctuations in emotional state, whereas *mood* usually refers to the relatively enduring emotional state (or tone) that often characterizes an individual's temperament or personality. In this usage, mood is to climate as affect is to weather. Since clinical states of depression and mania usually involve persistent and enduring states, it is probably more appropriate to call these mood disorders.

As noted above, the term *emotion* refers to a range of states. Although there is controversy over the concept of fundamental emotions and their number, clinicians often recognize states of anxiety and fear, sadness and depression, anger, rage and hostility, guilt, and shame and embarrassment. Ideally, a comprehensive classification of emotional disorders would include categories for disorders of anger, hostility, and rage, as well as disorders of guilt and shame. In current clinical practice, however, the term "mood disorder" almost always refers to states of depression and elation. Aubrey Lewis (1967) discussed the possible desirability of subsuming anxiety disorders along with depression, because of their frequent clinical coexistence and related features. Most nomenclatures, however, distinguish between mood disorders and anxiety disorders.

In ambulatory patients with nonpsychiatric conditions, anxiety and depression frequently coexist, and it is often difficult to distinguish which is the major symptom. Thus, terms such as "mixed anxiety-depressive states" are common. Goldberg (1980) has argued that the differentiation of anxiety from depressive states is more in the psychiatric theorist's experience than in the patient's experience. Early factor-analytic efforts to separate anxiety from depression frequently produced mixed factors.

This chapter reviews the current controversies in the diagnosis and classification of these two major groups of disorders with special reference to the development of the ICD-10.

AFFECTIVE (MOOD) DISORDER

The DSM-III was the first official nomenclature to include a separate category of affective disorders. The draft proposal for ICD-10 also includes a category of mood disorders.

The Group of bipolar affective disorders

In 1959, Leonhard (Leonhard, Korff & Schulz, 1962) proposed a modification of Kraepelin's (1921) concept of manic-depressive insanity, distinguishing conditions with recurrent episodes of only depression or only manic states (which he called "monopolar") from those conditions which had both mania and depression. This latter group he called "bipolar." Leonhard's monopolar concept has not been widely accepted, but the validity and utility of the concept of bipolar disorder have become one of the major areas of consensus in the classification of mood disorders. The term "unipolar" has subsequently been applied to Leonhard's monopolar recurrent depressions, but has not gained acceptance in official nomenclatures.

In the 1960s, three research groups simultaneously undertook family-genetic studies. Perris (1966) in Sweden, Angst (1966) in Switzerland and Winokur, Clayton, and Reich (1969) in St. Louis reported high levels of familial aggregation, suggesting the validity of separating the bipolar disorders from others.

Further evidence for the validity of this concept followed the demonstrated efficacy of lithium not only in the treatment of acute manic episodes, but in long-term maintenance treatment to prevent recurrence of depressive and manic episodes in bipolar patients.

Despite wide acceptance of the basic concept, there is considerable disagreement as to the range of conditions to be subsumed under the category of bipolar mood disorders (Klerman, 1981).

A large number of conditions have been proposed as belonging to a bipolar cluster or bipolar spectrum (Klerman, 1981; Akiskal, 1983). Bipolar II disorder, hypomania, cyclothymia, recurrent mania, and conditions involving manic and excited reactions to tricyclic MAO inhibitors have been considered part of this group. The greatest consensus surrounds cyclothymia; family-genetic, developmental, and treatment studies indicate a close relationship between cyclothymia and depression.

In conclusion, the bipolar concept seems highly accepted and merits a special place. Yet to be determined is how extensive to make its boundaries. Cyclothymic personality and hypomanic personality, traditionally considered personality disorders, are now increasingly regarded as variants of bipolar disorder.

The problem of classifying depressive disorders

The draft of ICD-10 includes a number of depressive disorders in Section F-3. I believe that this would benefit from a grouping together, in particular, to distinguish between acute, chronic, and recurrent forms. It is notable that the endogenous-neurotic distinction does not appear prominently in Section F-3.

Endogenous versus reactive depression

The concept of endogenous depression has been a central feature of European thinking about affective disorders since the time of Kraepelin. In its broader sense, it refers to an etiologic principle for grouping disorders within the so-called functional psychoses. Some investigators and clinicians emphasize a cyclical course with defined episodes and clearly demarcated periods of return to normal premorbid functioning. Other clinicians and theorists emphasize the absence of precipitating events.

Of all subtypes of depression, endogenous depression has been considered the most biological. In view of this assumption, it is surprising how little validation has emerged from recent research studies. Studies of life events show no discrimination between endogenous and situational categories (Hirschfeld, 1981). Most surprisingly, family aggregation studies do not support a genetic basis for endogenous depression. If there was a subtype of depression in which one might expect to have familial aggregation, one would usually use the term "endogenous." Furthermore, there is considerable overlapping between the concepts of endogenous and severe. The question often arises as to whether a severity judgment would suffice in place of what is usually a qualitative judgment of endogeneity.

The problem of classifying psychotic features of affective disorders

Although the psychotic versus neurotic distinction as a basis for a classificatory system has not been validated, clinical and research evidence indicates the special importance of delusions and other psychotic features in depressive states. In the DSM-III, this is handled by a qualifying category "with psychotic features" that are "mood congruent" and another with those that are "mood incongruent."

In the ICD-10, perhaps an additional digit could be used to subdivide the categories of recurrent depressive disorders and single depressive episode into the following types: without psychotic features; with psychotic features – mood congruent; and with psychotic features – mood incongruent.

Conclusion

The comments made above are mainly aimed at refining the subclassifications within F-3. Basically, I strongly endorse the decision to create a broad category or section of affective (mood) disorders.

ANXIETY DISORDERS

The situation of the draft of ICD-10 with regard to anxiety disorders is, however, less satisfactory. This draft contains a section, F-4, encompassing neurotic, stress-related, and somatoform disorders. I would have recommended that a separate section for anxiety disorders include phobic disorders, anxiety states, and obsessive-compulsive disorders, but the alphabetical-numerical system adopted for ICD-10 restricts the number of major categories or sections of mental disorders in Section F. Therefore, anxiety disorders must be combined with other conditions.

A radical proposal would be to combine anxiety disorders with affective disorders in Section F-3. The theoretical justification for this would be that depression and mania, on one hand, and anxiety states, on the other hand, are variations of emotional disorders. Empirically, there is much overlapping between anxiety disorders and depression. Approximately 60 percent of depressive patients also have anxiety states, and the clinical distinction is often difficult.

If combining anxiety disorders with affective disorders in Section F-3 is too radical a proposal, I would recommend that Section F-4 be retitled "anxiety, stress, and adjustment disorders."

Phobic conditions

Within Section F-4, the categories for phobic disorders and obsessive-compulsive disorders are well delineated and in line with current clinical practice and research knowledge.

Within the phobic disorders, it may be an advantage to delineate subcategories within social phobia, particularly for the fear of public speaking, since this phobia responds differently to drug treatment than the other social phobias, and appears to be more related to performance anxiety than other phobias.

Similarly, under *isolated phobias*, it may be useful to create a subcategory for fear of blood, since research, particularly that by Marks (1985) and others, indicates that the psychophysiologic response in this phobia involves predominantly parasympathetic responses, including fainting, whereas most other phobias are characteristically associated with sympathetic arousal.

Panic anxiety and generalized anxiety

Serious problems were noted with the subsection, "other anxiety states." An early draft of ICD-10 failed to incorporate recent advances in psychopathology and therapeutics that support the separation of panic anxiety from generalized anxiety, also known as free-floating or anticipatory anxiety.

Extensive research on psychopathology, epidemiology, and family studies indicate the validity of the separation of panic disorder from other forms of anxiety. Phenomenologically, the experience of panic disorder is unique: It occurs in surges with rapid onset of associated dread and foreboding, and bodily symptoms suggestive of autonomic arousal. There is a high affinity between panic disorder and agoraphobia, and one prominent theory regards agoraphobia as a reaction to the avoidance response initiated by the aversive nature of the panic attacks. Studies, particularly those by Torgesen (1984) in Norway, by Crowe, Noyes, Pauls, and Slymen (1983) in Iowa, and by Weissman (1988) at Yale, indicate that panic and agoraphobia occur together, and aggregate separately from generalized anxiety disorder. In addition, psychophysiological studies reported by Barlow et al. (1984), and the response to lactate, yohimbine, and other challenge tests (Gorman, 1984) further supports the separation. Moreover, therapeutically, panic disorder with or without agoraphobia responds to MAO inhibitors, tricyclic antidepressants, and triazolobenzodiazepines.

Conclusion

ICD-10 should have a subsection entitled "anxiety disorders" and subdivided into "generalized anxiety disorders (free-floating or anticipatory anxiety)" and "panic anxiety disorder."

Criteria would have to be developed to distinguish panic anxiety and generalized anxiety from stress reactions and adjustment disorders in which anxiety symptoms frequently occur. In stress reactions and adjustment disorders, the anxiety usually occurs in conjunction with other affective states, such as guilt, fear, depression; and more important, usually occurs immediately after a traumatic event that preoccupies the consciousness and memory of the patient. In contrast, generalized anxiety conditions are usually chronic in duration and the patient reports varying amounts of fear, worry, and dread in anticipation of possible future adversities, rather than in response to a prior traumatic event, as is the case in post-traumatic stress disorder or adjustment disorder.

RECOMMENDATIONS

Comparing the ICD-10 draft with previous classifications demonstrates the advances in knowledge of psychopathology, epidemiology, genetics, and therapeutics of mental disorders, in general, and in the mood (affective) disorders and states related to anxiety and phobia, in particular. These advances have led to a consensus on the desirability of a category for affective (mood) disorders; less evident is the consensus on how to classify anxiety disorders.

Recommendations regarding affective (mood) disorders

The following recommendations apply to the proposed section of affective disorders:

1. Consideration should be given to retitling this category as "mood disorders."
2. The category of bipolar disorder should include a subcategory for "other forms of bipolar disorder."
3. Cyclothymic disorder should be placed in a position adjacent to bipolar disorder.
4. The depressive disorders would benefit from being grouped together.
5. Although there is no longer a clear distinction between neurotic and psychotic depression, some form of subcategory "with psychotic features" would have clinical, diagnostic, and predictive value.
6. Subclassification within the depressive disorder category remains a source of controversy.

Recommendations regarding the anxiety disorders

1. Ideally, there should be a category of anxiety disorders in parallel with the category of affective disorders. Epidemiologic research indicates that these conditions are highly prevalent, particularly in primary care, and that they bear

certain theoretical unity, although no presumption as to etiology should be inferred.

2. One possibility would be to move the group of anxiety disorders to Section F-3, thus combining them with depression and bipolar disorder into a new category of mood and anxiety disorders.
3. If anxiety disorders remain in Section F-4, a new title for Section F-4 is needed. Neither the term "emotional" nor "neurotic" is satisfactory. Instead, I suggest using the term "anxiety, stress, and adjustment disorders."
4. The distinction among the phobias proposed by Marks (1985), in terms of simple phobias, social phobias, and agoraphobia, has stood up well in clinical care, research, and epidemiologic studies.
5. The subsection on anxiety disorders should include subdivisions for panic anxiety disorder and chronic generalized anxiety.
6. Obsessive-compulsive disorder remains an important clinical condition, and is probably best classified along with the anxiety disorders.

REFERENCES

Akiskal, H. 1983. Dysthymic disorder: Psychopathology of proposed chronic depressive subtypes. *Am. J. Psychiatry* 120: 11–20.

Angst, J. 1966. *On the Etiology and Nosology of Endogenous Depressive Psychoses*. Berlin: Springer-Verlag.

Angst, J. 1973. The etiology and nosology of endogenous depressive psychoses: a genetic, sociological, and clinical study. *Foreign Psychiatry* 2: 1–108.

Barlow, D. II. Cohen, A. S., Waddell, M. T., Vermilyea, B. B., Klosko, J. S., Glanchard, E. B., and Dinardo, P. A. 1984. Panic and generalized anxiety disorders: nature and treatment. *Behav. Therapy* 15: 431–449.

Crowe, R. R., Noyes, R., Pauls, B. L., and Slymen, D. 1983. A family study of panic disorder. *Arch. Gen. Psychiatry* 40: 1065–1069.

Goldberg, D. 1980. Training family doctors to recognize psychiatric illness with increased accuracy. *Lancet* 6: 521–523.

Gorman, J. M. 1984. Biology of anxiety. In *Psychiatry Update*, vol. 3, ed. L. Grinspoon, pp. 467–481. Washington, D.C.: American Psychiatric Press.

Hirschfeld, R. M. 1981. Situational depression: validity of the concept. *British Journal of Psychiatry* 139: 297–305.

Klerman G. L. 1981. The spectrum of mania. *Compreh. Psychiatry* 22: 11–20.

Kraepelin, E. 1921. *Manic Depressive Insanity and Paranoia*. Trans. M. Barclay. Edinburgh: Livingstone.

Leonhard, K., Korff, I., and Schulz, H. 1962. Temperament in families with monopolar and bipolar psychoses. *Psychiat. Neurol.* 143: 416–434.

Lewis, A. 1967. *Inquiries in Psychiatry: Clinical and Social Investigators*. New York: Science House.

Marks, I. 1985. *Fears, Phobias, Rituals*. New York: Oxford University Press.

Perris, C. 1966. A study of bipolar (manic-depressive) and unipolar recurrent depressive psychoses. *Acta Psychiatr. Scand.* 194 (suppl.): 1.

Torgesen, S. 1984. Genetic and nosological aspects of schizotypal and borderline personality disorders: a twin study. *Arch. Gen. Psychiatry* 41: 546–554.

Weissman, M. M. 1988. The epidemiology of panic disorders and agoraphobia. In *APA Annual Review of Psychiatry*, vol. 7, ed. H. A. Frances, and R. E. Hales. *Section I. Panic Disorders*, ed. K. Shear, and D. Barlow. Washington, D.C.: American Psychiatric Press.

Winokur, G., Clayton, P., and Reich, T. 1969. *Manic Depressive Illness*. St. Louis: C. V. Mosby.

14 *International views on somatoform, hysterical, and related disorders*

MAURICE DONGIER (Canada)

The somatoform disorders constitute a new category in the third edition of the *Diagnostic and Statistical Manual of Mental Disorders* (DSM-III) (American Psychiatric Association, 1980). "Somatoform" is a hybrid adjective (half Greek and half Latin) adopted by the authors of DSM-III to designate disorders that suggest physical illness but for which there are no demonstrable organic findings.

This terminology is another attempt – there have been many in the history of psychiatry – to do away with the word "hysteria," which has been with us for more than three thousand years and has been repeatedly found to represent an inappropriate concept. Babinski (1901) said that "the definition of hysteria has never been given and will never be." However, Aubrey Lewis (1975) wrote that "hysteria will survive its obituarists." DSM-III ranks among the obituarists by fragmenting hysteria into a number of syndromes, which traditionally were linked with one another under the name of "hysteria." Some of these syndromes are included in the "somatoform" group; some are not.

The International Classification of Diseases, ninth edition (ICD-9), issued by the World Health Organization (1978), provides the following definition of "hysteria":

Mental disorders in which motives, of which the patient seems unaware, produce either a restriction of the field of consciousness or disturbances of motor or sensory function which may seem to have psychological advantage or symbolic value. It may be characterized by conversion phenomena or dissociative phenomena. In the conversion form, the chief or only symptoms consist of psychogenic disturbance of function in some part of the body, e.g., paralysis, tremor, blindness, deafness, seizures. In the dissociative variety, the most prominent feature is a narrowing of the field of consciousness which seems to serve an unconscious purpose and is commonly accompanied or followed by a selective amnesia. There may be dramatic but essentially superficial changes of personality sometimes taking the form of a fugue (wandering state). Behaviour may mimic psychosis or, rather, the patient's idea of psychosis.

Table 14.1 lists the five somatoform disorders and a number of other disorders that DSM-III, unlike ICD-9, does not consider at the present time as having any relationship with the somatoform disorders.

In this chapter I review the essential features of each of the five somatoform

143

Table 14.1. *Histerical conditions in DSM-III*

---

1. Somatoform disorders in DSM-III
Somatization disorder
Conversion disorder
Psychogenic pain (or idiopathic pain, or pain-prone) disorder
Hypochondriasis
Atypical somatoform disorder

2. Separate or unrelated hysterical conditions in DSM-III
Hysterical (histrionic) personality
Dissociative disorders
   Psychogenic amnesia
   Psychogenic fugue
   Multiple personality
   Depersonalization disorder
Schizophreniform psychosis (Ganser's syndrome, hysterical type) (hysterical
   psychosis)

---

disorders, then discuss the pros and cons of the stance taken by DSM-III, particularly from an international and transcultural viewpoint.

SOMATIZATION DISORDER

DSM-III lists as essential features "recurrent and multiple somatic complaints of several years duration for which medical attention has been sought but which apparently are not due to any physical disorder." The diagnostic criteria are

(a) A history of physical symptoms beginning before the age of 30.
(b) Complaints of at least 14 symptoms for women and 12 for men, from the 37 symptoms listed below. To count a symptom as present, the individual must report that the symptom caused him or her to take medicine other than aspirin, alter his or her life pattern, or see a physician. The symptoms, in the judgment of the clinician, are not adequately explained by physical disorder or physical injury, and are not side effects of medication, drugs, or alcohol. The clinician need not be convinced that the symptom was actually present, e.g., that the individual actually vomited throughout her entire pregnancy; report of the symptom by the individual is sufficient.
Sickly: Believes that he or she has been sickly for a good part of her life.
Conversion or pseudoneurological symptoms: Difficulty swallowing, loss of voice, deafness, double vision, blurred vision, blindness, fainting or loss of consciousness, memory loss, seizures or convulsions, trouble walking, paralysis or muscle weakness, urinary retention or difficulty urinating.
Gastrointestinal symptoms: Abdominal pain, nausea, vomiting spells (other than during pregnancy), bloating (gassy), intolerance (e.g., gets sick) of a variety of foods, diarrhea.
Female reproductive symptoms: Judged by the individual as occurring more

frequently or severely than in most women: painful menstruation, menstrual irregularity, excessive bleeding, severe vomiting throughout pregnancy or causing hospitalization during pregnancy.

Psychosexual symptoms: For the major part of the individual's life after opportunities for sexual activity: sexual indifference, lack of pleasure during intercourse, pain during intercourse.

Pain: Pain in back, joints, extremities, genital area (other than during intercourse); pain on urination; other pain (other than headaches).

Cardiopulmonary symptoms: Shortness of breath, palpitations, chest pain, dizziness.

Most of these symptoms were described by Briquet (1859) in his treatise on hysteria. Unlike the DSM-III system, he related somatic symptoms to hysterical personality features (temperament generally impressionable and hyperemotional, propensity to involuntarily imitate others' symptoms).

Guze (1967, 1970, 1975) has contributed to the refinement of diagnostic criteria and to procedures leading to the validation of the syndrome. It is remarkable that DSM-III limits the diagnostic criteria for somatization disorder (or "multiple somatoform disorder," which is the more precise term proposed by a group gathered by the World Health Organization to prepare ICD-10) to a list of somatic symptoms (including conversion) and ignores psychogenic aspects (primary gain, secondary gain, and personality traits) as predisposing factors, whereas they are mentioned for the following disorder (conversion). More empirical research is obviously necessary in this respect.

CONVERSION DISORDER

DSM-III proposes the following diagnostic criteria:

A) The predominant disturbance is a loss of or alteration in physical functioning suggesting a physical disorder.

B) Psychological factors are judged to be etiologically involved in the symptom, as evidenced by one of the following:
   (1) There is a temporal relationship between an environmental stimulus that is apparently related to a psychological conflict or need and the initiation or exacerbation of the symptom.
   (2) The symptom enables the individual to avoid some activity that is noxious to him or her.
   (3) The symptom enables the individual to get support from the environment that otherwise might not be forthcoming.

C) It has been determined that the symptom is not under voluntary control.

D) The symptom cannot, after appropriate investigation, be explained by a known physical disorder or pathophysiological mechanism.

E) The symptom is not limited to pain or to a disturbance in sexual functioning.

F) Not due to Somatization Disorder or Schizophrenia.

This definition is unique in DSM-III in that it implies specific psychological mechanisms to account for the disturbance, namely primary and/or secondary gain:

  a) A wish or internal conflict is kept out of awareness (initiation or exacerbation of the symptom is in temporal relationship with an external event: e.g., aphonia, paralysis, blindness follows an occasion of rage).
  b) The conversion symptom provides satisfaction of a wish for dependency or avoidance of a noxious activity.

The authors of the DSM-III system are going out of their way to accept unconscious motivations as diagnostic criteria: "The symptom has a symbolic value that is a representation and partial solution of the underlying psychological conflict" (DSM-III, p. 244).

One must stress that primary gain, secondary gain, and personality are not even mentioned in other somatoform disorders except pain disorder. Why these two disorders are singled out remains unclear, and we believe this would have to be discussed in revisions of the DSM-III (DSM-III-R). We cannot but agree with Cloninger (1983) and with Raskin, Talbott, and Meyerson (1966) that secondary gain is observed as often in patients coping with physical disorders as in patients coping with conversion symptoms. One should, therefore, reconsider its value as a diagnostic criterion.

Finally, one may wonder whether the status of conversion should not revert from disease to symptom, as conversion is common not only in hysteria, but also in schizophrenia, obsessive-compulsive neurosis, and many other categories of mental illness. In particular, it often seems to be associated with physical disorders (Slater & Glithero, 1965; Whitlock, 1967; Engel, 1968).

HYPOCHONDRIASIS

According to DSM-III, the essential features of hypochondriasis are as follows:

  A) The predominant disturbance is an unrealistic interpretation of physical signs or sensations as abnormal, leading to preoccupation with the fear or belief of having a serious disease.
  B) Thorough physical evaluation does not support the diagnosis of any physical disorder that can account for the physical signs or sensations or for the individual's unrealistic interpretation of them.
  C) The unrealistic fear or belief of having a disease persists despite medical reassurance and causes impairment in social or occupational functioning.
  D) Not due to any other mental disorder such as schizophrenia, affective disorder, or somatization disorder.

Considering hypochondriasis a discrete diagnostic entity is problematic. Many authors view it as a symptom or a syndrome occurring as part of disorders such as schizophrenia, depression, anxiety state or personality disorders. Kenyon (1964, 1965, 1976) concluded from exhaustive studies that hypochondriasis does not exist as a primary state and suggested its use as a descriptive adjective when there is a "morbid preoccupation with health or body," which can occur in depressions, anxiety states, personality disorders, or paranoid states, including monosymptomatic hypochondriasis.

PSYCHOGENIC PAIN DISORDER

The major diagnostic criteria in DSM-III for psychogenic pain disorder are:

A) Severe and prolonged pain is the predominant disturbance.

B) The pain presented as a symptom is inconsistent with the anatomic distribution of the nervous system; after extensive evaluation, no organic pathology or pathophysiological mechanism can be found to account for the pain; or, when there is some related organic pathology, the complaint of pain is grossly in excess of what would be expected from the physical findings.

C) Psychological factors are judged to be etiologically involved in the pain, as evidenced by at least one of the following:

  (1) A temporal relationship between an environmental stimulus that is apparently related to a psychological conflict or need, and the initiation or exacerbation of the pain.

  (2) The pain's enabling the individual to avoid some activity that is noxious to him or her.

  (3) The pain's enabling the individual to get support from the environment that otherwise might not be forthcoming.

D) Not due to another mental disorder.

As seen in conversion disorder, there is recognition of a psychological etiology.

Blumer and Heilbronn (1982) suggest changing the name of the disorder to "pain prone disorder," to avoid the term "psychogenic," and propose that it be reclassified as a subtype of major depression, as complaints of pain are common in depressed patients and many such patients have a relative with a depressive disorder. Williams and Spitzer (1982) disagree and point out that the course of pain-prone disorder is usually chronic over many years and differs from the course of major depression, which is episodic in nature most of the time. They agree that the adjective "psychogenic" should be dropped and propose "idiopathic pain disorder" as the replacement.

As pointed out in regard to conversion disorder, secondary gain is equally common in patients with physical disorders and is therefore an unspecific criterion for psychogenic or idiopathic pain.

ATYPICAL SOMATOFORM DISORDERS

The DSM-III classification system reserves this residual category for cases that meet the general description of somatoform disorders and are apparently linked to psychological factors but do not fit one of the four previous categories. One example given is dysmorphophobia. Cloninger (1983) points out that many such patients are delusional and should not be categorized as having somatoform disorders.

CATEGORIES UNRELATED TO HYSTERIA IN DSM-III

The categories listed below have been classically considered forms of hysterical syndromes, and that is the way they are considered in ICD-9. In DSM-III they are described as follows:

(1) *Psychogenic Amnesia*
   A) Sudden inability to recall important personal information that is too extensive to be explained by ordinary forgetfulness.
   B) The disturbance is not due to an Organic Mental Disorder (e.g., blackouts during alcohol intoxication).
(2) *Psychogenic Fugue*
   A) Sudden unexpected travel away from one's home or customary place of work, with inability to recall one's past.
   B) Assumption of a new identity (partial or complete).
   C) The disturbance is not due to an Organic Mental Disorder.
(3) *Multiple Personality*
   A) The existence within the individual of two or more distinct personalities, each of which is dominant at a particular time.
   B) The personality that is dominant at any particular time determines the individual's behavior.
   C) Each individual personality is complex and integrated with its own unique behavior patterns and social relationships.
4) *Depersonalization Disorder*
   A) One or more episodes of depersonalization sufficient to produce significant impairment in social or occupational functioning.
   B) The symptom is not due to any other disorder, such as schizophrenia, affective disorder, organic mental disorder, anxiety disorder, or epilepsy.

HYSTERICAL PERSONALITY

DSM-III does not include histrionic personality features among the diagnostic criteria for somatoform disorders. As mentioned earlier, this is not the case in ICD-9, which gives the following description of hysterical personality disorder: "characterized by shallow, labile affectivity, dependence on others, craving for appreciation and attention, suggestibility and theatricality. There is often sexual immaturity, e.g., frigidity and overresponsiveness to stimuli. Under stress, hysterical symptoms (neurosis) may develop."

The features of the traditional "hysterical personality" are spread into various categories of personality disorders in the DSM-III, as summarized in Table 14.2.

The extent of association between personality disorders and somatoform disorders is a controversial and unresolved issue. What has been established is that conversion symptoms appear not only in typical histrionic personalities, but also in other personality disorders and other diagnostic categories, such as schizophrenia, melancholia, obsessive-compulsive neurosis, Alzheimer's disease, etc.

Table 14.2. *Four categories of personality disorders that include classical features of the traditional "hysterical personality"*

---

1. Borderline
   Impulsivity, unpredictability
   Unstable and intense interpersonal relationships
   Lack of control of anger
   Identity disturbance
   Affective instability
   Intolerance of being alone

2. Avoidant
   Hypersensitivity to rejection
   Desire for affection and acceptance
   Low self-esteem

3. Dependent
   Inability to function independently
   Lack of self-confidence

4. Histrionic
   Self-dramatization
   Overreaction to minor events
   Drawing of attention
   Shallow, lacking genuineness
   Egocentric
   Manipulative suicidal threats

Note: In ICD-9, all of the above are part of "hysterical personality disorder" (also called psycho-infantile personality).

Only "en passant," at the end of the pages devoted to histrionic personality, does the DSM-III system note that "in many cases somatization disorders and histrionic personality disorders coexist." Chodoff and Lyons (1958) reported only three hysterical personalities in 17 patients with conversion disorder. They noted, however, that "psycho-infantile personality" (a term listed in ICD-9 as related to hysterical personality disorder) was found in a number of those patients. It is noteworthy that psychological infantilism includes 8 of the 10 behavioral components of the DSM-III criteria for histrionic personality disorder. In fact, immaturity is a major feature of the latter. Also exemplifying a controversial conclusion, Stephens and Kamp (1962), upon studying a series of patients with conversion disorder, reported "no predominance of hysterical personalities, but rather passive dependent traits." With Marmor (1953) and others, I submit that oral receptivity, passivity, and dependency should actually be included as part and parcel of histrionic personality features. It seems premature to conclude with Cleghorn (1969) that personality has no valid relationship with conversion, or with other somatoform and dissociative disorders.

DISCUSSION AND INTERNATIONAL PERSPECTIVES

The above review leads us to three avenues that I would select as suggestions for promising research:

The etiological issue: psychogenic and organic components

The DSM-III system of classification leaves its usual atheoretical attitude and takes psychological etiology into account, as mentioned earlier, when conversion disorder and idiopathic pain are concerned. This amounts to a theoretical bias, as there is no mention of organic components. To balance psychological causation, there should be room for Paul Schilder's (1939) concept of "organic repression," "a phenomenon which at the structural level repeats what is going on in other repressions in the so-called psychic level." Schilder considers that the same conversion symptom may be the end result of either an organic cerebral illness or a psychological disturbance on a background of cerebral immaturity. "The conversion is based on childhood experiences, but the later organic trauma may be the nucleus and pattern for the final formation of the symptom" (Schilder, 1939). The finding of concomitant organic disease and hysterical symptoms has been repeatedly pointed out in the last few decades. A cerebral organic syndrome may change the functions of the brain in such a way as to provoke neurotic attitudes. This is true for multiple sclerosis, brain tumors, cerebral arteriosclerosis, sequelae of encephalitis, and so on (Slater & Glithero, 1965; Whitlock, 1967; Engel, 1968).

Ellenberger (1968) expresses a similar view on hysteria when he defines it as a psychopathological reaction due to the effect of a psychic trauma upon a constitutionally predisposed central nervous system. We may add that acquired organic lesions may be part of the predisposition.

Transcultural and historical perspectives

Nowhere in psychopathology do we find a more elusive entity than hysterical disorders, owing to interpersonal and cultural influences. In few areas in psychiatry are symptoms created and modified to such an extent by society's expectations and, in particular, by the doctor-patient relationship, as already pointed out by Briquet (1859). We cannot expect the list of symptoms listed by Guze (1975) in the course of their work in the United States to be valid for all countries and all times. This is of special importance as DSM-III seems to be on its way to being used all over the world. In France, for instance, fits and other paroxysmal symptoms were more frequent in the days of Briquet and Charcot than in Babinski's era, when more permanent neurological symptoms, such as paralysis and anesthesia, predominated. Nowadays, following the "repression" exercised against conversion, an increase in psychosomatic illnesses (psychophysiological disorders) is noted by Brisset (1970) with a "progressive burying of symptoms inside the body." More specifically, what one would say, using DSM-III terminology, is that conversion disorders have decreased to give way to somatization disorders (Briquet's Syndrome), personality disorders (Axis II), and concomitant organic illnesses (Axis III).

Although statistical data are not available, hysteria seems to be more repressed by North American culture and physicians than by their French, Italian, Spanish, South American, or other counterparts. The hypothesis proposed by Brisset (1970) is that in a given society there is an inverse proportion of cases of conversion hysteria and of psychophysiological disorders. Repression of hysteria leads to psychosomatic illness. The joint influence of culture and of the physician leads to internalization of hysteria. For instance, patients with war hysteria were flooding hospitals during World War I, but the corresponding rates were exceptionally low during World War II, when peptic ulcers were proliferating. Mesmer, writes Brisset (1970), was attracting hysterics, Charcot was cultivating them, Babinski repressed them, and we continue the repression. The development of the nomenclatures and criteria for DSM-IV and ICD-10 is certainly in need of reliable studies of somatoform and hysterical disorders in various countries.

Links between somatoform disorders and other aspects of "hysteria"

What Briquet described in his *Treatise* is an association of four syndromes: hysterical personality, conversion phenomena, somatization disorder, and dissociative states (Dongier, 1983). No one, including Briquet, doubted that this association is far from constant, but there indeed appears to be an overlap in the prevalence of the four. Opinions differ about the importance of the overlap, how often are they associated, and how often they are not. The DSM-III system should perhaps mention somewhere the frequent coexistence of somatoform and dissociative states. The legitimacy of restricting the field of hysteria to one of these syndromes and giving it the name of Briquet or somatization disorder is questionable. It means limiting the field to a group of severe cases (several years duration, rare spontaneous remission, frequent unnecessary surgery, often chaotic life). Many of the patients described by Briquet (1859) did not have the chronic and malignant course described by Guze (1970) that limits hysteria to somatization disorders and restricts it to one end of the spectrum. There seems to be a conceptual and phenomenological impoverishment in the fragmentation introduced by DSM-III. This is, however, a clinical intuition shared by many clinical psychiatrists that remains to be documented. Many more empirical studies are needed to validate, if feasible, the unity of what we used to call hysteria.

REFERENCES

American Psychiatric Association 1980. *Diagnostic and Statistical Manual of Mental Disorders*. 3rd ed. (DSM-III). Washington, D.C.: American Psychiatric Press.

Babinski, J. 1901. Definition de l'hystérie *C. R. Soc. Neurol.* Paris, 7 novembre.

Blumer, D., and Heilbronn, M. 1982. Chronic pain as a variant of depressive disease: the pain-prone disorder. *J. Nerv. Ment. Dis.* 170: 381–406.

Briquet, P. 1859. *Traité de l'hystérie.* Paris: Baillière et Fils.

Brisset, C. H. 1970. Hystérie et psychosomatique: les rapports de la structure et de l'histoire. *Evol. Psychiatr* 377–404.

Chodoff, P., and Lyons, H. 1958. Hysteria, the hysterical personality and "hysterical" conversion. *Am. J. Psychiatry* 114: 734–740.

Cleghorn, R. A. 1969. Hysteria – multiple manifestations of semantic confusion. *Can. Psychiatr. Assoc.* 14: 539–551.

Cloniger, C. R. 1983. Diagnosis of somatoform disorders: a critique of DSM-III. In *Diagnosis and Classification in Psychiatry. A Critical Appraisal of DSM-III*, ed. G. L. Tischler. Cambridge: Cambridge University Press.

Dongier, M. 1983. Briquet and Briquet's Syndrome viewed from France. *Can. J. Psychiatry* 28: 422–427.

Ellenberger, H. F. 1968. *Aspects ethnopsychiatriques de l'hystérie. Confrontations psychiatriques.* Paris: Specia.

Engel, G. L. 1968. A reconsideration of the role of conversion in somatic disease. *Compreh. Psychiatr.* 9: 316–326.

Guze, S. B. 1967. The diagnosis of hysteria: What are we trying to do? *Am. J. Psychiatry* 124: 77–84.

Guze, S. B. 1970. The role of follow-up studies: their contribution to diagnostic classification as applied to hysteria. *Semin. Psychiatr.* 2: 392–402.

Guze, S. B. 1975. The validity and significance of the clinical diagnosis of hysteria (Briquet's Syndrome). *Am. J. Psychiatry.* 132: 138–141.

Guze, S. B., Woodruff, R., Clayton, P. 1975. The significance of psychotic affective disorders. *Arch Gen. Psychiatry* 32: 1147–1150.

Kenyon, F. E. 1964. Hypochondriasis. A clinical study. *Br. J. Psychiatr.* 110: 478–488.

Kenyon, F. E. 1965. Hypochondriasis: a survey of some historical, clinical and social aspects. *Br. J. Med. Psychol.* 38: 117–133.

Kenyon, F. E. 1976. Hypochondrical states. *Br. J. Psychiatr.* 129: 1–14.

Lewis, A. J. 1975. The survival of hysteria. *Psychol. Med.* 5: 9–12.

Marmor, J. 1953. Orality in the hysterical personality. *J. Amer. Psychoanal. Assoc.* 1: 656–671.

Raskin, M., Talbott, J. A., and Meyerson, A. T. 1966. Diagnosis of conversion reactions: predictive value of psychiatric criteria. *J.A.M.A.* 197: 102–106.

Schilder, P. 1939. The concept of hysteria. *Am. J. Psychiatry.* 98: 1389–1413.

Slater, E., and Glithero, E. 1965. A follow-up of patients diagnosed as suffering from "hysteria." *J. Psychosom. Res.* 9: 9–14.

Stephens, J. H., and Kamp, M. 1962. On some aspects of hysteria: a clinical study. *J. Nerv. Ment. Dis.* 134: 305–310.

Whitlock, F. A. 1967. The aetiology of hysteria. *Acta Psychiatr. Scand.* 43: 14.

Williams, J. B. W., and Spitzer, R. L. 1982. Idiopathic pain disorder: a critique of pain-prone disorder and a proposal for a revision of the DSM III category psychogenic pain disorder. *J. Nerv. Ment. Dis.* 170: 415–419.

World Health Organization 1978. *Manual of the International Classification of Diseases, Ninth Revision (ICD-9).* Geneva.

15 Adjustment disorder as a nosological entity in DSM-III

A cultural analysis

HORACIO FABREGA, JR. (USA), JUAN E. MEZZICH
(USA and Peru), AND ADA C. MEZZICH (USA and Peru)

ILLNESS FROM A HISTORICAL, CULTURAL, AND CLINICAL STANDPOINT

Problems of illness are ubiquitous in human recorded and unrecorded history. Members of all social groups, it is safe to assume, have experienced and will continue to experience periodic outbursts of health problems that thwart their capacity to function and that can prove lethal to them. The evidence available to paleopathologists, physical and cultural anthropologists, and comparative social historians attest to these generalizations (Boyd, 1970). Basic tenets of the general theory of evolution provide the conditions for the ubiquity of interferences in health and well-being. The concept of illness as a negatively valued discontinuity in the functioning of the individual, a discontinuity giving rise to a need for corrective action, has proved to be of enormous use to scholars and scientists of various persuasions (Fabrega, 1972). The concept refers to a disorder of functioning of the whole person, and thus embraces social, psychological, and biological spheres. In this general frame of accounting, all people develop illnesses (along with any number of additional natural and man-caused catastrophes or disasters) but differ in the way they name, classify, explain, and deal with them. Thus, all people studied possess a vocabulary about illness, along with nosologies and theories of illness that explain causation. The ideas of "theories of illness" and "systems of medicine" (or "medical-care systems") have proved useful to scientists who study medical phenomena from a general and comparative point of view (Fabrega, 1974).

THE THEORY OF ILLNESS IN WESTERN MEDICINE

The theory of illness of late modern and especially contemporary Western Europe and of societies dominated by its cultural assumptions (i.e., based on its symbols about the nature of reality, about its religion, morality, subsistence and economic practices, family and kinship organization, etc.) has been termed biomedical because of the central role played in the theory by modern biological science. This theory is linked to the highly technical and technological view of man that is dominant in contemporary society and excludes factors that

153

involve spirituality. Interesting questions that require further research are those that ask exactly how, when, and why in the course of modern Western European history the societies influenced by this "culture" evolved the theory referred to as "biomedical." Certainly, there is much in the practice of medicine of the Greeks and Romans that can be linked to the contemporary biological approach to man, just as one can find analogous inklings of such an approach in other great civilizations and corresponding traditions of medicine (Phillips, 1913; Scarborough, 1969; Leslie, 1976). Such "biological" assumptions, however, were linked to magical and "religious" beliefs, and the quintessentially technical and machinelike view of man and disease never arose (Dijksterhuis, 1961). In the *biomedical theory of illness*, a set of preexisting *causal* factors are held to produce a condition of *disease* that consists of a dysfunction in the structure and/or functioning of the various systems of the body (Fabrega, 1980). The condition of disease is measurable through operations and investigations performed on the body and its various parts and products. A condition of disease, in turn, produces a condition or state of illness, which consists in subjective and objective changes in a person's concrete behavior and actions in the world.

BEHAVIORAL CHANGES AS THE CONCRETE DATA OF ILLNESS

It is important to emphasize that subjective and objective or concrete changes in behavior and adaptation are integral to a condition of illness and that this is true in all branches of modern biomedicine as it is, indeed, in all societies regardless of the kind of theory of illness that prevails. Congestive heart failure exists as a behavioral profile consisting of changes in subjective well-being and in objective changes in the activities of the individual. The same is true of diabetes, cerebral vascular accidents, and, indeed, any medical condition. Someone, either the person afflicted or a significant other, notices a behavioral discontinuity that in turn leads to a medical inquiry. The task of the physician is to explain the behavioral change (which constitutes the illness) as a transformation out of an altered bodily state of disease, and he or she accomplishes this by various means of investigation and examination. The account given here is based on the *biomedical theory of illness* that underlies the practice of the Western trained physician. The fact that such a physician can diagnose a state or condition of disease in an individual in the absence of a state or condition of illness (the "asymptomatic" individual) in no way invalidates the theory. Indeed, a reasonable goal in biomedical policy is to prevent or eliminate states of disease before they eventuate into states of illness (i.e., symptoms, morbidity, etc.).

THE BIOMEDICAL PHYSICIAN AS A DECULTURATING AGENT

The task of the physician can be conceptualized as requiring him or her to inquire about the behavioral functioning of a potential patient and through an analysis of this functioning, uncover clues that suggest an underlying state or condition of disease. A potential patient submits to this inquiry and describes his or her subjective and objective behavioral state; that is, he or she relates his or her recent illness or symptom, or complaint. The patient relates this account in terms of his or her own assumptions and beliefs and grounds his or her description of behavior in social contexts that have personal meaning to him or her. Stated differently, one could say that (1) the patient gives a *culturally laden* account of illness or behavioral change, "culture" here denoting the symbol systems the patient draws on from his or her social and ethnic background, and that (2) the physician abstracts out of the patient's account a relatively "objective" or "culture-free" account that is maximally useful in his or her attempt to arrive at clues about a possible underlying state or condition of disease. The physician, in short, is filtering or parceling out cultural symbols and translating a cultural account into possible culture-free symbols of illness that may in turn allow for the diagnosis of disease. In this sense, the physician is a "de- or unculturating" agent.

PSYCHIATRIC ILLNESS IN THE BIOMEDICAL FRAMEWORK

The account given in the preceding sections has been explicated with reference to general medical practice and is easily applied to the practice of psychiatry. To a psychiatrist, it makes obvious sense that a patient's illness picture or set of complaints consists of "altered" or "disordered" behavior. Behavior has a special and traditional link to psychiatry and a useful way of describing it is to draw attention to its psychosocial and neurovegetative features. In the contemporary theory of psychiatry, a condition or state of (psychiatric) illness entails a negative discontinuity or disvalued change in subjective behavior (thinking, feeling, willing, etc.), social behavior (working, relating to others, etc.), and/or neurovegetative behavior (sleep, sexuality, appetite, etc.). The various theoretical schools of psychiatry can all be seen as providing the psychiatrist with a schema or language with which to describe and explain the behavioral change of illness in ways not unlike the way the general physician approaches illness. The phenomenologic, psychoanalytic, behavioristic, and biologistic psychiatrist all proceed, as indicated above, as "deculturating agents." First of all, they reduce the personalized and culturally contextualized behavioral data of personal illness to categories and rubrics that leave out the cultural colorations of the patient's account of a possible "actual," "observed" change in behavior. Thus, the phenomenologist searches for such things as changes in form and structure of experience; the psychoanalyst for expressions of unconscious conflicts, ego-defense profile, impulse control; the behaviorist for stimuli acting as reinforcers and for types of reinforcing schedule that promote maladaptive behavior, and the biologist for any of the preceding plus aspects of behavior that reflect mood, motivational, and attentional changes correlated with changes in brain function. Second, although this may seem more controversial, all types of psychiatrists would probably acknowledge that well-specified changes in behavior presenting as illness phenomena are the expression of or correlated with specified changes in the organization and functioning of the central nervous system. A general postulate in psychiatric theory, in short, is that many, if not most, psychiatric illnesses constitute transformations of (disease) changes in the central nervous system. Only the biological psychiatrist, of course, explicitly searches for "biological markers" (i.e., measures that reflect presumed states of central nervous disease). Nonetheless, it is unlikely that empirical support for such markers will dissuade the behaviorist, psychoanalyst, or phenomenologist from continuing to seek clarification of their concepts and theories that after all address the domain of behavior and not the neural sciences per se. In many respects, the focus of psychiatrists can be viewed as levels or types of discourse that are logically and not necessarily empirically disconnected. Thus, the concepts of illness and of disease as stipulated in the biomedical theory have an obvious relevance to all types of psychiatrists, and the same can be said of the concept of antecedent causes (e.g., social stressors, genetic loadings, etc.).

DSM-III AS AN EXPRESSION OF BIOMEDICAL THEORY

A characteristic feature of the contemporary approach in clinical psychiatry is the emphasis on diagnosis. In the practice of psychiatry, "diagnosis" has broadened to embrace additional parameters of illness that reflect clinically significant facts necessary for a full understanding of a psychiatric condition. The multiaxial approach to diagnosis that is linked to DSM-III constitutes a procedure that enables the clinician to specify a number of fundamental facts of a psychiatric illness condition (Mezzich, 1983, 1985). Because of its intrinsic connection to many domains of scientific knowledge and research within psychiatry, the multiaxial approach as articulated in DSM-III is also a theory, the axes of which articulate and measure parameters that explain an illness as an occurrence and trajectory having social, biological, and temporal parameters as well as strictly clinical ones. This is to say that etiologic, descriptive, prognostic, and treatment consequences are implied by a multi–DSM-III "diagnosis" of an illness condition. The determination of Axis I constitutes a basic imperative and it is this enterprise that characteristically involves the clinician in the task of decontextualizing (i.e., "deculturating") parameters of the individual's adjustment so as to address behavioral and related clinical criteria. Such criteria are framed in abstract language referring to objective parameters. Typically obtaining data from Axes IV and V is more likely to involve the clinician in the immediate psychosocial and cultural circumstances of the individual's situation.

CULTURAL RELATIVISM AND DSM-III UNIVERSALISM

The categories, rationale, and general content of DSM-III may be seen as an expression of the evolving biomedical theory of illness applied to psychiatry. To repeat, the biomedical theory looks for phenomena that lie "underneath" illness in the apparatus of the person; it seeks to uncover biological indicators that are distinct and removed from manifest illness; that is, phenomena distinct from manifest behavior. Furthermore, application of the biomedical theory and of DSM-III can be seen as reducing the symbolic and cultural richness of an illness picture to behavioral phenomena that are culturally uniform and hopefully universal. Indeed, an implicit assumption is that DSM-III (like similar diagnostic schemas in general medicine) should be applicable anywhere and in any era. This means that the categories, rationale, and general indicators of psychiatric disorders of DSM-III are not anchored in behaviors that are culturally or historically specific. The material of DSM-III is couched in abstract and "objective" language; moreover, its substance or content is drawn from various supporting theoretical schools of psychiatry mentioned earlier, which themselves eschew culturally and/or historically specific features of human behavior. The modern "biomedic" user of DSM-III believes that through clinical inquiries in relevant *natural language*, it is possible to elicit material that would lead to a suitable diagnosis in the more abstract and objective language of DSM-III. In this endeavor, the clinician is essentially translating the content of an individual's illness into the culture-free and universalistic system or code of DSM-III (i.e., he or she is again acting as a deculturating agent). Examples of just such efforts are illustrated in the work of Morice and of Orley and Wing. Whether attempting to diagnose Western-specified psychiatric disorders or to explicate the (Western) nosologic significance of culture-bound syndromes, these researchers seem to implicitly rely on notions about the universal applicability of contemporary psychiatric diagnosis and the theoretical assumptions and parameters about behavior, all of which are also reflected in DSM-III (Morice, 1978; Orley & Wing, 1979).

ADJUSTMENT DISORDER AS A TRANSITIONAL CATEGORY OF ILLNESS: CONCEPTUAL ISSUES

The DSM-III criteria for a mental disorder, as stated on page 6 of its manual, involve the following: "a clinically significant behavioral or psychological syndrome or pattern . . . associated with either a painful symptom . . . or impairment in one or more important areas of functioning." These criteria are compelling and useful and embody considerable face validity; however, they are also vague and difficult to measure. For example, no guidelines are offered for quantifying the level of "painful symptom" or degree of impairment (nor in which area[s] of functioning). The preceding are critical for demarcating a state of illness from that of social maladaptation or merely a problem in morale that is common in the population. The criteria also indicate "there is an inference that there is a behavioral, psychological, or biological dysfunction, and that the disturbance is not only in the relationship between the individual and society"; this implies that the illness condition is somehow lodged in the individual and/or has a natural history of some sort. But how and on what basis this is to be decided is left unspecified. Lack of specificity regarding issues such as these presumably disqualify states of social deviance; but given the potential for controversies across theoretical schools and cultures, greater rigor than that the scientific community will agree upon is desirable for specifying that a referral condition truly constitutes a condition of illness (Moore, 1977; Stone, 1984). Psychiatry is currently one of the more politicized medical disciplines, and to ensure its medical integrity, the measurable criteria for illness should be emphasized. Social and philosophical issues related to the topic of general criteria for illness are not dealt with further in this chapter. We assume that a practicing clinician implicitly draws on his/her criteria for illness as versus nonillness when a diagnosis is stipulated, and our task is to clarify what the correlates of these implicit criteria might be. The DSM-III criteria for adjustment disorder (AD) add to the above general criteria for illness ideas of (1) *maladaptive reaction* to (2) an *identifiable* psychosocial *stressor* that (3) *occurs within three months after the onset of the stressor*, (4) it being assumed that the *disorder will remit* after the stressor ceases and that (5) the disturbance *does not meet the criteria for any other specific disorder*.

In order to reach a diagnosis through the use of DSM-III, an evaluating clinician is most likely to focus on presenting signs and symptoms, in particular, the extent and duration of these and their impact on the person's adjustment; and he/she will attempt to "match" the clinical facts with the criteria for specific named psychiatric disorders. In this evaluation, the clinician is likely to learn about environmental happenings; for example, stressors and social supports. It is in light of this analysis that the diagnosis of adjustment disorder is made. By the definition, specific and named psychiatric disorders have priority in the diagnostic process based on DSM-III.

This means that the use of the adjustment disorder label approximates that of a diagnosis by exclusion. The clinician, in other words, judges the patient in some way ill, but cannot fit the symptom picture to a named illness condition, and thus relates the illness to the social circumstances of the individual. Given the general significance that adaption theory has in human biology and medicine, any named illness condition can be expected to be produced by an identifiable stressor or constellation thereof. One is tempted to postulate that conditions such as post-traumatic stressor disorder, generalized anxiety disorder, dysthymic disorder, somatization (and conversion) disorder, and brief reactive psychosis are most likely to arise as possibilities in the diagnostic inquiry, but resolution of this issue is obviously best left to empirical studies.

It is clear that a "theory" about human social behavior and functioning is implicit in the DSM-III rationale for adjustment disorders. This theory may be termed "the coping and adaptation theory," which relates as well to crisis theory (Selye, 1946; Caplan, 1964; Coelho, Hamburg & Adams, 1974).

Such a theory stipulates that individuals encounter any number of challenges and stressors in the pursuit of tasks and goals devolving from their social situation and environment. Social supports of various kinds help to "buffer" the "stress" that the individual experiences, thus improving the individual's ability to function in the face of environmental stressors. Even an adequate number (and/or quality) of supports, however, may fail to prevent psychological symptoms and/or impairments in social functioning. In this theory, successful coping involves mastery of these environmental contingencies. A certain level of "stress," reflected subjectively, psychophysiologically, and/or in terms of social functioning, is to be expected in association with coping efforts. Presumably, such a level of stress is natural if not "adaptive" (as versus "maladaptive"). Some of these challenges and stressors, however, can overwhelm the individual's resources and capacities and lead to a "maladaptive stress reaction." Environmental challenges (i.e., stressors) that overwhelm the individual and lead to maladaptive changes in the person and in his/her ability to function are said to "produce" an adjustment disorder.

The terms "adaptive" and "maladaptive" are obviously problematical in this theory. The terms appear to presuppose (1) what level or type of reactions a given stressor (or constellation of stressors) can be expected to produce in a hypothetical individual, for it would then be possible (2) to decide what level or type of stress reaction is adaptive as opposed to maladaptive. Normative data on stressor-response patterns are not in any rigorous way available at present. Moreover, it is not clear how the root form "adaptive" is to be construed in this theory. Does "adaptive" mean a level or type of stress reaction that is natural or expectable or healthy or constructive or noninterfering, given the stressor (and/or other contingencies) that impact on the individual? From a purely medical standpoint, this could very well be a moot point: Maladaptive could be defined purely in terms of subjective symptoms and/or a decrement in social functioning, instilling an obvious circularity in the definition. But, if this is so, symptoms/social functioning criteria would be sufficient, and criteria involving stressors would be relaxed considerably, if not entirely. From a strictly logical standpoint, it would be difficult to exclude the possibility that "stressors" are not always acting on individuals, given the vicissitudes, complexities, and problems attendant on living and the vagaries of personal psychologies. But, if stressors are always acting, why bother to require them in the definition, leaving inquiries tied to Axis IV and V to handle the problem? In the last analysis, of course, stressors are (intuitively) what "stress" the individual and one can expect profound individual differences regarding what types of stressors can affect adaptation and coping. In this regard, the term "identifiable" (used to qualify stressor) among the criteria of adjustment disorders is ambiguous. Does it refer to anything the clinician or the individual identifies or only to the types of stressors included as common, recurring, and likely to negatively affect the individual, as explicated by adaptation and crisis theories?

All of the preceding issues raise the following question: By the use of adjustment disorder, is one labeling particularly healthy or unhealthy persons? Thus, how will an individual with a personality disorder or a vulnerability for a specific psychiatric disorder respond to a stressor or constellation of stressors that in another individual produces an adjustment disorder? Such individuals may, of course, respond with specific named conditions or with an adjustment disorder, but it would not be clear what clinical significance one could place on such eventualities. An individual without a personality disorder or vulnerability to a specific named psychiatric condition would presumably respond to such stressors with an adjustment disorder, but what if a named condition does develop? Does this render the stressor greater or reflect a constitutional weakness? These logical and conceptual quandaries are perhaps to be expected given our level of knowledge of human behavior functioning and psychiatric disorders. Moreover, it is only by accumulating data on adjustment disorder and related illness and nonillness categories that one can be expected to resolve the logical and conceptual dilemmas (Andreasen & Wasek, 1980; Andreasen & Hoenk, 1982). Presumably, it is the careful assessment of Axes IV and V in individuals receiving diagnosis of named illness conditions (as well as ancillary data about treatment response, future course, etc.) that would help clarify these issues.

Issues discussed so far involving the wide applicability of adaptation theory and, in particular, its obvious relevance to name illness conditions of DSM-III (concretely demonstrated in Axes IV and V formulations) as well as to adjustment disorder, suggest the following issues. A key feature in the judicious application of the adjustment disorder label might involve people who are showing symptoms and/or decrements in social functioning and about whom the clinician judges that the balance of factors in the environment/person equation that leads to the production of a potential illness is to be found in the environment. In other words, people showing symptoms and/or decrements in social functioning and about whom the clinician concludes (after detailed anamnesis) that stressors in the physical and social environment are most heavily influential in a clinical sense as compared to relevant features of the individual (e.g., his personality style, his adjustment/coping history, etc.) are the ones to be favored with the adjustment disorder category. This would, of course, render post-traumatic stress disorder (PSD) an important contrastive category for studies of clinical validity. It should be noted that adjustment disorder and PSD both include stressors in the criteria entailed for diagnosis, the entities differing in that identifiable versus recognizable are used, respectively, to qualify stressors. Moreover, PSD explicitly includes the stipulation that the stressor would lead to symptoms in almost anyone (an issue that raises obvious problems, as already noted) and the additional factor of a *characteristic symptomatic profile* (a factor common to other named illness conditions and accounting for the marginal status of an AD, i.e., a diagnosis by exclusion).

A host of problems is raised by stipulations number three and four mentioned in the criteria of definition, namely, that the clinical condition arises within three months after the onset of the stressor and it being assumed that the clinical condition will remit after the stressor ceases. One involves ascertainment of when a stressor "begins." Clearly, stressors entailed by events in the social and physical environment can be dated precisely, although even here when an individual (a) *learns of the stressor* or (b) *evaluates* (or feels the impact of) the stressor could raise knotty issues. However, stressors not entailed by events but by such things as situations, deadlines (e.g., regarding career plans/goals), and finally by social relationships are likely to prove even more problematic when the matter of ascertainment of the duration of the stressor is to be assessed. How a time interval of three months is to be applied in these latter instances is difficult to specify and, given the imprecision one is likely to encounter as opposed to stressors entailed by events, it is difficult to be certain how empirical data related to validity studies will be interpreted. Moreover, obvious deficiencies in the utility of the AD category devolve from a definitional criterion that specifies a clinician's assumption as to the course of the condition should the stressor cease. A clinician may not have information on how long stressors act on individuals (even if it should be available) and/or may not be in a position to apply it in making a diagnosis, since this requires him or her to know a great deal more than is reasonable to expect about the person he or she is evaluating. Finally, it is not at all clear when a stressor "ceases" to be a stressor, an issue obviously related to the matter of ascertainment of time, duration (of three months) in the definition mentioned earlier.

ADJUSTMENT DISORDER AS A TRANSITIONAL CATEGORY OF ILLNESS: EMPIRICAL ISSUES

The preceding analysis has presented reasons why adjustment disorder may be viewed as a marginal or transitional category of illness within DSM-III. To date, there is very little literature of a theoretical or empirical nature that explicates factors of importance linked to this marginal or transitional illness category of DSM-III. In this segment, we summarize the results of a study of individuals falling within this category of illness (Fabrega, Mezzich & Mezzich, 1987). A group meeting criteria for "adjustment disorder" was compared to one meeting criteria for the logically complementary category, namely, those that can be referred to as "named illness conditions" (NIC). The sample of individuals studied was drawn from a population of individuals seeking care in a major metropolitan psychiatric facility. This psychiatric population encompasses all age groups, and it experiences a wide variety of forms and levels of psychopathologic symptoms; it is served through specialized child, adolescent, adult, and geriatric clinical programs (Mezzich, Coffman & Goodpastor, 1982). Patient evaluations were conducted using the Initial Evaluation Form (IEF), a semistructured assessment procedure having mutually complementary narrative and standardized components (Mezzich et al., 1981).

Results showed that compared to AD, individuals of NIC tended to show higher measures on all indicators of psychopathology. On the other hand, AD tended to receive higher measures on a variety of different types of stressors, on overall level of stressor severity, and on level of adaptive functioning during the year predating the evaluation and on current functioning. Thus, although rated as more highly "stressed," the AD group also appears to be rated as "healthier" (symptomatically and functionally) than the group of NIC subjects.

A lower level of psychopathology in the AD group was expected: The NIC group was, after all, a composite of all commonly recognized clinical entities and insofar as the indicators of these entities are being tapped by the IEF, the result of averaging symptom/sign levels across entities could be expected to produce a profile of higher percentages. Nonetheless, not all sets of indicators, nor all of the items of any one set, necessarily constitute components of named illness conditions, and insofar as AD subjects may represent early "cryptic" forms of named illness conditions, the AD group as a whole could very well have shown significantly higher values on some indicators, which was not the case. We concluded that levels of recognized indicators of psychopathology are lower in the AD than in the NIC group and that this points to the descriptive validity that AD possesses when the IEF and DSM-III systems are applied. The data support the notion that, although judged as ill by clinicians, AD subjects are also judged as "healthier" than NIC subjects, and results argue for the usefulness within DSM-III of this particular transitional category of illness.

Although the presence of stressors is on logical grounds a property of AD, there are no theoretical reasons for anticipating that empirically clinical influence of stressors is less in NIC subjects. The stress/coping and adaptation theory that underlies the stipulation of AD is *general* in its scope and is assumed to be equally relevant to all psychiatric illnesses (as well as medical illnesses, for that matter). A level of stress in the AD group not different from that of NIC subjects, with otherwise the same pattern of results, would have suggested that the AD group was somehow more prone to careseeking: That is, a group that in the context of fewer recognized symptoms and higher social functioning, but no higher measures of stress, had sought psychiatric evaluation. The pattern of results that was actually obtained does not allow one to conclude that a special "proneness towards helpseeking" is operating: Clearly, it appears that AD subjects are burdened by a higher level of "stress." Longitudinal studies and/or retrospective data allowing one to uncover duration, course, and social impact of illness across time would clarify further the significance of the higher level of stress in the context of the results obtained. Also, the higher level of stressors in AD versus non-illness conditions offered evidence of its special role in AD. The finding of greater stress in AD, however, could result from observer bias supporting the idea that a circularity in the method of evaluation accounts for it. This possibility is being examined in current studies at the Western Psychiatric Institute and Clinic of the University of Pittsburgh.

ADJUSTMENT DISORDER AND CULTURAL VARIABILITY

A host of problems can be anticipated in the cross-cultural and cross-national application of DSM-III with respect to the entity of adjustment disorder. For purposes of discussion, we adopt here the widest possible application, namely, that geared to the evaluation of nonliterate peoples residing in communities where non-Indo-European languages are spoken. Among "cultures" such as these one is likely to encounter people very different from those of Western nations, wherein ideas of mental health and illness have developed and hence can be applied more appropriately and easily. For the sake of conciseness, only general factors are covered. It can be assumed that problems touched on here are complex and difficult to solve but that in most settings where DSM-III researchers are likely to work (urban communities populated by Western-educated peoples), the problems are not as likely to prove as difficult.

A basic problem in the diagnosis of AD is that of establishing that general criteria for psychiatric illness are met; namely, that of the presence of psychiatric symptoms or impairment. The domain of "psychiatric symptoms" obviously encompasses bodily and mental referents, and an unambiguous labeling as "psychiatric" presupposes the exclusion of general medical pathology that cannot always be accomplished in field situations. The problems of somatization and the cultural variability in expressions about the body will plague the researcher/clinician. Even if subjective distress is singled out for analysis and organic medical pathology can be ruled out, the researcher is confronted with definitional problems devolving from notions of personhood, emotion (including type, level, evoking situations, social appropriateness, etc.) and sense of well-being that are inextricably colored by varieties of terminologies and worldviews that are culturally conditioned. All of this needs to be untangled in order to get a good handle on what individuals report about mental phenomena, such as sadness, concentration, dysphoria, and anxiety. With regard to the criterion of social impairment, a similar degree of sensitivity to cultural variability will be required, since the clinician or researcher is forced to seek documentation of kinds of formal and informal social situations (such as, work, family, institutional) and the individual's accustomed mode and levels of functioning in them. In summary, the assessment of subjective well-being and social functioning/impairment (general criteria of psychiatric illness) necessarily involves careful analysis of language, symbols, and standards of behavior that are by definition permeated with culture, and applying ideas and rationales embodied in DSM-III will pose conceptual and linguistic difficulties. The manifestations are permeated by the cultural background of the person.

As already indicated, the special criteria stipulated for AD arise out of stress/coping and adaptation theory, and a number of problems are tied to application of this theory cross-culturally. In the broadest sense, a culture is a conglomeration of systems of *symbols*; and such symbols include beliefs and values that condition how individuals judge and evaluate social situations and happenings that encompass so-called stressors. Cultures also provide individuals with strategies for coping with or managing stress as defined culturally, and these strategies involve distinctive styles of instrumental activities. In other words, the kinds of instrumental actions dictated in the setting of "stressors" will obviously vary cross-culturally, so that the appropriateness or inappropriateness of the individual's solution to the stress as defined by him or her and comembers of the group needs to be assessed carefully. Norms exist regarding constructive and unconstructive solutions to stressors. Some norms stipulate styles of emotionality; thus, emotional control and inhibition may be emphasized or alternatively, passive resignation and/or fatalism. In some communities, the correct way to deal with a stressor may involve the ritualized expression of emotion in an individualistic or interpersonal sense. The researcher needs to be acquainted with all of these patterns of behavior before making a judgment of "maladaptive stress reaction" as stipulated in DSM-III. In short, it is important to emphasize that besides "creating" and defining the "stressful," the culture of a social group provides (1) different types of ways of handling emotion and relating interpersonally in the context of stress, (2) a number of formal and informal mechanisms or processes, and different types of support groups, that members can turn to and use in coping with problems, and (3) a set of institutions that teach individuals all of the above. The rudiments of appropriate coping, in other words, are learned by individuals from his/her group and are not just social facts, or psychological traits everyone learns in the same way. Moreover, all of these factors are *culturally conditioned* and hence variable and can be expected to pose empirical problems in the cross-cultural assessment of stress/coping, and hence application of the AD label. In summary, the two basic tasks of a coping strategy – handling emotions and handling problematic situations – will differ in societies governed by different systems of social symbols, and the AD entity that is grounded in constructs pertaining to stress/coping needs to be applied with an awareness of this fact.

In the light of factors touched on in this section, one is entitled to ask whether some of the so-called culture-bound syndromes described in the literature in anthropology and cultural psychiatry are in actuality illness entities or merely culturally conditioned types of unusual adjustment disorders. Some culture-bound syndromes no doubt qualify as unusual or brief reactive psychoses and others as major psychiatric disorders, all of these conditioned by patterns of central nervous system activation that are culturally influenced. Some, however, may best be analyzed as culturally modeled and hence standard ways of coping behaviorally and interpersonally with recurring and also culturally structured stressors.

REFERENCES

Andreasen, N. C., and Joenk, P. R. 1982. The predictive value of adjustment disorders: A follow-up study. *American Journal of Psychiatry* 139: 584–590.

Boyden, S. V. 1970. *The Impact of Civilization on the Biology of Man.* Toronto: University of Toronto Press.

Caplan, G. 1964. *Principles of Preventative Psychiatry.* New York: Basic Books.

Coelho, G. V., Hamburg, D. A., and Adams, J. 1974. *Coping and Adaptation.* New York: Basic Books.

Dijksterhuis, E. J. 1961. *The Mechanization of the World Picture.* New York: Oxford University Press.

Fabrega, H., Jr. 1972. Concepts of disease: logical features and social implications. *Perspectives in Biology and Medicine* 15: 583–616.

Fabrega, H., Jr. 1974. *Disease and Social Behavior: An Interdisciplinary Perspective.* Cambridge, Mass.: Massachusetts Institute of Technology Press.

Fabrega, H., Jr., 1980. The position of psychiatric illness in biomedical theory: a cultural analysis. *Journal of Medicine and Philosophy* 5: 145–168.

Fabrega, H., Jr., Mezzich, J. E., and Mezzich, A. C. 1987. *Archives of General Psychiatry* 44: 567–572.

Leslie, C. 1976. *Asian Medical Systems: A Comparative Study*. Berkley: University of California Press.

Mezzich, J. E. 1983. New developments in multiaxial psychiatric diagnosis. *Psychiatric Annals* 15: 793–807.

Mezzich, J. E. 1985. Multiaxial diagnostic systems in psychiatry. In *Comprehensive Textbook of Psychiatry*. 4th ed. Ed. H. I. Kaplan and B. J. Sadock. New York: Wilkins.

Mezzich, J. E., Coffman, G. A., and Goodpastor, S. M. 1982. A format for DSM-III formulation. Experience with 1,111 consecutive patients. *American Journal of Psychiatry* 139: 591–596.

Mezzich, J. E., Dow, J. T., Rich, C. L., Costello, A. J., and Himmelhoch, J. M. 1981. Developing an efficient clinical information system for a comprehensive psychiatric institute. II. Initial Evaluation Form. *Behavioral Research Methods and Instrumentation* 13: 464, 478.

Moore, M. S. 1977. Legal conceptions of mental illness. In *Philosophy and Medicine*. Vol. 5. The Netherlands: Reidel.

Morice, R. 1978. Psychiatric diagnosis in a transcultural setting: The importance of lexical categories. *British Journal of Psychiatry* 132: 87–95.

Orley, J., and Wing, J. K. 1979. Psychiatric disorders in two African villages. *Archives of General Psychiatry* 36: 513–520.

Phillips, E. D. 1913. *Greek Medicine*. London: Thames and Hudson.

Scarborough, J. 1969. *Roman Medicine*. London: Thames and Hudson.

Selye, H. 1946. General adaptation syndrome and diseases of adaptation. *Journal of Clinical Endocrinology* 6: 117–230.

Stone, A. A. 1984. *The Political Misuse of Psychiatry: A Tale of Two Generals, Law, Psychiatry and Morality*. Washington, D.C.: American Psychiatric Press.

16 *Issues on diagnosing and classifying personality disorders*

MASAAKI KATO (Japan)

HISTORICAL BACKGROUND

As far as the diagnosis and classification of personality disorders are concerned, nonsystematic, descriptive types of classification have been more popularly used than systematic ones. For instance, those classifications by Eysenck (1952, 1953; extrovert and introvert), Kretschmer (1922; schizoid, cycloid, and epileptoid), and Sheldon (1942; endomorphic, mesomorphic, and ectomorphic) are examples of systematic classifications, and those by Leonhard (1948) and Schneider (1923) – as well as those traditionally found in the various editions of the International Classification of Diseases and the U.S. *Diagnostic and Statistical Manual of Mental Disorders* (e.g., American Psychiatric Association, 1968, 1980) – are nonsystematic ones.

In the past, the most commonly used classification of personality disorders in Japan was that of Kurt Schneider (1923). His classification included the following types: (1) hyperthymic, (2) depressive, (3) insecure (anankastic), (4) fanatic, (5) attention-seeking, (6) labile, (7) explosive, (8) affectionless, (9) weak-willed, and (10) asthenic.

The classification by K. Leonhard (1948) contained the following types: (1) epileptoid, (2) anankastic, (3) hysterical, (4) paranoid, (5) reactive-labile, (6) cyclothymic, (7) subdepressive, (8) hypomanic, (9) anxious, and (10) mixed.

In ICD-8 (World Health Organization, 1965), the following classification was used: (1) paranoid, (2) cyclothymic, (3) schizoid, (4) explosive, (5) obsessive-compulsive, (6) hysterical, (7) asthenic, (8) antisocial, (9) other, and (10) unspecified.

DSM-II (American Psychiatric Association, 1968) added two subcategories to ICD-8, "passive-aggressive" and "inadequate" personalities.

The classification of ICD-9 (World Health Organization, 1977) on personality disorders reflected a modification of ICD-8 and included the following categories: (1) paranoid, (2) affective, (3) schizoid, (4) explosive, (5) anankastic, (6) hysterical, (7) asthenic, (8) with predominantly sociopathic or asocial manifestations, (9) other, and (10) unspecified.

The most remarkable modification in ICD-9 was the change from "antisocial personality disorder" to "personality disorder, with predominantly sociopathic or asocial manifestations." The perception that the "antisocial" category was based on social rather than medical criteria provided the main justification for this change.

Later, DSM-III (American Psychiatric Association, 1980) readopted "antisocial" within the following typology: (1) paranoid, (2) schizoid, (3) schizotypal, (4) histrionic, (5) narcissistic, (6) antisocial, (7) borderline, (8) avoidant, (9) dependent, (10) compulsive, (11) passive-aggressive, and (12) atypical, mixed or other.

The classification contained in an early draft for ICD-10 (World Health Organization, 1987) included the following: (1) paranoid, (2) schizoid, (3) Dyssocial, (4) impulsive, (5) histrionic, (6) anankastic, (7) anxious, (8) dependent, (9) other, and (10) unspecified.

The main difference between ICD-9 and the proposed ICD-10 in the classification of personality disorders was that "affective" and "aesthenic" were eliminated, "explosive" was changed to "impulsive," and "dependent" and "anxious" were added. The relationships among the various nosologies reviewed – ICD-10, that of Schneider, ICD-9, and DSM-III – are shown in Table 16.1.

Those categories that were consistently used in the classifications of Schneider, Leonhard, ICD-8, ICD-9, the 1984 draft of ICD-10, DSM-II, and DSM-III were "paranoid," "hysterical (or histrionic)" and "anankastic (insecure or obsessive)." Other categories have varied from one classification to the next.

THE 1971 WHO SEMINAR ON THE DIAGNOSIS OF PERSONALITY DISORDERS AND DRUG DEPENDENCE

The seventh WHO Seminar on Standardization of Psychiatric Diagnosis, Classification, and Statistics, which dealt with personality disorders and drug dependence, was held in Tokyo in December 1971 (World Health Organization, 1972). Diagnostic exercises with 10 case histories and two videotaped interviews were carried out by 12 members of a "nuclear" group of international experts and 14 members of a "local" group of psychiatrists from the Western Pacific and Asia.

Among several categories of psychiatric diagnoses (i.e., schizophrenia, reactive psychosis, childhood mental disorders, mental disorders in the aged, mental retardation, neurosis, and personality disorders) that were discussed in WHO seminars on ICD-8 from 1965 to 1972, clinician concordance was lowest with respect to diagnoses in the area of the personality disorders (see Table 16.2). Some of the problems found can be illustrated by the case summary depicting a "culture-bound" personality disorder in Japan, called *Shinkeishitsu*, that was presented at the Tokyo seminar. The case may be summarized as follows:

Male, 28 years, sought psychiatric help because he was unable to meet people and had a tremor of his hands. He came from a middle-class rural family and had a protected

Table 16.1. *Interrelations among the ICD-10 (1987 draft), Schneider, ICD-9, and DSM-III classifications of personality disorders*

ICD-10 (1987 draft)	Schneider	ICD-9	DSM-III
1. Paranoid	Fanatic	Paranoid	Paranoid
2. Schizoid	n.a.	Schizoid	Schizoid
			Schizotypal
3. Impulsive	Explosive	Explosive	n.a.
4. Anankastic	Anankastic	Anankastic	Compulsive
5. Histrionic	Attention-seeking	Hysterical	Histrionic
6. Dependent	n.a.	n.a.	Dependent
7. Dyssocial	n.a.	With predominantly sociopathic or asocial manifestations	Antisocial
n.a.	Depressive	n.a.	n.a.
n.a.	Labile	n.a.	n.a.
n.a.	Affectionless	n.a.	n.a.
n.a.	Weak-willed	n.a.	n.a.
n.a.	Hyperthymic	Affective	n.a.
n.a.	Asthenic	Asthenic	n.a.
n.a.	n.a.	n.a.	Narcissistic
n.a.	n.a.	n.a.	Borderline
8. Anxious	n.a.	n.a.	Avoidant
n.a.	n.a.	n.a.	Passive-aggressive
9. Other		Other	
10. Unspecified		Unspecified	

Note: n.a. = Not applicable.

childhood, graduating from a university at the age of 22. He became a government official but had a strong fear of social contacts. On examination, he was found to be unable to look the examiner in the eye. This patient improved on Morita Therapy and was subsequently able to function more effectively.

This case was assigned to more than 10 different diagnostic categories of personality disorder, including dependent personality, schizoid personality, and passive personality. Clinically, it is important to discuss the definitions of the various categories of personality disorder, although many statistical problems remain on their interrater reliability.

ON EVALUATION OF SEVERITY AND MULTIAXIAL FORMULATION

The severity of personality disorders is emerging as an important issue. The report from the seventh WHO Seminar on Standardization of Psychiatric Di-

Table 16.2. Concordance of diagnoses among WHO seminar members in 1971

Seminar members	Reactive psychosis	Childhood mental disorder	Mental disorder in aged	Mentally retarded	Neurosis	Personality disorder	Average
United States (I)	28	55	31	39	47	24	37.3
Japan	28	53	39	27	49	23	36.5
Switzerland	24	51	40	—	42	25	36.4
United States (II)	19	57	42	38	32	24	35.3
Norway	33	57	49	16	31	29	35.8
Peru	19	47	38	27	—	—	32.8
France	33	35	49	16	31	31	32.5
United Kingdom	33	51	32	24	35	31	34.3
USSR	—	42	46	20	38	24	34.0
Austria	—	40	—	9	47	30	31.5
Average of international panel	27	48	40	24	39	27	
Average of regional panel	23	46	35	25	37	19	
Mean average	25	47	37.5	24.5	38	23	

— Insufficient data.

Source: Adapted from Brooke (1972).

agnosis, Classification and Statistics of Personality Disorders and Drug Dependence, in 1971, contains some pertinent recommendations:

For more effective use of the existing classification, it may be necessary to consider the possibility of recording the severity of the abnormality, particularly in personality disorders.

Personality is more logically considered in terms of a continuum than of a disease state that is present or absent. The glossary must therefore be explicit on how severe an abnormality of personality must be present for 301 to be coded. Some participants suggested that only extreme departure from normality should be coded, as the diagnosis of minor abnormalities is likely to be unreliable, but there was no unanimity on this point.

This discussion led to a consideration of the value of noting the degree of abnormality of personality, especially for forensic work, where some studies have shown the predictive formulation and that it is desirable to include severity in the ICD coding. In view of the lack of knowledge at present on how to measure this, WHO should undertake research into this topic. It was appreciated that this is a task for the future and that it is impossible to code severity at the present time.

In ICD-9, the coding for the etiology of mental retardation and borderline mental retardation that had been utilized in ICD-8 was excluded because medical evaluation had suggested that such codings were unreliable. As previously mentioned (WHO Seminar Recommendations, 1971), the application of an index for the severity (or degree of abnormality) of personality disorders might be more useful than the definition of subcategories of personality disorders, if the severity could be evaluated objectively. Schneider defined his term "psychopathic personality" as denoting "those who disturb themselves [*such leidend*] or disturb others [*sozial stoerend*] because of their abnormality in terms of personality."

One approach to the evaluation of severity of abnormality in personality disorders might be to introduce a classification similar to that used for mental retardation, namely, mild and other specified (moderate, severe, and profound). In the case of mental retardation, the following guidelines have been proposed: "The assessment of intellectual level should be based on whatever information is available, including clinical evidence, adaptive behaviour and psychometric findings," and "the IQ levels given are provided only as a guide and should not be applied rigidly." In the case of personality disorders, the evaluation of severity might be visualized as the coordinates of two dimensions: "self-disturbed" and "other-disturbed." For either dimension, assessments of the severity of abnormality should be based on whatever information is available, including clinical evidence, adaptive functioning, and psychometric findings.

Another problem is whether personality disorders and traits belong with the clinical syndromes. Formulating personality disorders in an Axis II, as DSM-III does, seems appropriate. This axis should also include "personality traits of psychiatric significance." As to the so-called enduring personality changes, some of them may belong to Axis I, and some others may more properly be located in Axis II.

If a fifth-character subdivision of personality disorders could be applied, it would provide a means of recording the severity of abnormality in personality disorders. Furthermore, it is important that any proposed changes be discussed and clarified, such as the reasons for excluding "affective" and "asthenic," for changing "explosive" to "impulsive," and for adding "anxious" and "dependent."

COMMENTS

In line with these considerations, I propose that the category of personality disorders be assigned to an Axis II together with personality traits of psychiatric significance, rather than be formulated with other clinical syndromes in Axis I.

Another issue to be considered is the possibility of recording the severity of abnormality in personality disorders. Clinically (i.e., to understand and treat patients properly), it is very important to consider subcategories of personality traits and disorders. Statistically, however, as was demonstrated during the WHO Seminar on Standardization of Psychiatric Diagnosis, Classification and Statistics of Personality Disorders and Drug Dependence, in 1971, clinician concordance was lowest with respect to diagnosis in the area of the personality disorders – particularly among psychiatrists from developing countries (Thailand, Indonesia, Philippines, Singapore, India, the Republic of Korea, Taiwan, Hong Kong, Malaysia, and Ceylon). The results of this seminar suggested that the definition of personality disorders is strongly influenced by sociocultural background; for example, during an exercise with a case history of *Shinkeishitsu*, more than 10 different diagnoses were assigned by participating psychiatrists from both developed and developing countries.

A final recommendation of the WHO seminar in 1971 was that the psychiatric profession should undertake "research into measuring the severity of abnormality of personality disorders as an important parameter." One possible way to accomplish this goal would be to index the severity of personality disorders on two coordinate dimensions: "self-disturbed" and "other-disturbed." Such an approach might lead to more effective use of existing classifications for this important and problematic area of psychopathology.

REFERENCES

American Psychiatric Association. 1968. *Diagnostic and Statistical Manual of Mental Disorders*. 2nd ed. (DSM-II). Washington, D.C.

American Psychiatric Association. 1980. *Diagnostic and Statistical Manual of Mental Disorders*. 3rd ed. (DSM-III). Washington, D.C.

Brooke, E. M. 1972. Paper presented at WHO Meeting on International Diagnosis, Classification, and Statistics, Geneva.

Eysenck, H. J. 1952. *The Scientific Study of Personality*. London: Routledge & Kegan Paul.

Eysenck, H. J. 1953. *The Structure of Human Personality*. London: Routledge & Kegan Paul.

Kretschmer, E. 1922. *Körperbau und Charakter*. Berlin: Springer.

Leonhard, K. 1948. *Grundlage der Psychiatrie*. Stuttgart: Ferdinand Enke Verlag.

Schneider, K. 1923. Die Psychopathische Persönlichkeiten. In *Handbuch der Psychiatrie*, ed. G. Achaffenburg. Leipzig: F. Deuticke.

Sheldon, W. H. 1942. *The Varieties of Temperament: A Psychology of Constitutional Differences*. New York: Harper.

World Health Organization. 1965. *The Eighth Revision of International Classification of Diseases*, (ICD-8). Geneva.

World Health Organization. 1972. *The Seventh Seminar on Standardization of Psychiatric Diagnosis, Classification and Statistics of Personality Disorders and Drug Dependence, Tokyo, 8–14 December 1971*. Report MH/ 72.2.

World Health Organization. 1977. *The Ninth Revision of International Classification of Diseases*, (ICD-9). Vol. 1. Geneva.

World Health Organization. 1987. *Draft of ICD-10 Chapter V (Mental, Behavioural and Developmental Disorders) Clinical Descriptions and Diagnostic Guidelines*. Geneva.

PART III

Developments in diagnostic nomenclature and assessment

17 *The lexicon and issues in the translation of psychiatric concepts and terms*

ERIK STRÖMGREN (Denmark)

Psychiatry has traditionally been accused of availing itself of a terminology that is far too large, difficult to understand, and often even contradictory. These accusations are only partly correct. The psychiatric vocabulary is by no means more extended than vocabularies in other specialties of medicine. What is true, however, is that there are confusing differences and contradictions between terminologies in different psychiatric schools. Why are these weaknesses especially spectacular within psychiatry? The main reason is probably that during the long time in which psychiatric therapy was not very efficient, the ambitions of those doing research in psychiatry usually expressed themselves in diagnostic and terminological endeavors. During the last few decades, in which progress in psychopharmacotherapy has been so remarkable, a tendency in the opposite direction has appeared, namely, toward giving up making diagnoses, and toward disregarding exact and meaningful terminology. Instead, such terms as "antipsychotic drugs," "antidepressant drugs," and other pharmacomorphic labels have come into use. Nevertheless, most psychiatrists feel that clear and informative terminology and well-defined classifications are necessary tools for research in psychiatry and for the formulation of indications for adequate therapy. Often it has turned out that contradictions between results of research can be explained as consequences of comparisons between patient groups that are not comparable in spite of sharing the same diagnostic label, which had been used with different meanings or delimitations in selecting the different groups.

It has naturally always been one of the most important tasks of the World Health Organization to create an internationally accepted and understandable system of classification of diseases. Although the eighth and ninth editions of the International Classification of Diseases (ICD) has been accepted by the majority of United Nations member states, it has been obvious that the section on mental disorders is far from ideal. It was, therefore, fortunate that the Division of Mental Health of the World Health Organization (WHO) engaged in a Joint Project with the U.S. Alcohol, Drug Abuse and Mental Health Administration (ADAMHA) on Diagnosis and Classification of Mental Disorders and Alcohol- and Drug-Related Problems (World Health Organization, 1985). The first joint conference took place in 1980, and on this occasion a number of scientific working groups were formed, one of which had "Standard-

175

ization of Nomenclature and Terminology in the Mental Health Field" as its subject. This working group met in Mannheim in April 1980. The report from this meeting described the outstanding problems in psychiatric nomenclature and terminology and agreed on suggestions for a number of activities during the years to follow (World Health Organization, 1981).

First, the group agreed on the formulation of certain essential distinctions:

Psychiatric *terminology* comprises all the words used for psychiatric concepts. The systematic arrangement of such terms together with their definitions would form a dictionary or lexicon.

Psychiatric *nomenclature*, on the other hand, is a systematically arranged set of names of the various psychiatric diseases, syndromes, and other identifiable conditions. A nomenclature is an open-ended system of terms to which new names may be added as new diseases or syndromes are identified.

A *classification* is the arrangement of the names of diseases, syndromes, and other conditions according to specified rules that conform to defined principles. Most classifications are closed systems, in the sense that the total number of the major categories within which all existing entities must be subsumed, is a fixed one.

A psychiatric *glossary* is a list of selected words and terms with definitions and explanatory notes on the composition and uses of the categories and concepts included in the classification.

The group identified a number of major categories of problems and issues that need further attention and collaboration.

First, the lack of uniformity in the definition and use of key terms in clinical psychiatry is not just a problem of language, since even people who speak the same language use psychiatric terms differently.

Second, some psychiatric schools use concepts and terms that do not have readily available counterparts in other psychiatric traditions. One famous example is the concept behind the term *bouffée délirante*. To those who want to know which concept is hidden by this term, which has been so helpful to psychiatry in francophone countries, little help can be obtained by consulting an ordinary dictionary, which will merely translate the word *bouffée* as "gust of wind" or "puff of air." Closer study of the literature and the kind guidance of French colleagues make it clear that the concept behind the word has no equivalents in the terminologies of other schools. It is, nevertheless, necessary to understand this concept.

A further difficulty arises from the fact that many terms used by psychiatrists are derived directly from popular language but gradually acquire a specific professional meaning. Correct translation of psychiatric terms can, therefore, be made only by translators who are familiar with psychiatric concepts.

Another problem is that certain psychiatric syndromes appear only in particular culture groups in which these syndromes have special names. These names cannot readily be translated into ordinary psychiatric terms, and some of the syndromes are so specific that they do not fit into any class in existing international classifications. A nomenclature and a glossary of culture-bound psychiatric disorders are thus very much needed.

Some terms that belong to popular language also have a tendency to creep in among professional people who are not particularly interested in classification and terminology. Examples of these terms are depression, breakdown, and crisis. Therefore, a question to be resolved is whether such terms should be used at all in professional technical language. They tend to be used by nonpsychiatrists in particular, who for some reason see psychiatric patients; for instance, neurologists have been known to invent such terms as "slow cerebration," an expression that is an insult to all bearers of this maximally organized and refined organ.

A special type of terminology seems to appeal to many professional people. One derives from the habit of attaching people's names to certain syndromes. Even if such names do not say anything about the nature of the disorder, they seem to stick to them forever, especially if the names are French. A French name seems to draw attention to the syndromes in question, with the result that they appear in the literature much more frequently than their true incidence could possible entitle them to. Examples of these names are Gilles de la Tourette, Capgras, and the like. Some such nominal designations can be directly misleading, for instance when, as has happened recently, the name "Briquet" came to be attached to a certain subtype of hysteria, without regard to the fact that a hundred years ago Briquet wrote a classic work on hysteria describing *all* types of hysteric disorders. Another example involves the attachment of the name of Baron Münchhausen to a certain type of factitious disorder arising in individuals with personalities very different from that of the historical person who carried the name. In addition, this name is invariably misspelled in the psychiatric literature. The history of psychiatric terminology is full of similar tragedies.

The scientific working group on standardization of nomenclature and terminology in the mental-health field made a number of recommendations to WHO and the steering committee of the joint program. Among these was the suggestion to set up a *lexicology task force*. This task force includes Erik Essen-Möller, Michael Shepherd, and Erik Strömgren.

The work of this group has included several steps. The first was a consequence of the fact that the glossary of ICD, ninth edition, was incomplete. Not all terms used in ICD-9 appeared in the glossary, and the remaining terms would have to be defined. Next, during the preparatory work for ICD-10, it would be necessary to provide definitions of all terms suggested for this edition.

Finally, it should be a goal to create a comprehensive lexicon of psychiatric terms, including those of importance for psychiatry from adjacent fields. This lexicon would have a different scope from that guiding existing psychiatric dictionaries. Whereas such dictionaries have been created primarily for professionals in the country in which the lexicon was authored, the WHO lexicon would be intended for all users of ICD, regardless of their country or psychiatric school. It should serve the purpose of creating a truly international psychiatric language.

The lexicon group started work in 1980. First, a number of terms relevant to ICD-9 were defined and discussed at meetings. Next, Michael Shepherd, with the assistance of the WHO's Division of Mental Health, collected a lexicon draft (World Health Organization, 1983). The preface of this draft states that "the definitions are intended to be neither encyclopedic nor operational. They are essentially a set of explanatory notes on the various categories and concepts employed in chapter V of ICD-9, designed to facilitate the use of the earlier group of terms by providing definitions, synonyms, and cross-references."

The draft contains more than two hundred items, some of which are, however, just cross-references. All terms are translated into Arabic, Chinese, French, Russian, and Spanish.

The draft was sent to a great number of experts in different countries for comments. About 75 responses, some very extensive, were obtained. Within the Division of Mental Health these comments were edited by J. van Drimmelen. The result was a volume of several hundred pages containing a wealth of information. There were comments referring to many of the items included in the draft. In addition, many general viewpoints were expressed concerning the desirable structure and content of the lexicon.

In conclusion, I present an enumeration of some of the ingredients that appear appropriate for inclusion in the lexicon:

1. The lexicon should define all terms mentioned in ICD-9.
2. All terms from DSM-III should be included, and it should be stated on which points the definitions of these terms may differ from identical or similar terms in ICD.
3. Terms from current classifications in wide use in different countries should be included and defined.
4. Also to be considered are terms from special schools of psychiatry and related disciplines, among them the psychoanalytic world of concepts and terms.
5. Relevant terms in popular language, including designations of culture-bound syndromes, should be candidates for inclusion.

In all cases, the relationship of such concepts and terms to those used in the ICD should be described and discussed, and it should be indicated why the ICD-terms are preferred. The use of especially ambiguous, controversial, or misused terms should be discouraged.

During this work, the editors of the lexicon had to comply with a set of general rules determined by the WHO Technical Terminology Service in cooperation with the Council of the International Organization of Medical Societies (CIOMS). These guidelines are of great value for the editors but, naturally, also imply some restrictions.

REFERENCES

World Health Organization. 1981. *Current State of Diagnosis and Classification in the Mental Health Field.* A report from the WHO/ADAMHA joint project on diagnosis and classification of mental disorders and alcohol- and drug-related problems. Geneva.

World Health Organization. 1983. *Lexicon of Psychiatric and Mental Health Terms. Diagnosis and Classification of Mental Disorders and Alcohol- and Drug-Related Problems.* Geneva.

World Health Organization. 1985. *Mental Disorders; Alcohol- and Drug-Related Problems: International Perspectives on Their Diagnosis and Classification.* International Congress Series 669. Amsterdam: Excerpta Medica.

18 AMDP in multiaxial classification

R.-D. STIEGLITZ, E. FÄHNDRICH, AND
HANFRIED HELMCHEN (Federal Republic of Germany)

INTRODUCTION

The concept of psychiatric multiaxial diagnostics has a long tradition beginning with the work of Essen-Möller and Wohlfahrt (1947), although this basic idea can already be detected in classical German psychopathology (Helmchen, 1983).

According to Mezzich (1979) a multiaxial diagnostic model includes the systematic formulation of patients' characteristics in the form of different variables, aspects, or so-called axes. These variables are supposed to reveal significant clinical information and be independent of one another. Therefore, the goal of multiaxial diagnostics is an explicit, systematic, and mutually independent record of data about various aspects of the patient (Helmchen, 1983).

Although one can find various alternative terms for the concept "multiaxial" in the literature (see Mezzich, 1983) and various problems are connected with this in regard to both language and content (Berner and Katschnig, 1983), the concept has gained acceptance.

A total of 15 multiaxial systems can be differentiated today (see Mezzich, 1985), which differ particularly in regard to the number of axes used. The individual axes can be subsumed mainly under the areas of phenomenology, etiology, time, and "adaptive functioning" (Mezzich, 1979). The majority of the approaches contain five axes, and some systems also include subaxes. Corresponding to the scaling, one can differentiate between typological or categorial and dimensional axes, and in most cases one finds a mixed model containing both types of axes (Mezzich, 1979).

According to Mezzich, Fabrega, and Mezzich (1985), the various multiaxial approaches all purport to describe clinically significant factors comprehensively and make them useful for various purposes (e.g., clinical description, treatment, prognosis, research). The following are the main arguments given in the literature for developing multiaxial diagnostics (see Helmchen, 1980, 1983; Mezzich et al., 1985; Mezzich, 1983; Kendell, 1984):

1. Diagnoses in the traditional sense implicitly consist of various elements representing different aspects of the psychic disorder.

180

2. A multiaxial classification reflects the complexity of psychiatric diagnosis better, that is, more explicitly.
3. A multiaxial classification corresponds more closely to the assumptions of a multiconditional etiopathogenesis.
4. Clinically more significant information is contained in a multiaxial diagnosis than in individual diagnostic categories.
5. Contamination of observable symptomatology and of hypothetical assumptions about etiology is prevented.
6. It is possible to examine individual aspects empirically (including their reliability).
7. The prediction of specific outcome criteria can be improved.
8. One can make falsifiable hypotheses about causal relationships.
9. It is possible to design new nosological constellations.

However, one must not forget the educational value of such a classificatory system in the area of training (Helmchen, 1980).

In establishing the number of axes, Spitzer and Forman (1979) remind us that a system should be limited to a small number of axes if it is to be useful and applicable. According to previously defined information, this number of axes should represent a maximum of clinical usefulness for the largest possible number of cases. The establishment and selection of the number of axes for a multiaxial system are critical steps as they always constitute a compromise between the need for a comprehensive description and the demand for parsimony and simplicity (Mezzich, 1979, 1983).

A survey of 175 experts from different countries that was carried out by Mezzich et al. (1985) showed that 83 percent of the sample had had experience with multiaxial concepts, and 67 percent of this group found them to be highly useful. The critical point for the acceptance of a multiaxial system by clinicians will be found in the empirical evidence that the descriptive and predictive validity as well as the practicability is better than the traditional procedure involved in making a diagnosis (Helmchen, 1983).

In the following sections we present our own views about multiaxial diagnostics and studies concerning it using the AMDP-system. First, we briefly discuss the AMDP-system as described in previous studies. The axes that we designed from the AMDP-system are also introduced, along with information from validation studies on these axes.

THE AMDP-SYSTEM

The AMDP-system (Association for Methodology and Documentation in Psychiatry, 1979; Baumann and Stieglitz, 1983; Bobon et al., 1983; Guy and Ban, 1982) is a documentation system that contains predominantly general information and data recorded using ratings at the start of treatment. Through repeated use, one can also illustrate, for example, the course of the treatment.

The system consists of the following parts, ready for electronic data processing:

1. Anamnesis – demographic data (e.g., education, level of employment)
2. Anamnesis – life events (e.g., death of spouse/partner, shop/business defunct)
3. Anamnesis – psychiatric history (e.g., birth and childhood, previous psychiatric episodes)
4. Psychopathological symptoms (100 items) (e.g., incoherence, delusional ideas, depressed mood)
5. Somatic Signs (40 items) (e.g., interrupted sleep, nausea, dizziness).

All available objective and subjective information is used in rating the individual symptoms. These data are collected in an open interview with no time limit. If a symptom is considered to be present, then the rater is required to quantify the characteristic ("mild," "moderate," or "severe").

A manual with explanations of the anamnestic sheets and definitions of the psychopathological symptoms and somatic signs is available as an aid to the user. There are numerous translations (e.g., French, English, Japanese) available both in Europe and elsewhere. Besides the standard version, there are some documentation sheets comparable to the AMDP-system in their formal structure, which can be used for further documentation (e.g., documentation of EEG findings, documentation of suicide attempts, documentation for epilepsy, gerontopsychiatry).

Many evaluation studies, as well as studies concerning reliability and validity (see, Baumann and Stieglitz, 1983), show the AMDP-system to be a practicable documentation system, the application of which is not limited to the psychiatric area only (e.g., examinations of cardiac patients; see Baumann and Stieglitz, 1983).

In particular, the formation of syndromes (e.g., paranoid-hallucinatory syndrome, manic syndrome, depressive syndrome) by means of mathematic-statistical approaches can be regarded as an advantage of an economical description of the psychopathology. Empirical studies stress the reliability and validity of these syndrome scales as well (Gebhardt et al., 1983; Pietzcker et al., 1983; Gebhardt & Pietzcker, 1983). Whereas the AMDP-system was previously used primarily for documentation, especially in studies of psychopharmacologic drugs, the next step should be to make it useful for diagnostic purposes. The following studies concerning multiaxial diagnostics represent the first attempts in this direction.

MULTIAXIAL CLASSIFICATION WITH THE AMDP-SYSTEM

In accordance with analyses of existing multiaxial systems (see Mezzich, 1979, 1983), the areas of symptomatology, etiology, and time are frequently illustrated in individual axes. Since statements are also made about these areas in the AMDP-system, these axes were first defined a priori and then the various items assigned to them were identified. To be more precise, one can subdivide the procedure involved, with regard to contents and methods, into three steps:

1. Definition of the axes from the anamnestic sheets (Parts 1–3) as well as from the psychopathological symptoms and somatic signs (Parts 4 and 5)
   Axis 1: symptomatology
   Axis 2: etiology
   Axis 3: time
2. Validation of these axes regarding their capacity to make descriptive differentiations (criterion: ICD-diagnoses)
3. Validation of these axes with respect to their predictive power (criteria: length of hospital stay, positive change in psychopathology, and assessment of the success of treatment)

Consider the individual axes.

Axis I: symptomatology. Table 18.1 contains the seven syndromes subsumed under this axis, consisting of items from the psychopathological symptoms and somatic signs (Parts 4 and 5). Gebhardt et al. (1983) obtained these syndromes using factor analytic procedures with two independent samples. The syndromes have satisfactory reliabilities (internal consistency; Cronbach $\alpha = .65 - .86$), show slight intercorrelations ($r = .04 - .37$), and permit a satisfactory division of clinical groups diagnosed according to ICD-9 (discriminant analysis; see Gebhardt and Pietzcker, 1983).

Axis II: etiology. Table 18.1 also contains 11 etiologically relevant items from the anamnestic sheets 3 and 4, such as somatic or psychological problems present during the three weeks preceding the onset of the present illness, life events, family psychiatric history, birth and childhood, and suspected precipitating factors.

Axis III: time. Eleven items from anamnestic sheet 3 are included among the temporal aspects (see Table 18.1). The data here include the course of illness, psychiatric episodes, the duration of the present episode, and suicide attempts.

Like most other multiaxial systems, this is a mixed model, that is, a combination of typological and dimensional axes. Note the larger number of subaxes in comparison with previously published multiaxial approaches. As these are the first analyses with the AMDP-system, we consider this procedure appropriate at present. Empirical studies have yet to show whether it is wise to reduce the number of subaxes.

VALIDATION STUDIES

Sample

The sample underlying the following empirical analyses comprises 1,107 inpatients of the Psychiatric Clinic of the Free University of Berlin (West) from 1983 and 1984 (discharges in the years 1983 and 1984).

Table 18.2 displays the age distribution. The mean age is 42.6 years ($s = 16.7$; median: 39.3; mode: 28). More women (639) are represented in the sample than men (468): $\chi^2 = 26.41$, $df = 1$, $p < .01$.

Table 18.1. *Axes of the AMDP-system*

Axis I, symptomatology[a]	Axis II, etiology	Axis III, time

Paranoid-hallucinatory syndrome (PARHAL)	22[b] Precipitating factors
	    answered by patient
	    answered by psychiatrist
	    divergency between patient and
	        psychiatrist
		24 Present illness
		    First manifestation
		    Age at first manifestation

Psychoorganic syndrome (PSYORG)	23 Life events	25 Characteristics of previous illness
		    Course since first manifestation
		    Intermittent or chronic
		    Full or partial remission

Manic syndrome (MANI)	23 Other current illnesses	Severity (increased, decreased, constant, or fluctuating)

Depressive syndrome (DEPRES)	26 Present episode
	    Somatic problems
	    Psychological problems
		Changes in symptomatology

Hostility syndrome (HOST)	27 Birth and childhood
	    Pathological pregnancy and/or birth
	    Motor and/or speech delay
	    Childhood neurotic symptoms
		26 Present episode
		    Duration of present episode

Apathy syndrome (APA)	28 Family psychiatric history	31 Suicide attempts (patient)
		    The number of confirmed attempts
		    The time in relation to the
		        present admission

Autonomic syndrome (AUT)		32 Previous psychiatric episodes
		33 Number of previous psychiatric admissions

[a] Syndromes of Gebhardt et al. (1983), Pietzcker et al. (1983).
[b] Item number (see Association for Documentation and Methodology in Psychiatry, 1979; Guy & Ban, 1982)

Table 18.2. *Age distribution of the total sample (N = 1107)*

Age	f	f%
under 20	36	3.3
20–29	247	22.3
30–39	276	24.9
40–49	219	19.8
50–59	118	10.7
60–69	98	8.9
70–79	99	8.9
80–89	12	1.1
90–99	2	.2

Note: Mean = 42.6; mode = 28; median = 39.3; s = 16.7.

Table 18.3. *Final diagnosis (ICD-9) of the total sample (N = 1107)*

ICD-9	f	f%
290–294	91	8.2
295	407	36.8
296	227	20.5
297	40	3.6
298	5	0.5
299	1	0.1
300	153	13.8
301–316	148	13.4
317–319	1	0.1
Others	34	3.0

The distribution according to diagnoses (ICD-9; World Health Organization, 1978) is presented in Table 18.3. The schizophrenic psychoses represent the most frequent diagnostic group (ICD 295, N = 407), followed by affective psychoses (ICD 296, N = 227) and neurotic disorders (ICD 300, N = 153). The numerically largest subgroups are schizophrenic psychoses of the paranoid type (ICD 295.3, N = 264), manic-depressive psychoses of the depressed type (ICD 296.1, N = 134), and neurotic depressions (ICD 300.4, N = 89).

Descriptive validity

By descriptive validity we mean that aspect of validity that allows statements to be made about whether the chosen subsection (here, axes and corresponding subaxes) is relevant for illustrating the intended object. Since customary psychiatric diagnoses contain at least the three axes that we have proposed (symptomatology, etiology, and time), ICD-diagnoses are chosen as criteria, and the relationships between the axes or the subaxes and ICD-diagnoses are explored.

To carry out the comparison between the internally homogeneous groups, we selected the three numerically largest ICD-groups: 295.3 (schizophrenic psychosis paranoid form, N = 264); 296.1 (manic-depressive psychosis depressed type, N = 134); and 300.4 (neurotic depression, N = 89).

Axis I: symptomatology

COMPARISONS OF MEANS. In comparing the ICD-diagnoses 295.3, 296.1, and 300.4, we computed one-way analyses of variance and subsequent Scheffé-tests (McNemar, 1969) for the admission data. The statistical analyses were performed using the SPSS procedures, "Oneway," "Discriminant," "Crosstabs," and "Regression" (Nie et al., 1975).

The results are summarized in Table 18.4, which shows that the three diagnostic groups differ significantly in all seven syndromes ($F(2, 484)$, $p < .01$). In addition, the subsequently selected contrasts show that the significant differences between the groups lie in the expected direction. For example, ICD 295.3 differs from the other two groups particularly in the prominence of the paranoid-hallucinatory syndrome, the autonomic syndrome, and the hostility syndrome. ICD 296.1 differs from the others in the prominence of the depressive and apathy syndromes. Seen as a whole, the differences between ICD 296.1 and 300.4 are less striking than those between ICD 296.1 or 300.4 and 295.3.

Figure 18.1 displays these results graphically. The ICD-groups 296.1 and 300.4 have profiles of a relatively similar shape ($r_s = .86$, $p < .05$). They are clearly different from that of group 295.3 ($r_s = -.67$ and $-.53$, respectively, $p > .05$). These contrasts are particularly conspicuous with regard to the paranoid-hallucinatory, depressive, autonomic, manic, and hostility syndromes.

DISCRIMINANT ANALYSES. Discriminant analyses for the multivariate separation of diagnostically relevant groups can provide further statements about the validity of the subaxes of axis I, "symptomatology" (Table 18.5). Here the ICD-groups 295.3, 296.1, and 300.4 were also selected. The samples were randomly divided in half for these computations. The computation of the first discriminant analysis was made on the first random split-half (analysis sample). The classification was cross-validated on the second random split-half (validation sample). A second discriminant analysis was subsequently computed on the second random split-half and validated on the first random split-half. Two significant discriminant factors emerged in both samples. The proportions of variance accounted for by the first factor in the two samples were 91 percent and 88 percent, respectively, and in the second sample 9 percent and 12 percent, respectively. Consequently, the first discriminant factor was the one that contributed most to the separation of the three groups.

Table 18.4. *One-way analysis of variance and selected contrasts (Scheffé tests) of the ICD-9 diagnostic groups 295.3, 296.1, and 300.4, on Axis I (symptomatology) subaxes*

Axis I subaxes	Means at admission (T-scores)			$F (2,484)$	p	Scheffé tests $(p < .05)$
	295.3 (N = 264)	296.1 (N = 134)	300.4 (N = 89)			
Paranoid-hallucinatory syndrome	61.8	47.9	43.4	217.3	≤.01	295.3 > 296.1 > 300.4
Psychoorganic syndrome	49.1	50.3	45.0	11.4	≤.01	295.3 = 296.1 > 300.4
Manic syndrome	52.8	49.2	47.6	13.4	≤.01	295.3 > 296.1 = 300.4
Depressive syndrome	49.4	59.8	56.1	90.2	≤.01	296.1 > 300.4 > 295.3
Hostility syndrome	54.8	49.9	48.0	25.6	≤.01	295.3 > 296.1 = 300.4
Apathy syndrome	52.5	56.5	51.3	12.5	≤.01	296.1 > 295.3 = 300.4
Autonomic syndrome	46.6	52.3	52.8	25.3	≤.01	296.1 = 300.4 > 295.3

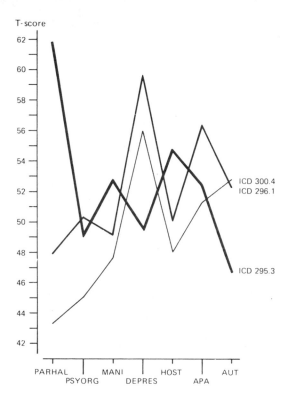

Figure 18.1. Syndrome profiles of schizophrenic psychosis, paranoid type (ICD 295.3; N = 264), manic-depressive psychosis, depressed type (ICD 296.1; N = 134) and neurotic depression (ICD 300.4; N = 89)

In the first as in the second random split-halves, the first discriminant function (standardized discriminant function coefficients > .50) is characterized by the paranoid-hallucinatory syndrome (.81 and .75, respectively) and by the depressive syndrome (− .53 and − .63, respectively).

The second discriminant function is characterized in both random split-halves by the depressive syndrome (.62 and .56, respectively) and by the apathy syndrome (.53 and .51, respectively).

These analyses led to the correct classification of 70 percent and 75 percent of the patients, respectively. These figures are somewhat lower than, but within the same order of magnitude as, the findings in the study carried out by Gebhardt and Pietzcker (1983).

In both analyses the best correspondence was shown for the ICD-group 295.3 (87.8 percent and 85.6 percent) and the poorest for 300.4 (44.7 percent and 63.0 percent), whereby – as can be expected from the profiles of means – "mix-ups" with the 296.1 group are most apt to be obtained.

Seen as a whole, the results in this section indicate the considerable capacity

Table 18.5. *Discriminant analyses for classification of cases*

Actual group	Predicted group			
	295.3	296.1	300.4	Σ
A. First discriminate analysis				
Analysis sample, 1st random split-half				
295.3	101 (87.8%)	8	6	115
296.1	14	41 (58.6%)	15	70
Validation sample, 2nd random split-half				
300.4	2	24	21 (44.7%)	47
Σ	117	73	42	232
Correctly classified: 70%				
B. Second discriminate analysis				
Analysis sample, 2nd random split-half				
295.3	119 (85.6%)	14	6	139
296.1	6	40 (60.6%)	20	66
Validation sample, 1st random split-half				
300.4	1	16	29 (63.0%)	46
Σ	126	70	55	251
Correctly classified: 75%				

Note: Variables: subaxes of Axis I, symptomatology. Groups: ICD diagnostic groups 295.3, 296.1, and 300.4.

Table 18.6. *Comparison of frequencies of the ICD-9 diagnostic groups 295.3, 296.1, 300.4, on the subaxes of Axis II, etiology*

Axis II subaxes	Percentage present			χ^2 (df = 2)	p
	295.3 (N = 264)	296.1 (N = 134)	300.4 (N = 189)		
Life events (in recent years)	69.8	50.4	81.3	22.3	≤.01
Other current illnesses	32.9	31.1	48.0	6.8	≤.05
Family psychiatric history (illnesses among family members)	14.0	23.5	21.3	5.5	≤.10
Precipitating factors patient	49.5	50.4	85.3	31.5	≤.01
Precipitating factors psychiatrist	67.1	68.9	90.7	16.1	≤.01
Precipitating factors: divergency between patient and psychiatrist	69.4	72.3	90.2	13.5	≤.01
Somatic problems	9.3	17.9	15.9	4.8	≤.10
Psychological problems	42.6	46.2	67.6	12.6	≤.01
Pathological pregnancy and/or birth	10.2	3.2	13.8	6.2	≤.05
Motor and/or speech delay	7.4	2.1	6.2	3.3	>.10
Childhood neurotic symptoms	21.1	8.5	25.0	8.9	≤.01

of the subaxes of axis I "symptomatology" for differentiating among the ICD-diagnostic groups 295.3, 296.1, and 300.4.

Axis II: etiology

COMPARISONS OF FREQUENCIES. To examine the descriptive significance of the individual subaxes of axis II, "etiology," we set up contingency tables between the dichotomous subaxes and the ICD-diagnostic groups 295.3, 296.1, and 300.4. In addition, the differences in frequency were computed using χ^2 (see Siegel, 1956).

Table 18.6 presents the results. The following differences became apparent (χ^2 at $p \leq .10$):

1. Paranoid schizophrenics and neurotic depressives more frequently had problems from current life events than endogenous depressives did.

2. Neurotic depressives suffered from additional current illnesses (e.g., chronic somatic illnesses) more frequently than endogenous depressives and paranoid schizophrenics did.
3. Neurotic depressives had a higher frequency of precipitating factors (by self-report and by rating) than the other two groups.
4. The difference of opinion between physician and patient with respect to the kind of precipitating factors were greater in the group of neurotic depressives than in the groups of endogenous depressives and paranoid schizophrenics.
5. Somatic problems before the onset of illness and a psychiatric history in the family were more frequently present in endogenous and neurotic depressives than in paranoid schizophrenics.
6. For neurotic depressives, psychological problems were also more frequently present.
7. Paranoid schizophrenics and neurotic depressives reported previous psychic disorders more frequently (pathological pregnancy and/or birth, childhood neurotic symptoms) than endogenous depressives did.

COMPARISONS OF MEANS. In addition, one-way analyses of variance and subsequent Scheffé tests were computed for some subaxes, when the level of measurement made this possible. Table 18.7 summarizes the results. These are in line with the χ^2 results. The neurotic depressives were the highest group in current life events and in current illnesses. Furthermore, neurotic depressives again obtained higher ratings in precipitating factors, and in divergency with regard to the kind of precipitant.

Axis III: time

COMPARISONS OF FREQUENCY. The results regarding the comparisons of frequency for axis III "time" are summarized in Table 18.8. Differences appear in the following subaxes (χ^2 at $p \leq .05$):

1. More neurotic depressives and paranoid schizophrenics exhibited a chronic course than endogenous depressives did.
2. More endogenous depressives had a full remission, whereas more paranoid schizophrenics and neurotic depressives had a partial remission.
3. More paranoid schizophrenics and endogenous depressives showed a change in symptomatology than neurotic depressives did.
4. The duration of the present episode was shorter in paranoid schizophrenics than in patients of the other two groups.
5. More neurotic depressives had attempted suicide than patients of the other two groups.
6. A suicide attempt was apt to lie further in the past for more paranoid schizophrenics compared with the endogenous or neurotic depressives.

No significant differences appeared for the subaxes "severity since first manifestation" and "first manifestation."

Table 18.7. One-way analysis of variance and selected contrasts (Scheffé tests) of the ICD-9 diagnostic groups 295.3, 296.1, and 300.4 on Axis II (etiology) subaxes

| Axis II subaxes | Means | | | F (2,484) | p | Scheffé tests ($p < .05$) |
	295.3 (N = 264)	296.1 (N = 134)	300.4 (N = 89)			
Life events (in recent years)	2.0	1.1	2.8	21.0	≤.01	300.4 > 295.3 > 296.1
Other current illnesses	.4	.4	.8	7.6	≤.01	300.4 > 295.3 = 296.1
Precipitating factors: patient	.9	.9	2.0	27.1	≤.01	300.4 > 295.3 = 296.1
Precipitating factors: psychiatrist	1.3	1.3	2.4	27.8	≤.01	300.4 > 295.3 = 296.1
Precipitating factors: divergency between patient and psychiatrist	2.0	2.0	3.8	33.6	≤.01	300.4 > 295.3 = 296.1

Table 18.8. *Comparison of frequencies of the ICD-9 diagnostic groups 295.3, 296.1, 300.4, on subaxes of Axis III (time)*

| Axis III subaxes | Percentage present | | | χ^2 | df | p |
	295.3 (N = 264)	296.1 (N = 134)	300.4 (N = 89)			
First manifestation	23.6	19.7	30.3	3.3	2	>.10
Course of illness						
Intermittent	40.5	40.2	32.9	10.2	4	≤.05
Chronic	18.2	8.2	22.4			
Type of remission						
Full remission	25.6	49.2	18.4	31.2	4	≤.01
Partial remission	34.3	18.0	28.9			
Severity since first manifestation						
Increased	22.8	19.8	23.3			
Decreased	22.3	31.1	21.1	5.9	6	>.10
Constant	3.7	1.6	2.6			
Fluctuating	21.1	22.1	19.7			
Change in symptomatology	20.3	14.0	8.2	6.4	2	≤.05
Duration present episode						
About 1 month	59.9	30.4	30.8	29.2	4	≤.01
Over 1 month	39.5	69.6	69.2			
Suicide attempts	33.5	32.0	51.3	9.3	2	≤.01
Most recent attempt						
About 6 months	8.2	16.4	26.0	21.3	4	≤.01
Over 6 months	17.8	12.1	23.3			

COMPARISONS OF MEANS. One-way analyses of variance and Scheffé tests were performed for a few subaxes (Table 18.9) in the time domain. Here it became apparent

1. That endogenous depressives were the oldest and the paranoid schizophrenics the youngest of the groups at the time of first manifestation
2. That paranoid schizophrenics and endogenous depressives listed more definable manifestations and admissions to psychiatric wards than neurotic depressives did.

Summary. The above results yielded no surprises. They reflect, however, the experience and findings of psychiatric research and practice (e.g., the relationship between age and first manifestation) and thus have considerable descriptive validity for the subaxes (and therefore for the three axes) with respect to the ICD-9 reference criterion.

Table 18.9. *One-way analysis of variance and selected contrasts (Scheffé tests) of the ICD-9 diagnostic groups 295.3, 296.1, and 300.4 on Axis III (time) subaxes*

Axis III subaxes	Means at admission			F (2,484)	p	Scheffé tests (p ≤.05)
	295.3 (N = 264)	296.1 (N = 134)	300.4 (N = 89)			
Age at first manifestation	27.9	48.1	34.4	95.5	≤.01	296.1 > 300.4 > 295.3
Previous psychiatric episodes	3.8	4.0	1.9	7.9	≤.01	295.3 = 296.1 > 300.4
Number of previous psychiatric admissions	4.0	3.0	1.6	15.2	≤.01	295.3 > 296.1 > 300.4

Predictive validity

The relevance of a multiaxial diagnostic system becomes particularly apparent to the extent to which it allows the formulation of successful predictions (predictive or prognostic validity). The predictive validity of the axes was examined in relation to the following criteria:

1. Length of hospital stay, i.e., the number of days spent as inpatients from admission until discharge
2. Positive change in psychopathology (difference between admission and discharge data in the syndrome scores)
3. Assessment of success of inpatient treatment on the basis of the dimensions on symptomatology, achievement ability, social situation, social behavior and subjective feeling of well-being

Multiple regressions were computed with the stepwise inclusion of the AMDP-subaxes to determine their combined predictive power in regard to these three criteria. Using the multiple correlation technique, it is possible to examine relationships between several predictor variables and a single criterion variable.

The multiple correlation coefficient (R) represents the correlation between the predicted and the actual criterion scores. The multiple R square reflects the proportion of variance explained by the variables entered in the regression equation.

The significance of the individual predictor variables for predicting the criterion emerges from the standardized regression coefficients (Beta). The computations were first carried out separately for the axes "symptomatology," "etiology," and "time" and then for all three axes together. The obtained regression equations were statistically significant (F test; $p \le .05$).

Criterion "length of hospital stay." As can be gathered from Table 18.10, the multiple correlations (R) for individual axes fall between .19 and .29, when the statistically significant predictors ($p \le .05$) are taken into consideration.

AXIS I: symptomatology. Of the subaxes, the depressive, the apathy, the manic, and the paranoid-hallucinatory syndromes proved to be relevant for prediction. High values in these syndromes at admission point to a longer hospital stay.

AXIS II: etiology. Only 2 of the 11 subaxes here proved to be significant. An absence of psychological problems before clinic admission and a slighter incidence of stressful life events before the onset of illness are predictive of a longer hospital stay.

AXIS III: time. Three of the 11 axes here proved to be relevant. Older age at the time of the first manifestation, only partial remission, and absence of a recent suicide attempt were predictive of a longer clinic stay.

Table 18.10. *Stepwise multiple regression to predict length of hospital stay*

Predictors studied	Multiple R	Significant predictors ($p \leq .05$)	F to enter	p	Beta[a]
Axis I, symptoma- tology	.29	Depressive syndrome	58.4	≤.01	.17
		Apathy syndrome	23.2	≤.01	.14
		Manic syndrome	10.6	≤.01	.08
		Paranoid-hallucinatory syndrome	7.1	≤.05	.08
Axis II, etiology	.19	Life events (in recent years)	14.3	≤.01	−.14
		Psychological problems	8.5	≤.01	−.12
Axis III, time	.20	Age at first manifestation	5.9	≤.01	.13
		Most recent suicide attempt: under 1 month	5.7	≤.01	−.11
		Partial remission	4.6	≤.05	.11
Axes I to III Axis III	.44	Depressive syndrome	48.2	≤.01	.35
		Most recent suicide attempt: under 1 month	10.1	≤.01	−.14
		Psychoorganic syndrome	7.9	≤.01	.11
		Partial remission	5.3	≤.05	.12
		Age at first manifestation	6.7	≤.01	.13
		Psychological problems	5.4	≤.05	−.11

[a]Standardized regression coefficient.

ALL THREE AXES. If one includes all three axes in the analysis, the multiple correlation increases markedly ($R = .44$) as long as only the significant predictors are taken into consideration ($p \leq .05$).

A pronounced depressive and psychoorganic syndrome, a previous partial remission, older age at the time of first manifestation, the absence of a recent suicide attempt, and the absence of psychological problems were predictive of a longer clinic stay.

Criterion "positive change in psychopathology." The regression computation for Axis I must be omitted at this point, because the extent of positive change in psychopathology is determined on the basis of the difference between admission and discharge scored for the syndromes of Axis I.

AXIS II: etiology. Of the 11 subaxes, only one or two proved to be significant (see Table 18.11). When the statistically significant predictors were taken into account, the multiple correlations fell between .10 (psychoorganic

Table 18.11. *Stepwise multiple regression for predicting positive change in psychopathology with Axis II subaxes*

Reference syndromes	Multiple R	Significant predictors from Axis II (p ≤ .05)	F to enter	p	Beta[a]
Paranoid-hallucinatory syndrome	.14	Precipitating factors: divergency between patient and psychiatrist	3.9	≤.05	−.11
		Childhood neurotic symptoms	3.9	≤.05	.10
Depressive syndrome	.16	Childhood neurotic symptoms	6.5	≤.01	−.11
		Precipitating factors: psychiatrist	3.6	≤.05	−.09
Apathy syndrome	.16	Other current illnesses	6.8	≤.01	−.13
		Childhood neurotic symptoms	3.7	≤.05	−.10
Hostility syndrome	.19	Precipitating factors: psychiatrist	14.1	≤.01	−.19
Manic syndrome	.17	Precipitating factors: psychiatrist	11.1	≤.01	−.17
Psychoorganic syndrome	.10	Precipitating factors: psychiatrist	4.1	≤.05	−.10
Autonomic syndrome	—	—			—

— No significant regression equation.
[a]Standardized regression coefficient.

syndrome) and .19 (hostility syndrome). No significant predictors could be established for the *autonomic syndrome*. When the differences of opinion between physician and patient regarding suspected precipitating factors were less and childhood neurotic symptoms were present, the *paranoid-hallucinatory syndrome* decreased more intensely (R = .14). When there were no childhood neurotic symptoms and fewer suspected precipitating factors were reported by the physician, the *depressive syndrome* decreased more intensely (R = .16). When there were fewer other current illnesses and no childhood neurotic symptoms, the *apathy syndrome* decreased more intensely (R = .16). The fewer suspected precipitating factors reported by the physician, the greater was the decrease in the *hostility syndrome* (R = .19), the *manic syndrome* (R = .17) and the *psychoorganic syndrome* (R = .10).

AXIS III: time. When the significant predictors were taken into consideration, the multiple correlations fell between .15 (psychoorganic syndrome) and .31 (paranoid-hallucinatory syndrome). Of the 11 subaxes, between 2 and 6 proved to be significant (see Table 18.12). No significant predictors could be determined for the *autonomic syndrome*, which was also the case for the axis "etiology."

Table 18.12. *Stepwise multiple regression for predicting positive change in psychopathology wih Axis III subaxes*

Reference syndromes	Multiple R	Significant predictors from Axis III (p ≤ .05)	F to enter	p	Beta[a]
Paranoid-hallucinatory syndrome	.31	Duration present episode	13.9	≤.01	− .17
		Chronic course	11.2	≤.01	− .17
		Age at 1st manifestation	10.5	≤.01	− .17
		First manifestation	3.6	≤.05	.10
Depressive syndrome	.18	Age at 1st manifestation	10.2	≤.01	.17
		Full remission	3.6	≤.05	.09
Apathy syndrome	.27	Most recent suicide attempt: 1–5 years	8.7	≤.01	.16
		Age at 1st manifestation	11.7	≤.01	.16
		Full remission	4.0	≤.05	.11
		Severity since 1st manifestation: decreased	5.0	≤.05	− .11
Hostility syndrome	.19	Full remission	10.3	≤.01	.13
		Number of psychiatric admissions	4.1	≤.05	.10
Manic syndrome	.30	Number of psychiatric admissions	11.8	≤.01	.13
		Most recent suicide attempt: 1–5 years	5.6	≤.05	− .12
		Most recent suicide attempt: under 1 month	3.8	≤.05	− .11
		Severity since 1st manifestation: fluctuating	4.4	≤.05	− .17
		Severity since 1st manifestation: increased	7.1	≤.01	− .15
		Previous psychiatric episodes	3.9	≤.05	.13
Psychoorganic syndrome	.15	Chronic course	4.4	≤.05	− .11
		Most recent suicide attempt: under 1 month	4.2	≤.05	.10
Autonomic syndrome	—	—	—		

— No significant regression equation.
[a]Standardized regression coefficient.

The *paranoid-hallucinatory syndrome* decreased more intensely ($R = .31$) when the duration between onset of illness and clinic admission was short, the age at first manifestation was low, there was no chronic course, and a first manifestation was present. When the age at first manifestation was greater and a full remission was present, the *depressive syndrome* decreased more intensely ($R = .18$). The *apathy syndrome* decreased more intensely ($R = .27$) when a suicide attempt took place further in the past, when the age at first manifestation was greater, a full remission occurred previously, and the severity of the illness did not decrease.

If a full remission occurred previously and the number of psychiatric admissions was greater, the *hostility syndrome* decreased more intensely ($R = .19$). The *manic* syndrome decreased more markedly ($R = .30$) when there was a greater number of psychiatric episodes and psychiatric admissions as well as an absence of suicide attempts occurring either more recently or further in the past and an absence of a fluctuating or an increasing degree of severity. The *psychoorganic syndrome* decreased more intensely ($R = .15$) when a suicide attempt occurred more recently and there was no chronic course.

THE TWO AXES. The multiple correlations increased when the subaxes of both axes were included, except in the case of paranoid-hallucinatory syndrome. No significant regression equation could be determined for the autonomic syndrome here either (see Table 18.13).

The *paranoid-hallucinatory syndrome* decreased more intensely ($R = .30$) when the duration between onset of illness and clinic admission was short, when the course was not chronic, and when the age at first manifestation was lower. When the age at first manifestation was greater and fewer suspected precipitating factors were reported by the physicians, the *depressive syndrome* decreased more intensely ($R = .21$). The *apathy syndrome* diminished more intensely ($R = .33$) when a suicide attempt occurred farther in the past, the age at first manifestation was greater, a full remission occurred previously, the number of current illnesses was smaller, and there was no change in the symptomatology and no decrease in the degree of severity since the first manifestation. The *hostility syndrome* decreased more ($R = .27$) when a full remission and a change in symptomatology occurred, there were fewer suspected precipitating factors reported by the physician, and the patient's age at first manifestation was lower. The *manic syndrome* diminished more ($R = .31$) when there were no suicide attempts occurring either more recently or farther in the past, there was no increase or constancy in the degree of severity of the illness since the first manifestation, fewer suspected precipitating factors were reported by the physician, and there was a greater number of psychiatric admissions. The *psychoorganic syndrome* decreased more ($R = .22$) when there was no partial remission, no psychological problems and no chronic course, and a suicide attempt occurred more recently.

Criterion "assessment of success." After treatment was terminated, an assessment of success was made for each patient using five global scales (symptomatology, achievement ability, social situation, social behavior, and subjective feeling of well-being). To examine the connection among the individual measures of success their intercorrelations were determined first and a principal-component analysis (main diagonal = 1) was conducted.

Table 18.13. *Stepwise multiple regression for predicting positive change in psychopathology wih Axis II and III subaxes*

Reference syndromes	Multiple R	Significant predictors (Axes II & III) ($p \leq .05$)	F to enter	p	Beta[a]
Paranoid-hallucinatory syndrome	.30	Duration present episode	13.5	≤.01	−.16
		Chronic course	10.5	≤.01	−.19
		Age at 1st manifestation	11.2	≤.01	−.17
Depressive syndrome	.21	Age at 1st manifestation	11.5	≤.01	.17
		Precipitating factors: psychiatrist	5.9	≤.05	−.12
Apathy syndrome	.33	Most recent suicide attempt: 1–5 years	8.4	≤.01	.17
		Age at 1st manifestation	11.0	≤.01	.16
		Other current illnesses	9.1	≤.01	−.15
		Severity since 1st manifestation: decreased	4.2	≤.05	−.09
		Full remission	3.8	≤.05	.11
		Change in symptomatology	4.4	≤.05	−.12
Hostility syndrome	.27	Precipitating factors: psychiatrist	14.3	≤.01	−.15
		Full remission	7.0	≤.01	.12
		Age at 1st manifestation	4.7	≤.05	−.11
		Change in symptomatology	3.7	≤.05	.10
Manic syndrome	.31	Precipitating factors: psychiatrist	11.2	≤.01	−.11
		Number of psychiatric admissions	6.8	≤.01	.19
		Most recent suicide attempt: 1–5 years	4.8	≤.05	−.12
		Severity since 1st manifestation: increased	4.0	≤.05	−.15
		Severity since 1st manifestation: constant	6.3	≤.01	−.15
		Most recent suicide attempt: under 1 month	4.4	≤.05	−.11
Psychoorganic syndrome	.22	Partial remission	4.5	≤.05	−.11
		Psychological problems	5.0	≤.05	−.13
		Most recent suicide attempt: under 1 month	5.1	≤.05	.12
		Chronic course	4.9	≤.05	−.11
Autonomic syndrome	—	—			—

— No significant regression equation.
[a]Standardized regression coefficient.

Table 18.14. *Stepwise multiple regression for predicting success at termination of treatment*

Predictors studied	Multiple R	Significant predictors ($p \leq .05$)	F to enter	p	Beta[a]
Axis I, symptom- atology	.13	Paranoid-hallucinatory syndrome	5.4	≤.05	.13
Axis II, etiology	.23	Motor and/or speech delay	7.2	≤.01	−.16
		Precipitating factors: psychiatrist	6.1	≤.05	−.14
		Pathological pregnancy and/or birth	4.1	≤.05	.11
Axis III, time	—	—			—
Axis I to Axis III	.33	Full remission	9.2	≤.01	.14
		Most recent suicide attempt: under 1 month	7.7	≤.01	.15
		Motor and/or speech delay	5.8	≤.05	−.14
		Paranoid-hallucinatory syndrome	5.8	≤.05	.12
		Most recent suicide attempt: 1/2–1 year	4.9	≤.05	−.12
		Precipitating factors: psychiatrist	4.3	≤.05	−.11

— No significant regression equation.
[a]Standardized regression coefficient.

Only one eigenvalue greater than 1 ($\lambda_1 = 3.11$) emerged, which explained 62.3 percent of the total variance.

On the first unrotated factor, four of the five scales exhibited a loading of $a_i > .80$ (scale "social situation," $a = .41$). Consequently, one can speak of a common factor in the success rating. Therefore it appears to be meaningful to determine a total value for "success rating."

AXIS I: symptomatology. Of the seven subaxes, only the paranoid-hallucinatory syndrome ($R = .13$) proved significant (cf. Table 18.14). The assessment of success upon termination of treatment was more positive when the initial scores were higher in this syndrome.

AXIS II: etiology. Of the 11 subaxes, 3 proved relevant. The success rating was more positive when there was no motoric retardation or slowness of speech, when pathological pregnancy or birth anamnesis was present, and when fewer suspected precipitating factors were reported by the physician.

AXIS III: time. No significant predictors could be determined from this axis.

ALL THREE AXES. Here too, the multiple correlation increased when the subaxes of all three axes were taken into account ($R = .33$). A more positive success rating was predicted by the presence of a full remission, a more recent suicide attempt, a pronounced paranoid-hallucinatory syndrome, as well as the absence of motoric retardation or slowness of speech, no suicide attempts farther in the past, and fewer suspected precipitating factors reported by the physician.

DISCUSSION AND PERSPECTIVES

Starting with the assignment of AMDP-items to axes on "symptomatology," "etiology," and "time," the descriptive validity of these axes was investigated by means of comparative frequency and discriminant analyses. Prognostic validity was determined in relation to criteria involving duration of hospital stay, positive change in psychopathology, and assessment of success upon termination of treatment.

The results show that the axes and subaxes we selected from the AMDP-system differentiated with reference to the ICD-diagnoses. One should note, however, that the ICD-diagnoses do not represent an optimal criterion. Furthermore, they contain the risk of circularity given that some of the subaxes also play a part in the formation of the ICD-diagnoses.

Seen as a whole, however, one can conclude that the axes appeared to have descriptive validity. They are independent of each other with regard to the rating process, since no nosological diagnoses were entered. The axes represent a compromise between simplicity and comprehensive description.

Prognostic validity was determined with regard to duration of hospital stay, positive change in psychopathology, and assessment of success. It became apparent

1. That, seen as a whole, the variance explained by regression computations for the individual axes was only partly satisfactory (up to 10 percent of the variance was explained)
2. That it is possible to predict more successfully when items of two or three axes are taken into consideration (up to 20 percent explained variance)
3. That the subaxes have varying significance for the individual criteria (differential prognostic validity)
4. That some subaxes were not significant for any of the criteria (e.g., family psychiatric history or somatic problems from Axis II, "etiology," and should possibly be eliminated, or drastically revised in their measurement)

Consequently, the results emphasize the necessity and practicability of a multiaxial procedure for predicting clinically relevant events. But the findings obtained with the aid of the AMDP-system need to be systematically replicated and supplemented with further criteria (e.g., response to medication) with such goals as reducing the number of subaxes. Furthermore, the content of the axes need to be clarified using multivariate methods (e.g., cluster analyses).

One should not lose sight of the main task in all of these studies on multiaxial diagnostics. The point is to improve diagnosis with the goal of providing the physician with clear instructions regarding prognosis and therapy.

REFERENCES

Association for Methodology and Documentation in Psychiatry. 1979. *Das AMDP-System. Manual zur Dokumentation psychiatrischer Befunde.* 3rd ed. Berlin: Springer.

Baumann, U., and Stieglitz, R.-D. 1983. *Testmanual zum AMDP-System. Empirische Studien zur Psychopathologie.* Herausgegeben von der Arbeitsgemeinschaft für Methodik und Dokumentation in der Psychiatrie (AMDP). Berlin: Springer.

Berner, P., and Katschnig, H. 1983. Principles of "multiaxial" classification in psychiatry as a basis of modern methodology. In *Methods in Evaluation of Psychiatric Treatment*, ed. T. Helgason, pp. 71–79. Cambridge: Cambridge University Press.

Bobon, D., Baumann, U., Angst, J., Helmchen H., and Hippius, H. (ed.). 1983. *The AMDP-System in Pharmacopsychiatry.* Basel: Karger.

Essen-Möller, E., and Wohlfahrt, S. 1947. Suggestions for the amendment of the official Swedish classification of mental disorders. *Acta Psychiatrica Scandinavica, Suppl.* 47: 551–555.

Gebhardt, R., and Pietzcker, A. 1983. Zur Validierung der AMDP-Syndromskalen. *Archiv für Psychiatrie und Nervenkrankheiten* 233: 509–523.

Gebhardt, R., Pietzcker, A., Strauss, A., Stöckel, M., Langer, C., and Freudenthal, K. 1983. Skalenbildung im AMDP-System. *Archiv für Psychiatrie und Nervenkrankheiten* 233: 223–245.

Guy, W., and Ban, T. A. 1982. *The AMDP-system. Manual for the Assessment and Documentation of Psychopathology.* Berlin: Springer.

Helmchen, H. 1980. Multiaxial systems of classification. Types of axes. *Acta Psychiatrica Scandinavica* 61: 43–55.

Helmchen, H. 1983. Multiaxial classification in psychiatry. *Comprehensive Psychiatry* 24: 20–24.

Kendell, R. E. 1984. Reflections on psychiatric classification – for the architects of DSM-IV and ICD-10. *Integrative Psychiatry* 2: 43–47.

McNemar, Q. 1969. *Psychological Statistics.* 4th ed. New York: Wiley.

Mezzich, J. E. 1979. Patterns and issues in multiaxial psychiatric diagnosis. *Psychological Medicine* 9: 125–137.

Mezzich, J. E. 1983. New developments in multiaxial psychiatric diagnosis. *Psychiatric Annals* 13: 793–807.

Mezzich, J. E. 1985. Multiaxial diagnostic systems in psychiatry. In *Comprehensive Textbook of Psychiatry*, 4th ed., ed. H. I. Kaplan, and B. J. Sadock, pp. 613–616. Baltimore, Md.: Williams & Wilkins.

Mezzich, J. E., Fabrega, H., and Mezzich, A. C. 1985. An international consultation on multiaxial diagnosis. In *Psychiatry – The State of the Art*, ed. P. Pichot, P. Berner, R. Wolfe, and K. Thau. London: Plenum Press.

Nie, N. H., Hull, H., Jenkins, J. G., Steinbrenner, K., and Bendt, D. H. 1975. *SPSS. Statistical Package for the Social Sciences.* New York: McGraw-Hill.

Pietzcker, A., Gebhardt, R., Strauss, A., Stöckel, M., Langer, C., and Freudenthal,

K. 1983. The syndrome scales in the AMDP-System. In *The AMDP-System in Pharmacopsychiatry*, ed. D. Bobon, U. Baumann, J. Angst, H. Helmchen, and H. Hippius, pp. 88–99. Basel: Karger.

Siegel, S. 1956. *Nonparametric Statistics for the Behavioral Sciences*. New York: McGraw-Hill.

Spitzer, R. L., and Forman, J. B. W. 1979. DSM-III field trials: II. Initial experience with the multiaxial system. *American Journal of Psychiatry* 136: 818–820.

World Health Organization. 1978. *Mental Disorders: Glossary and Guide to Their Classification in Accordance with the Ninth Revision of the International Classification of Diseases*. Geneva.

19   An overview of the Diagnostic Interview Schedule and the Composite International Diagnostic Interview

LEE N. ROBINS (USA)

THE DIAGNOSTIC INTERVIEW SCHEDULE

The Diagnostic Interview Schedule (DIS) (Robins et al., 1979) was written at the request of the National Institute of Mental Health as an instrument to be used in the largest epidemiological study that had ever been launched in the United States. The study is known as the ECA, or Epidemiologic Catchment Area study (Regier et al., 1984), and has taken place at five sites in the United States, including New Haven, Baltimore, St. Louis, Los Angeles, and five counties in North Carolina. (First results from three of the sites have been reported [Robins et al., 1984; Myers et al., 1984; Shapiro et al., 1984].)

What the ECA required was an interview that could be administered by lay interviewers and could make diagnoses according to the official criteria of the American Psychiatric Association (1980) as published in its *Diagnostic and Statistical Manual of Mental Disorders*, third edition (DSM-III). It had to be usable with persons eighteen years of age or older, with no upper age limit and at all education levels. It had to cover the commonly used diagnoses in DSM-III. In order to cover those diagnoses, it had to review history as well as assess current status. And, finally, the total interview had to take an average of no more than an hour to carry out with a member of the general population.

The authors of this instrument reviewed the DSM-III, which was still in draft form at the time the interview was being written, and decided on those diagnoses for which criteria appeared to be sufficiently specific so that it was possible to write questions that could be asked and scored directly by lay interviewers without requiring considerable clinical judgment. Table 19.1 shows the diagnoses selected. Three of these diagnoses – bulimia, generalized anxiety, and post-traumatic stress – were added after the ECA began. The Folstein-McHugh Mini-Mental State Examination was incorporated to detect dementia. It does not produce a DSM-III diagnosis, because organic brain disorders in DSM-III require specifying the organic factors responsible, but it does indicate that some sort of organic impairment is probably present. It differs from other diagnoses in being restricted to a *current* assessment. The second version of the DIS (the first having been revised in response to last-minute changes in DSM-III and to critiques from colleagues who tried out the first version) was tested for validity

205

Table 19.1. *Representation in the DIS of Adult DSM-III diagnoses (excluding "atypical," "mixed," "other," "unspecified," V codes)*

	DSM-III	DIS
Eating disorders	3	2[a]
Organic mental disorders	44	1
dementias	4	1[b]
Substance use disorders	14	14
Schizophrenic	5	1[b]
Paranoid	4	0
Psychotic, NEC	3	1[a]
Affective	7	6[a]
Anxiety	10	10
Somatoform	4	1[a]
Dissociative	4	0
Gender identity	1	1
Paraphilias	8	0
Psychosexual dysfunctions	7	1[b]
Ego-dystonic homosexuality	1	1
Factitious disorders	2	0
Impulse control	5	1[a]
Adjustment disorder	7	0
Personality disorders	11	1[a]
Total	122[c]	40

[a]The diagnoses covered in these classifications are eating: anorexia, bulimia; psychotic: schizophreniform; affective: all except cyclothymic; somatoform: somatization; impulse control: pathologic gambling; personality: antisocial.
[b]Covers all but nonspecific. Dementia is ascertained by Folstein-McHugh Mini-Mental State Exam.
[c]Without subtypes not distinguished by the DIS ∴ total N = 109.

in a predominantly clinical sample (Robins et al., 1981; Robins et al., 1982). On the basis of that test and the experience in New Haven, the site in which the ECA began, the DIS was revised and used at all remaining sites (Version III). These two versions have also been used in many other epidemiologic and clinical studies.

Some of the ECA participants and other researchers who have used the DIS made their own adaptations of the interview. Some of these have been incorporated into subsequent revisions. The latest DIS edition is Version III-B. This version includes all the diagnoses noted in Table 19.1 and, in addition, ascertains recency and onset for each positive symptom.

A major challenge that the authors of the DIS faced was to decide how the presence of a psychiatric symptom could be assessed by a lay interviewer. Table

Table 19.2. *Assessment of dizziness in the St. Louis ECA*

Step 1: Was it ever present?		
"Have you ever been bothered by dizziness?"	Yes:	24%
Step 2: Did it fail to meet severity criteria?		
Not reported to doctor, no medication taken, and little interference with life.		− 7%
Step 3: Was it always explained by alcohol or drugs?		
"Yes."		− 1%
Step 4: Was it always explained by physical illness?		
"Yes."		−12%
Remainder: Possible psychiatric symptom		4%

19.2 shows the format used. First, a standard question is asked – in this example: "Have you ever been bothered by dizziness?" If the respondent answers yes to that question, the clinical significance of the symptom is assessed by means of a standard set of probes, which ask if the symptom was reported to a physician or other health professional, if the respondent has taken medication for the symptom more than once, and if the symptom has caused considerable interference with the respondent's life and functioning. If none of these occurred, the symptom is not considered clinically significant and is pursued no further. The interviewer does not always need to determine clinical significance. Some symptoms, such as suicide attempts, are considered intrinsically significant, and these probes are unnecessary.

Assuming the symptom is clinically significant, the next step is to use probes to learn whether there was always a physical explanation for it. Two kinds of physical explanations are considered: The symptom might be a side effect of consuming alcohol, medication, or illicit drugs, or it might be a symptom of a physical illness or of a physical condition such as pregnancy. If these physical explanations always accounted for the symptom, it is not considered a possible symptom of psychiatric disorder.

Through the probe structure, which determines whether a symptom is both clinically significant and does not have a purely physical explanation, the DIS overcomes one of the chief failings of earlier surveys by lay interviewers – their failure to distinguish possible psychiatric symptoms from the ordinary discomforts of everyday life and from signs of physical illness.

Table 19.2 shows what happened with a typical symptom in the St. Louis ECA study when this set of standard probes was applied. Dizziness was reported as having occurred at some time by 24 percent of the population, but it was clinically significant in only 17 percent; it was explained entirely by alcohol, drugs, or physical illness in 13 percent, leaving only 4 percent in whom it constituted a possible psychiatric symptom.

Symptoms that are considered possibly psychiatric are combined by computer

Table 19.3. *Varying ways of defining a lifetime diagnosis of major depressive episode, St. Louis household and institutional samples*

	Percent
Any depressive episode	5.7
Excluding:	
a. Those whose only episode was bereavement and	5.5
b. Those whose episode might be explained by dementia or psychosis and	4.9
c. Those who sought no medical advice, took no medication, and report little interference with life	3.9

to make a diagnosis. We also have provided directions for hand-scoring diagnoses for investigators and clinicians who do not have access to a mainframe computer. In the near future, it will be possible to score these interviews on a microcomputer.

For some diagnoses, our computer programs provide a number of options with respect to defining a disorder as present. An example is given in Table 19.3, which shows the definitions that have been developed for "major depressive episode" and their frequency in the St. Louis ECA sample. At least one depressive episode lasting two weeks or more had been experienced by 5.7 percent of the St. Louis sample. But if we exclude those cases whose only episode had been associated with bereavement, the figure drops to 5.5 percent. One coding option then is to include or exclude depressive episodes that occur only in connection with bereavement. The next coding option provides for attending to or not attending to the exclusion criteria in DSM-III with respect to dementia and psychosis. If we discount depressive episodes in persons who also had psychotic symptoms or who had positive scores on the Mini Mental State Exam, the prevalence of depression dropped from 5.5 percent to 4.9 percent. Finally, DSM-III is not entirely clear about whether or not a depressive episode must cause impairment in order to be counted. The text of DSM-III says impairment is almost always involved, but that requirement does not appear in the list of specific criteria for a depressive episode. Since we did not know whether or not to require impairment, we provided programs that scored the disorder both ways. If we do not count as cases persons whose episode never resulted in impairment by the criteria noted above for clinical significance, the frequency in the general population drops from 4.9 percent to 3.9 percent. Since these options provide widely differing estimates of diagnostic prevalence, it is important to report exactly which option was selected so that comparisons with other studies can be meaningful.

Programs for the DIS also provide flexibility in deciding whether a disorder is current or in remission. A current disorder can be one in which the recency of the last episode (for episodic disorders) or the last symptom (for other dis-

Table 19.4. *Flexibility in defining "current" diagnosis depressive episode, St. Louis (percent)*

	Varying definitions of "current"				
Varying definitions of episode	Last 2 weeks	Last month	Last 6 months	Last year	In remission
Any depressive episode	2.4	2.7	3.3	3.8	1.9
Any nonbereaved episode	2.4	2.6	3.1	3.6	1.9
Any nonbereaved episode not explained by dementia or psychosis	2.2	2.4	2.9	3.3	1.6
Any nonbereaved episode not explained by other diagnosis and not too mild	1.6	1.7	2.1	2.4	1.5

orders) is within the last two weeks, within the last month, within the last six months, or within the last year. In addition, for disorders such as alcohol and drug disorders and antisocial personality, in which it is common for brief symptom-free periods to be followed by relapse, there is a fifth option: any symptom within the last *three* years. Which of these definitions of currency is selected will depend on whether one is interested in short-term changes in course or in more long-term changes. As Table 19.4 shows, combining the 5 different definitions of a depressive disorder with the 4 options for defining currency provides 20 different answers to the question, "Does this person have a current depressive episode?" The rates of current disorder produced ranged from 3.8 percent to 1.6 percent, depending on which pair of options was selected. Again, the advantages of this flexibility are accompanied by the danger of misunderstanding unless the options selected are clearly stated in reports of results.

In addition to ascertaining currency of the disorder, the DIS ascertains age at which the first symptom occurred and whether or not any symptom of the disorder was reported to a physician. This makes it possible to study the order in which multiple disorders appear and remit and helps us to understand clinical course and to decide which of the multiple disorders might be considered primary and which secondary. See Table 19.5 for an illustration of change in depressive episode status.

The DIS also provides information at levels other than the diagnostic level. Each symptom is rated as to its presence, its clinical significance, and whether it was always explained by physical causes. The computer then provides a total count of psychiatric symptoms across diagnostic boundaries. Within each diagnostic category, a count of the symptoms of that diagnosis ever experienced is provided, whether or not the individual met criteria for the diagnosis. The earlier versions of the DIS obtained the age at which the first symptom of each diagnosis was experienced, the age at which the last symptom of each diagnosis was experienced, and whether any of them was discussed with the doctor. In

Table 19.5. *Change in depressive episode status*

	At first interview		
	Had never had an episode (2,281)	Last episode more than one year ago (53)	Episode within last year (118)
Percentage *with* depressive episodes in year following first interview:			
Incident cases	2		
Relapse cases		11	
Continuing cases			27
Percentage *without* depressive episodes in year following first interview:			
No disorder	98		
Remission continued[a]		89	
Remitted[a]			73
	100	100	100

[a]Includes cases who deny having ever had an episode at second interview, but reported one at first interview.

the most recent version, 3B, age at first and last experience is provided for *every* psychiatric symptom.

The computer programs to make diagnoses follow the decision structure of DSM-III, combining symptoms to evaluate each diagnostic criterion labeled with a capital letter, and assigning the diagnosis if all are met. The intermediate decisions with respect to each criterion are saved. For people who do *not* meet diagnostic criteria, this makes it possible to learn which criteria have and have not been met. With the building blocks for diagnoses (both symptoms and criteria) preserved by the computer, it is possible to learn a great deal about the relative frequency of symptoms and criteria and their intercorrelations. One can determine which symptoms are commonly medically explained and which ones are almost always psychiatric. Because the onset and offset of each symptom are dated, it is also possible to learn the order in which symptoms typically appear and disappear.

The fact that so much detailed information is available in addition to diagnoses means that it is possible to apply diagnostic systems other than DSM-III to DIS protocols, since most diagnostic systems tend to employ the same symptoms, although they may assign them to different diagnoses.

In addition, symptom data may be interesting in their own right as illustrated in Table 19.6, which shows that the median number of depressive symptoms among persons with at least one depressive symptom is only two. Therefore, it

Table 19.6. *Information at the symptom level: depression, St. Louis*

Median number of symptoms, if any	2
Most common symptom: dysphoria	26%
Least common symptom: loss of sexual interest	2%
Occurrence of suicidal thoughts	10%
Suicide attempt	3%
Discussed depressive episode with doctor	6%

is common to have just a few depressive symptoms without coming close to meeting criteria for the disorder. It also shows that the most common depressive symptom is dysphoria and the least common is loss of sexual interest. Ten percent of this general St. Louis population have had suicidal thoughts and 3 percent have actually made a suicide attempt. A slightly higher proportion of individuals discussed a depressive episode with the doctor than met criteria for a depressive episode. This indicates that the DSM-III criteria for depressive episodes by no means capture all of the people who are concerned about their depressive symptomatology.

The DIS has now been translated into many languages and has been used in clinical studies of psychiatric and medical patients, in genetic studies of the relatives of patients, in disaster victims, in Cambodian refugees, in prisoners, in American Indians, and in general populations in the United States, French Quebec, Shanghai, Portugal, Hong Kong, the Republic of Korea, Peru, Puerto Rico, Greece, Lebanon, and the Philippines. Although there have been some problems in adapting it for use in other cultures, the difficulties have not been major, and it seems to have been well received by respondents everywhere. No researcher has reported a problem with breakoffs or refusals to answer any sections of the interview. Many of the researchers have attended a one-week training session in St. Louis, where they were given lectures, watched videotapes, did written exercises, and conducted practice interviews under supervision. A comprehensive training manual, along with videotapes, has been prepared with the assistance of the Veterans Administration and awaits printing.

From data collected with the DIS, Version III, a screening interview for 12 of the longer diagnostic sections has been constructed. In collaboration with Drs. Marjorie Klein and John Greist of the University of Wisconsin, we are testing the administration and scoring of the DIS and its screening interview by microcomputer.

THE COMPOSITE INTERNATIONAL DIAGNOSTIC INTERVIEW

The Composite International Diagnostic Interview (CIDI) was written at the request of the ADAMHA/WHO Task Force on Psychiatric Assessment

Instruments. It was designed to compare different diagnostic systems in epidemiologic and clinical studies. The construction of this instrument was prompted by the impending rewriting of diagnostic formulations for ICD-10. Decisions about diagnostic categories and criteria for the mental disorder section of previous editions of this international classification system had been made by expert panels, whose members were influenced by their respective national traditions of psychiatric diagnosis, and who often lobbied for categories of disorder with which they were familiar.

The ADAMHA/WHO Task Force felt that the time had come to collect empirical data that could settle arguments among these experts. The data could be provided by the simultaneous application of multiple diagnostic schemes to patients in various cultures to learn whether the international nomenclature had lacunae that prevented their classifying culture-specific disorders, and whether categories that sounded similar across systems were actually applied to the same kinds of cases. To carry out this enterprise, a structured interview was needed that would cover the criteria for multiple systems and could be translated into many languages.

This approach to the problem of understanding national differences in classification had been used previously in the US-UK comparison of patients in mental hospitals (Cooper et al., 1972), a study that showed that the differences were more in ways of classifying patients than in the patients' symptom patterns. Although this study compared diagnostic traditions in two English-speaking cultures, the WHO had also had a successful experience with translating the interview used into many languages to compare symptom patterns cross-culturally in the International Pilot Study of Schizophrenia (IPSS) (World Health Organization, 1973).

These two studies had been carried out by clinicians interviewing patients. To settle the issues still outstanding, information would be needed not only about patients, but also about unreferred cases in the general population that practitioners would agree had a mental disorder, since referral practices were likely to differ across cultures. Therefore, the task force wanted an instrument that would be appropriate for epidemiologic as well as clinical studies.

In epidemiologic studies, the yield of cases is expected to be low and therefore the sample needs to be large if representative examples of all the diagnoses of interest are to be examined. Large samples require an interview that can be administered successfully by lay interviewers and that can be scored for diagnosis by computer. Further, it must be short enough so that it can be administered in a single sitting to avoid problems of attrition between interviews, and it must rely entirely or principally on information the respondent can supply to avoid problems of getting permission to talk to relatives or physicians.

An obvious model for such an interview was the DIS (Robins et al., 1980). That interview had been designed to incorporate three diagnostic systems simultaneously, DSM-III (American Psychiatric Association, 1980), RDC (Spitzer, Endicott & Robins, 1978), and Feighner et al. (1972). And, as we have noted, it had been used with apparent success in developing countries as well as in industrialized ones. It was reasonably brief, and lay interviewers could be trained to use it reliably in one to two weeks. These characteristics fit the task force's needs. In addition, since it incorporated questions to make 40 DSM-III diagnoses, it covered much of one of the principal diagnostic systems to be compared with the international classification.

The decision, then, was to preserve the DIS and add to it questions needed to cover other diagnostic systems. The most important was the current ICD–9 (World Health Organization, 1979). This presented problems, however, because the criteria for ICD-9 were less specific than those for DSM-III, and it was therefore difficult to phrase questions in a way that would be broadly accepted as ascertaining whether its criteria had been met.

The solution decided on was to incorporate the Present State Examination (PSE) (Wing, Cooper & Sartorius, 1974) as the best and most widely used structured interview representing mainstream international diagnosis, and used in both the US-UK study and the IPSS. Dr. John Wing decided which PSE items were already adequately covered by the DIS, and then selected other items to be translated into DIS format and added. Enough PSE items were added to allow the major PSE syndromes to be scored, but not enough to allow syndromes to be divided into their subtypes. The questions to be added were integrated alongside DIS questions on similar topics to make the flow of questions natural.

Other questions were added to assess the Edwards-Gross criteria for alcohol dependence written for the WHO (Edwards & Gross, 1976) and to make the interview more suitable than the DIS for use in nonindustrialized settings. For example, accidents as a criterion for alcohol disorders were broadened to include falls and getting cut with a knife in addition to the traffic accidents mentioned in DSM-III; poor work performance as a result of drinking was broadened to include failure to get work or chores done, problems that might pertain to self-employed farmers, in addition to the absenteeism and firing that are criterion problems for the salaried worker. Long questions were divided into parts to make them easier to understand and easier to translate. In addition, a separate drug module that assesses the severity and duration of dependence on specific drugs was written to be used when detailed information about substance abuse was wanted.

Table 19.7 shows the format of a typical CIDI question, Question 31. The left margin contains an index of the computer programs that use answers to this question. It is used for PSE Item 3, for the DSM-III diagnosis of somatization disorder (DSMSOM), and for the Feighner diagnosis of hysteria (FGNHYST). These program names are mnemonics because the computer limits us to eight characters for a name.

The right margin shows the possible scores for each question. The "PRB" score indicates whether or not the response is to be counted as evidencing a psychiatric symptom, and if not, the reason why not. If the response is to be counted as a psychiatric symptom, it is coded 5. This is determined by the set of standard probes described above for the DIS. The underlined portions of the question provide a short version of the symptom to be inserted by the

Table 19.7. *A CIDI symptom question*

PSE 3	31. Have you ever had *a lot of trouble with excessive*	PRB: 1 2 3 4 5
DSMSOM	*gas* or bloating of your stomach or abdomen?	
FGNHYST		
		ONS: 1 2 3 4 5 6
		AGE ONS: __/__
		REC: 1 2 3 4 5 6
		AGE REC: __/__
	MD:_____ OTHER:_____	SEV: 1 2

interviewer into the standard probes. The lines below the question provide a space on which to write the causes to which the symptom was attributed, so that a clinician can review the interviewer's scoring if necessary.

If the symptom was clinically significant and not every occurrence could be accounted for by physical causes, a 5 is coded, and the interviewer proceeds to ask about the onset date (ONS), and the most recent date (REC) at which the symptom was experienced. Both recency and onset are scored as within the last two weeks, two weeks to a month ago, a month to six months ago, six months to a year ago, within the last year but exactly when is not recalled, or more than a year ago. If the first or last occurrence was more than a year ago, the respondent's age at the time is requested; if the occurrence was within the last year, the respondent's current age will be inserted by computer. When an occurrence within the last month is discovered for a PSE item, its severity (SEV) during that period is ascertained. The standard criterion for severity is that the symptom bothered the respondent a lot most of the time during the last month. When the PSE uses a different criterion for severity, a special probe is added to be used only for the designated symptom.

This complex decision process executed by the series of standard probe questions is shown schematically in Figure 19.1. What it can produce in the way of describing symptomatology and the natural history of the disorder will become clear when we look at the summary statistics that can be generated by computer from the interview.

Table 19.8 shows what this decision tree produces for an individual symptom. The data come from a study of the effects of natural (flood and tornados) and man-made (dioxin and radioactive wells) disasters in the general population conducted while the CIDI was being written and used as a testing ground for its questions (Smith, Robins & Przybeck, 1986). The question being assessed is CIDI Question 16, "Have you ever had *a lot of trouble with abdominal or belly pain* (not counting times when you were menstruating)?" The top of Table 19.8, like Table 19.2, shows the progress of the question through the standard probes. An affirmative answer was given by 22.5 percent of the sample. A very small proportion of those answering yes then denied all four criteria for clinical significance, and a very small proportion of those for whom the symptom was

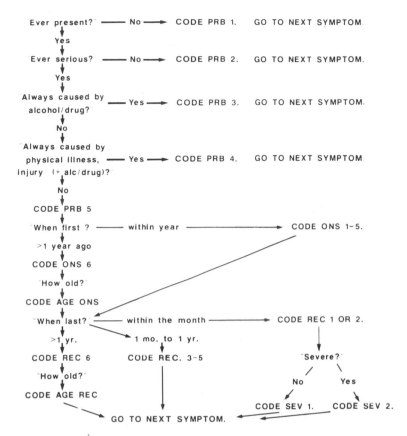

Figure 19.1. Coding a CIDI symptom

clinically significant attributed their pain entirely to alcohol or drugs. But almost three-quarters of those reporting the symptom attributed it entirely to physical illness. Thus, at the end, only 5 percent reported abdominal pain that was both clinically significant and possibly of psychiatric significance.

The sample of 538 had an average age of 41. The median age of onset for this symptom was 22 years, and for two-thirds onset was before age 30, the age by which somatization disorder must begin according to DSM-III. No new case of belly pain had appeared in the six months before interview, but a few cases had had an onset six months to a year before interview.

The median age at which the symptom had last occurred was 33. Subtracting the median age of onset from the median age at last occurrence gives an average duration of 11 years. (Since this is a cross-sectional study, age of onset, age at last symptom, and duration all depend on the sample's age distribution. To get lifetime expectancies for each of these figures, respondents would have to be followed until the symptom ended or death. Figures for lifetime expectancies would be higher than the cross-sectional figures for all three estimates.)

Table 19.8. *CIDI products: A. Individual Symptom, disaster study* (*N* = 538)

Q.16. "A lot of trouble with abdominal pain"	
Percentage of population ever positive, but	22.5%
not severe	−0.4%
explained by alcohol or drugs	−0.2%
explained by physical illness	−16.9%
Possible psychiatric symptom	5.0%
First occurrence, if psychiatric (N = 27)	
Median age	22
Before age 30	67%
Within last year	15%
Within last 6 months	0%
Last occurrence, if psychiatric (N = 27)	
Median age	33 years
Within last year	67%
Within last 6 months	52%
Within last month	41%
Within last fortnight	37%

Remission rates are modest, as shown by the fact that two-thirds of those who ever had the symptom have had it in the last year. Almost half (41 percent) of those who ever had the symptom have suffered from it within the last month, making them eligible for having a PSE symptom. Since PSE probes for severity were not incorporated into this study, we cannot give the final bit of information the CIDI will provide, the proportion of persons with this PSE symptom who had a severe symptom.

Table 19.9 moves from data for a single symptom to data summarizing all 37 symptoms used in the DSM-III diagnosis of somatization disorder. First we note that more than half the sample met criteria for at least one of these symptoms, and that the maximum number reported by any one person was 16. However, very few persons even approached a positive diagnosis. Only 3.5 percent had had as many as 6 positive symptoms, and only 0.2 percent had 12, the minimum number needed to get a positive DSM-III diagnosis. The average number of symptoms per person was 1.3, and the average number occurring in the last year was 0.8. This example shows that the CIDI does not overdiagnose somatization disorder in the community. In fact, the rates of diagnosable disorder are so low that one might consider recommending that DSM-III reduce the number of symptoms required.

Table 19.10 shows what would have happened if the diagnostic criteria had been reduced to 6 symptoms instead of the 12 required for men and the 14

Table 19.9. *CIDI products: B. Symptom level, disaster study* *(N = 538)*

Percentage with any somatic symptom	56.1%
Percent with 6 or more	3.5%
With 12 or more (DSM criteria for men)	0.2%
Maximum symptoms (out of 37) per respondent	16
Cross-sectional frequencies, average number	
In lifetime	1.3
In last year	0.8
In last 6 months	0.7
In last month	0.5
In last fortnight	0.5
Number new symptoms appearing	
In last year	0.12
In last 6 months	0.04
In last month	0.01
In last fortnight	0.00

Table 19.10. *CIDI products: C. Diagnostic level, disaster study* *(N = 538; modified somatization disorder; 6 or more somatic* *symptoms)*

Cross-sectional diagnosis:	
percentage with 6 or more somatic symptoms in	
Lifetime	3.5%
Last year	1.9%
Last 6 months	1.5%
Last month	0.7%
Last fortnight	0.7%
Crossing the diagnostic threshold:	
when the 6th positive symptom appeared	
Mean age	33.3 years
This year	32%
Within last six months	16%
Within last month	0%

required for women in DSM-III. As noted in Table 19.10, 3.5 percent of the sample would have met the criteria for having sufficient symptoms at some time in their lives. While their age of onset of the first symptom was typically early (not shown), the mean age at which their sixth symptom appeared was 33.3 years. Thus typically a number of years would have elapsed between the time the diagnosis might have been first suspected, at about age 22 according to Table 19.8, and the time at which a diagnosis could be finally confirmed.

Once diagnostic criteria were met, the symptoms tended to persist. More than half of those ever affected would have met criteria on a cross-sectional basis within the past year. One-fifth of those ever affected would have met the criteria on a cross-sectional basis within the last month (or two weeks).

Table 19.10 illustrates the variety of diagnostic data the CIDI can produce: the number who have ever had sufficient symptoms to meet diagnostic criteria; the number who met criteria on a cross-sectional basis within the last year, the last six months, the last month, or the last two weeks; the timing of the first symptom; the date at which the diagnostic threshold was first crossed; whether onset was gradual or acute (determined by the difference between the date of first symptom and the date by which sufficient symptoms had been manifested to cross the diagnostic threshold); the frequency of remission; and the duration of the disorder. Duration can be calculated in four ways: from the first to the most recent symptom, from first meeting full diagnostic criteria to the most recent symptom, from first meeting full diagnostic criteria to the time when the diagnosis could last have been made on a cross-sectional basis, and from the first symptom to the last time a diagnosis could have been made on a cross-sectional basis. Computer programs have been written to produce each of these descriptions of the natural history of the disorder.

Table 19.10 presents results for a single diagnosis, but the CIDI can also provide information about the individual's total diagnostic history. Its programs report how many disorders an individual has ever experienced, whether they overlapped in time, and the order in which their onsets took place. If some have remitted, we can see the order in which they remitted.

Finally, and this is the most important contribution of the CIDI to resolving nosological problems, the diagnoses achieved by applying the rules of different diagnostic systems can be compared. We can learn whether two systems choose virtually identical sets of individuals when they use similar sounding diagnoses or whether one system is the stricter, picking cases that are a subset of cases chosen by the other system, or whether the persons identified as cases do not overlap fully, so that certain kinds of cases identified by each system are missed by the other. The detailed information produced by our probing structure tells us which rules account for the rejection by one diagnostic system of symptoms accepted by the other, and so clarifies what adjustments in the diagnostic criteria would reduce or eliminate differences between diagnostic systems. When symptom questions and diagnostic algorithms for culture-specific diagnoses are added, we shall also be able to learn whether persons with "culture-specific" diagnoses do or do not qualify for diagnoses in more widely used systems.

The CIDI materials now available include the interview itself, a set of computer programs for assessing it, a manual for training interviewers, and videotapes to demonstrate its use and test its interviewers. Although many of its component parts have had extensive testing as parts of other instruments used in a variety of studies, testing of the instrument in its present form still lies ahead. An earlier German version has been tested by Dr. H.-U. Wittchen's group at the Max Plank Institute in Munich, and some modifications in the PSE questions have been made on the basis of that experience. A reliability component of this study is presented in Chapter 20. The next stage will be a restest of the revised PSE questions against a standard PSE interview administered by a clinician, and a test of the reliability of the drug module. If the CIDI stands up well to these tests, it will be translated into more languages and tested in a variety of cultures. Undoubtedly, this exercise will raise new questions that will require resolution.

One concern certain to arise has to do with length. Adding questions necessary to accommodate systems not covered by the DIS has lengthened the interview, as has the decision to add recent and onset dates for every positive symptom to increase information about the natural history. One solution to the increased length is to use our screening interview for DSM-III diagnoses in those diagnostic sections in which the user's interest is lower. The screening interview can determine whether or not diagnostic criteria for a diagnosis have ever been met but it does not collect complete information about *which* symptoms are positive or their order of appearance. The interview can be shortened further by dropping questions needed only to make diagnoses in which users have no interest. The indexing of use of questions in the left margin allows them to be certain that they are not eliminating questions they will need.

If the DIS is found to work well under microcomputer administration, we look forward to adapting the CIDI to the microcomputer. The microcomputer can be programmed to present a menu from which interviewers choose the diagnostic systems they wish to cover and the diagnoses in which they are interested within those systems. For the duration of their study, the computer would present on the screen only those questions needed for their particular purposes. They would not need to eliminate questions manually or have an abridged question set printed. A diagnostic profile could be available within a few seconds of completing an interview. A computerized interview that could be tailored to suit a study's needs in this easy fashion would greatly increse the CIDI's potential usefulness.

REFERENCES

American Psychiatric Association. 1980. *Diagnostic and Statistical Manual. 3rd ed*. DSM-III Washington, D.C.

Cooper, J. E., Kendell, R. E., Gurland, B. J., Sharpe, L., Copeland, J. R. M., and Simon, R. 1972. *Psychiatric Diagnosis in New York and London*. Maudsley Monograph, no. 20. London: Oxford University Press.

Edwards, G., and Gross, M. S. 1976. Alcohol dependence: Provisional description of the clinical syndrome. *British Medical Journal* 1: 1058–1061.

Feighner, J. P., Robins, E., Guze, S. B., Woodruff, R. A., Jr., Winokur, G., and Muñoz, R. 1972. Diagnostic criteria for use in psychiatric research. *Archives of General Psychiatry* 26: 57–63.

Myers, J. K., Weissman, M. M., Tischler, G. L., Holzer, C. E., Leaf, P. J., Orvaschel,

H., Anthony, J. C., Boyd, J. H., Burke, J. D., Kramer, M., and Stoltzman, R. 1984. Six-month prevalence of psychiatric disorders in three communities. *Archives of General Psychiatry* 41: 959–967.

Regier, D. A., Myers, J. A., Kramer, M., Robins, L. N., Blazer, D. G., Hough, R. L., Eaton, W. W., and Locke, B. Z. 1984. The NIMH Epidemiologic Catchment Area (ECA) Program: Historical context, major objectives and study population characteristics. *Archives of General Psychiatry* 41: 934–941.

Robins, L. N., Helzer, J. E. Croughan, J., and Ratcliff, K. S. 1981. The NIMH Diagnostic Interview Schedule: its history, characteristics, and validity. *Archives of General Psychiatry* 38: 381–389.

Robins, L. N., Helzer, J. E., Croughan, J., Williams, J., and Spitzer, R. L. 1980. The NIMH Diagnostic Interview Schedule, Version II, 1979, ADM-42-12-79, with History and Introduction (1980), Instructions (1979), and Computer Programs (1980).

Robins, L. N., Helzer, J. E., Ratcliff, K. S., and Seyfried, W. 1982. Validity of the Diagnostic Interview Schedule, Version II: DSM-III diagnoses. *Psychological Medicine* 12: 855–870.

Robins, L. N., Helzer, J. E., Weissman, M., Orvaschel, H., Gruenberg, E., Burke, J., and Regier, D. A. 1984. Lifetime prevalence of specific psychiatric disorders in three sites. *Archives of General Psychiatry* 41: 949–958.

Shapiro, S., Skinner, E. A., Kessler, L. G., Von Korff, M., German, P. S. Tischler, G. L., Leaf, P. J., Benham, L., Cottler, L., and Regier, D. A. 1984. Utilization of health and mental health services in three epidemiologic catchment area sites. *Archives of General Psychiatry* 41: 971–978.

Smith, E. M., Robins, L. N., and Przybeck, T. R. 1986. Psychological impact of a double disaster. In *Disaster Stress Studies: New Methods and Findings*, ed. J. H. Shore and L. N. Robins. Washington, D.C.: American Psychiatric Press.

Spitzer, R. L., Endicott, J., and Robins, E. 1978. Research diagnostic criteria: Rationale and reliability. *Archives of General Psychiatry* 35: 773–782.

Wing, J. K., Cooper, J. E., and Sartorius, N. 1974. *Measurement and Classification of Psychiatric Symptoms*. Cambridge: Cambridge University Press.

World Health Organization. 1973. *Schizophrenia: Report of an International Pilot Study*. Geneva.

World Health Organization 1979. *Glossary of Mental Disorders and Guide to Their Classification*. Geneva.

20 The test-retest reliability of the German version of the Composite International Diagnostic Interview on RDC diagnoses and symptom level

GERT SEMLER, HANS-ULRICH WITTCHEN, AND
MICHAEL ZAUDIG (Federal Republic of Germany)

INTRODUCTION

Today's research in classification has as one of its primary focuses the reliability of diagnostic systems and of the related methods to assess mental disorders. Yet, this was not always so. Only as far back as the 1930s, there was little interest in evaluating the reliability of psychiatric diagnoses. Clinicians at that time actually were aware of the need to make diagnoses reproducible, but implicitly suggested their diagnoses were reliable without more exact scrutiny. Along with the first attempts to deal systematically with the question of diagnostic reliability (Masserman & Carmichael, 1938; Boisen, 1938), a remarkable change in the prevailing attitude toward this issue took place at the end of that decade. Although the above-mentioned studies suffered from severe methodological limitations (e.g., reliability was not assessed directly), their general conclusion that diagnostic reliability was not as high as supposed was widely accepted. They stimulated other scientists to go into a more detailed examination of diagnostic reliability. Ash (1949) performed the first systematic study of interclinician agreement, resulting in a general confirmation of the above-mentioned findings. More specifically, Ash concluded that, first, interrater reliability in general was poor and, second, reliability was higher in major categories than in more specific categories.

The increasing interest in reliability led to a flood of relevant publications between 1950 and 1970 (Hunt, Wittson & Hunt, 1953; Foulds, 1955; Schmidt & Fonda, 1956; Norris, 1959; Kreitman, 1961; Beck et al., 1962; Sandifer, Pettus, & Quade, 1964; Zubin, 1967). Besides evaluating reliability, more and more efforts were made to investigate reasons for unreliability (Ward et al. 1962; Spitzer & Fleiss, 1974). Ward and his colleagues (1962) highlighted sources of diagnostic variance on the part of the patients, the interviewers and the nosological system. They found that poor reliability was for the most part due to unclear criteria, unclear weighing of symptoms, too subtle distinctions between diagnostic categories, and the fact that the clinician was allowed to assign only one diagnosis. Although Ward et al.'s analysis was not uncontested (Blashfield,

1984), their conclusions were generally accepted and strongly influenced further developments in this field of research.

Compared with earlier studies, markedly higher reliability was obtained in studies performed in the 1970s (Helzer et al., 1977; Spitzer, Endicott & Robins, 1978; Spitzer, Forman & Nee, 1979). The success of these studies can hardly be explained without considering their nosologic basis. As a consequence of the critiques on traditional nosology, Feighner et al. (1972) were the first to consider proposals made by Ward et al. (1962) by creating a new diagnostic approach originally designed for research purposes. The Research Diagnostic Criteria (Spitzer et al., 1978) and the *Diagnostic and Statistical Manual of Mental Disorders*, third revision (DSM-III) (American Psychiatric Association, 1980), represent further developmental stages in this new approach, which is characterized mainly by the use of explicit diagnostic criteria. The clinician using these systems determines whether a given patient fulfills specific diagnostic criteria instead of determining which of the various diagnoses available is most appropriate, as had been done earlier (Spitzer & Fleiss, 1974).

Another major innovation of this era aimed at removing a further source of diagnostic variance by standardizing the way in which relevant information is gathered in the diagnostic process. The Present State Examination (PSE) (Wing, Cooper & Sartorius, 1974), the Schedule for Affective Disorders and Schizophrenia (SADS) (Endicott & Spitzer, 1978), and the Diagnostic Interview Schedule (DIS) (Robins et al., 1981) are the best-known interview schedules representing this new development. By asking each patient the same questions in the same order, these instruments achieved relatively high interrater reliability (Wing, et al., 1977; Spitzer et al., 1978; Robins et al., 1981). Their usefulness and applicability have been demonstrated not only in such studies as those subsumed under the Epidemiologic Catchment Area Program (Eaton et al., 1981) but also in various international comparisons such as the U.S.-U.K. project (Cooper et al., 1972) and the International Pilot Study of Schizophrenia (World Health Organization, 1973).

Although the question of international comparability of research findings has gained importance through the work of Kendell et al. (1971) and other scientists (e.g., Sandifer et al., 1968; Katz, Cole & Lowery, 1969; Cooper et al., 1972) who investigated the diagnostic habits of American and British psychiatrists, communication is still hampered by the fact that scientists on both sides of the Atlantic generally use differing diagnostic systems, DSM-III in the United States and ICD-9 in most European countries. In order to construct a "bridge" between the alternative classification systems, the major authors of the DIS and the PSE – Robins, Wing, and Helzer – made an attempt to combine the properties of both interviews in a new interview schedule, called the Composite International Diagnostic Interview (CIDI). Data on the reliability and validity of the original version of the CIDI are not yet available. A first test of the diagnostic reliability of the German version was conducted at the Max-Planck-Institut für Psychiatrie and at the Bezirkskrankenhaus Kaufbeuren as part of a major project on the comparability of different diagnostic systems. Study findings, with regard to the reliability of the CIDI on diagnostic and symptom level based on RDC, are presented in this chapter. Further results of this study will be published elsewhere.

THE INTERVIEW

The study was carried out with the German translation of the CIDI, based on the draft version of September 1983. The CIDI is a highly structured interview schedule that can be administered by physicians as well as by non-physicians. It is basically a version of the DIS (Robins et al., 1981) extended by the addition of items adapted from the PSE (Wing et al., 1974) to allow the derivation of many of the PSE-CATEGO classes. (For further details see Chapter 19.)

The translation of the original version of the CIDI into German was done by using a three-stage procedure, which included the development of two independent translations, which were then reduced to a single version, and an extensive final revision with the help of German-speaking specialists in the field of psychopathology and the authors of the instrument (Robins, Wing & Helzer). The version used in this study covers the whole range of diagnoses included in the original version, except for antisocial personality, tobacco use disorder, ego-dystonic homosexuality, pathological gambling, post-traumatic stress disorder, and trans-sexualism. The assignment of PSE-CATEGO classes was not yet feasible at this developmental stage of the CIDI.

Owing to the complexity of the instrument and the problems posed by its administration, intensive training is required, during which the interviewer becomes familiar with the rationale of the instrument and its specific interviewer rules. The interviewers who participated in the present study were given nine days of training, at the end of which each interviewer was also supervised in five live interviews.

METHODS

The test-retest reliability of the CIDI was assessed by means of a stringent experimental design, aimed at reducing design-related sources of discrepancies between interviews (a more comprehensive description of the methods used is being published elsewhere). Sixty psychiatric inpatients with various diagnoses (Table 20.1) were interviewed twice within four days of each other (mean 1.7 days) by two interviewers. Interviewer pairing was rotated so that each of the four interviewers (two psychiatrists in residency training and two psychologists) who participated in the study was a test-retest partner for each of his three colleagues across 10 subjects – for 5 of these he conducted the test interview, for the remaining 5 the retest interview. The sample, as well as the assignment of subjects to the interviewers, was balanced with respect to the sex of the patients, so that 15 males and 15 females were interviewed by each interviewer.

Table 20.1. *Diagnostic distribution: ICD-9 principal diagnoses* $(N = 60)$

ICD-9 Code	Diagnosis	Frequency (%)
291.x − 293.x	Organic psychoses	5 (8.3)
295.x	Schizophrenic psychoses	18 (30.0)
296.x	Affective psychoses	11 (18.3)
297.x, 298.x	Nonorganic psychoses	4 (6.7)
300.x, 309.x	Neuroses and adjustment reactions	9 (15.0)
303, 304.x	Alcohol/drug dependence	7 (11.7)
301.x, 302.x		
307.1, 317	Other, nonpsychotic mental disorders	6 (10.0)

To arrive at RDC diagnoses, relevant information gathered by means of the CIDI was translated by using a slightly modified computer program initially developed for the DIS, Version 3 (Boyd et al., 1985). The calculation of agreement between test and retest interviews was done by dichotomizing diagnostic information, indicating the presence or absence of illness. Exclusion criteria, which are optionally available in the program, were ignored. Variables on item level were also dichotomized, indicating "symptom present and psychiatrically significant" versus "symptom absent or psychiatrically not significant."

As a measure of concordance between interviewers, three different reliability coefficients were used: overall percentage agreement, kappa-coefficients (Cohen, 1960), and y-coefficients (Yule, 1912). In contrast to percentage agreement, kappa and Yule's y reflect the degree of concordance achieved through lower chance. In addition, the y-statistic is suggested to be less sensitive to low base rates than kappa (Spitznagel & Helzer, 1985) and thus yields a new perspective on the problem of base-rate-dependency of agreement measures in reliability studies. It has to be pointed out, however, that the calculation of y is relatively complicated when a single cell of the 2 × 2 classification becomes zero. For that case, Spitznagel and Helzer (1985) propose a pseudo-Bayes estimation using a procedure described by Bishop et al. (1975).

RESULTS

Test-retest reliability of the CIDI on RDC diagnoses

Table 20.2 summarizes the results of the test-retest comparisons for 60 psychiatric inpatients with respect to RDC lifetime diagnoses. It gives information on the diagnostic distribution, percentage agreement, k- and y-coefficients. In addition, it is indicated whether k-coefficients are significantly different from zero. In calculating concordance rates, diagnostic hierarchies were ignored; that is, illnesses were considered present regardless of whether exclusion criteria were met. In the case of organic brain syndrome, where dichoto-

Table 20.2. *Diagnostic concordance in the CIDI: RDC lifetime diagnoses (without exclusions)*

					Int. 1 −	Int. 1 +
RDC diagnosis	Agreement (%)	k	y	Interviewer 2	− A	B
					+ C	D
Organic brain syndrome	95	.70***	—		β)	
Manic disorder	96	.73***	.79		51	0
					2	3
Major depressive disorder	83	.63***	.66		30	7
					3	17
Schizophrenia	90	.78***	.79		30	3
					3	21
Schizoaffective disorder, manic	95	.55*	.65		50	0
					3	2
Schizoaffective disorder, depression	88	.29	.47		47	4
					3	2
Definite hypomanic disorder	93	.63***	.78		48	1
					3	4
Alcoholism	91	.79***	.84		35	4
					1	15
Drug use disorder	94	.81***	.84		43	0
					3	8

(Table continues on next page.)

mization did not seem to be meaningful because of the differentiations made by the computer program, the variable was trichotomized indicating "absent" versus "present" versus "uncertain."

Except for anorexia nervosa (the diagnostic criteria of which were not met in any case), concordance rates were computed for all RDC diagnoses covered by the German version of the CIDI. Percentage agreement varied in these diagnostic areas between 82 percent and 95 percent. Chance-corrected agreement, as measured by kappa, ranged from .19 to .81. Kappa-values were highly significant

Table 20.2 *(continued)*

RDC diagnosis	Agreement (%)	k	y	Interviewer 2	Int. 1 − A	Int. 1 + B
Obsessive-compulsive disorder	94	.70***	.81		47	1
					2	4
Phobic disorder	82	.57***	.66		34	8
					2	11
Agoraphobia	88	.65***	.75		40	7
					0	9
Social phobia	89	.44*	.61		46	4
					2	3
Simple phobia	82	.19	.34		44	7
					3	2
Panic disorder	88	.40*	.59		49	5
					2	3
Briquet's disorder	88	−.06	.00		52	3
					4	0
Any RDC diagnosis	90	.52**	.72		4	5
					1	48

Note: * p < .05; ** p < .01. *** p < .001. β) = 3 × 3 table with 7 cases out of 57; 3 discrepancies.

(p < .001) for 10 out of 16 diagnostic categories and not significant for three categories. As expected, the calculation of y-values resulted in overall higher values as compared with kappas. y-values ranged from .34 up to .84. Relatively low agreement between the interviewers was found for two of the three phobic subclassifications (simple phobia and social phobia), for panic disorder and for schizoaffective disorder, depressed type. The negative k-value calculated for Briquet's disorder indicated less than chance agreement. Alcoholism and drug use disorders displayed the highest degree of concordance with k-values of .79 and .81, respectively.

Test-retest reliability of the CIDI on RDC symptom level

Results presented here refer only to those CIDI symptom questions necessary to compute RDC diagnoses. Hence, items exclusively related to DSM-III, Feighner, or PSE-CATEGO classes as well as codable interviewer instructions and time-related criteria (e.g., "offset" questions), were not considered in these calculations. In addition, the number of positive answers to a specific question in at least one of the two interviews had to be greater than 3. Concordance among raters was measured with the y-coefficient, given that the prevalence rates of a number of symptoms were very low.

The distribution of the calculated y-values in the respective diagnostic sections is demonstrated by the boxplot method (Tukey, 1977). Each figure in Figure 20.1 shows the location of the median, the spread, the tail length, and outlying data points. The location of the median is shown by the crossbar inside the box. The length of the box indicates the fourth-spread, defined as the range of data between the 25th and 75th percentile. The total range of values is indicated by the end points of the tail or the outliers, respectively (see also Emerson & Strenio, 1983).

Briquet's disorder. In this diagnostic area, 75 percent of all 17 items considered were found to have y-values greater or equal to .43, which corresponds to the low end of the box. The median characterized by the crossbar in the box is .54. The total range of values is $-.001$ to .80, with two outliers (indicated by X in figure 1), namely, "trouble with abdominal or belly pain" ($y = .0$) and "painful sexual relations" ($y = -.001$), both displaying agreement not different from chance agreement. Twenty-five percent of all items showed y-values of .63 or above, two of which were .80. These were "pain in the back" and "trouble walking."

Panic disorder. For the panic section, calculation of concordance on item level revealed a total range of values between .27 and .78, with a median of .51. The box indicating the range from the 25th to 75th percentile covers values from .34 to .65. Surprisingly, the lowest reliability was found for "Did you tremble or shake during this spell?" with a y-value of .27. The core symptom of the panic section asking whether panic attacks had ever occurred displayed the highest degree of concordance, with a y-value of .78.

Phobias. In this section the Yule values varied between .0 and .76, with a median of .49. The range covered by the box went from .20 to .75. Items located in the lower fourth of the range were "fear of being in a closed place" ($y = .0$) and "fear of seeing blood or getting a shot or injection with a needle or going to the dentist" (.0). At the upper end of the range were "fear of being in a

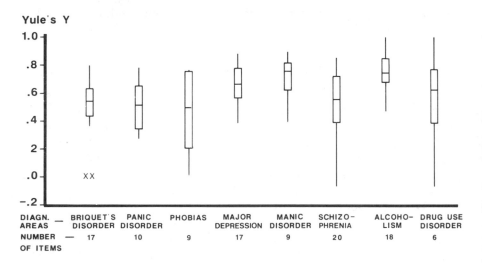

Figure 20.1. Distribution of y-values in specific diagnostic areas

crowd" (.75), "fear of being alone" (.75), and "fear of going out of the house alone" (.76).

Major depressive disorder. Among 17 calculated items in the depression section, the only one with a y-value lower than .40 was "gained weight" ($y = .38$). The fourth spread was between .56 and .77. The median was .66. Relatively high reliability was obtained for "feeling worthless" (.80), "thoughts of committing suicide" (.80), "trouble concentrating" (.81), and "attempted suicide" (.88).

Manic disorder. Compared with depression, slightly better results were obtained for items from the mania section. However, owing to the exclusion criteria applied for the selection of items, only nine mania items could be considered. These items displayed a median of $y = .75$, a total range of .39 to .89, and their fourth spread is located between .62 and .82. The lowest (.39) y-value obtained for "being easily distracted." Three items were at .81 and above: "feeling happy or excited or high over a period of one week or more," "going on spending sprees," and "lost interest in sex."

Schizophrenic disorder. y-values obtained for RDC schizophrenia items in the CIDI spread from a minimum of − .07 to a maximum of .85. The box is located between .38 and .72. The median is .55. One-third of 18 items calculated displayed y-values lower than .40, the lowest values being for "commenting voices" (− .07) and "someone was plotting against you" (.22). Approximately another third (seven items) showed y-values above .65. Among these were: "being bothered by strange smells" (.85), "feeling that someone put strange thoughts into one's mind" (.72) and "believes that special messages were being sent through television or radio" (.72).

Alcoholism. Overall highest values in the present study were obtained for items from the alcohol section. The values ranged from .47 to 1.0, with a median of .74. The box covers the range between $y = .67$ and $y = .85$. Except for two items with y-values of .47 and .50 ("being sweaty, sick to one's stomach" and "feeling depressed or irritable," respectively, both pertaining to waking up in the morning during times of daily drinking), all items attained values of at least .60. Perfect concordance ($y = 1.0$) was obtained for three items: "lose a job on account of drinking," "trouble driving because of drinking," and "arrested because of drinking."

Drug use disorder. Owing to low base rates in most of the items of this section, concordance was calculated for only six items, all of which related to problems caused by drug use in general, irrespective of the specific drug used. Very low reliability, at chance level, was found for "emotional or psychological problems from using drugs" ($-.07$), whereas, "felt like you needed drugs or were dependent on drugs" revealed perfect agreement. y-values for the remaining items lay between .53 and .69.

COMMENT

Skepticism concerning the utility of psychiatric diagnosis, which developed some decades ago among mental health professionals, especially in the United States, seems to be decreasing. As has been shown in recent publications, psychiatric diagnosis can be made with a satisfying degree of reliability (Helzer et al., 1977; Wing et al., 1977; Spitzer et al., 1979; Andreasen et al., 1981; Robins et al., 1981; Burnam et al., 1983; Semler & Wittchen, 1983). By using new diagnostic classifications models, including well-defined diagnostic criteria, and standardizing the way in which relevant information is gathered in the evaluation process, researchers have made vital contributions to this progress. A first test of the reliability of an extended version of the DSI and the CIDI further confirms the usefulness of the interview approach. Test-retest reliability appeared to be acceptable in almost all RDC lifetime diagnoses. Only in Briquet's disorder, in schizoaffective disorder, depressed type, and in the majority of anxiety disorders, especially in simple phobia, did the respective concordance rates indicate low reliability. Calculation of concordance rates on item level also yielded satisfying results in general, although some items appeared to be unreliable. It should also be mentioned that the base rates for several symptoms and some diagnostic areas (e.g., mania; schizoaffective disorder, manic type) were rather low, and therefore the respective concordance rates must be interpreted with caution. The results are nonetheless impressive as they were obtained in a sample with severely disturbed inpatients, 7 percent of whom had a diagnosis of schizophrenic disorders or other psychoses (see Table 20.1). In contrast to the expectation that patients with severe psychotic disorders can hardly be examined by means of a highly structured interview, it was shown that concordance rates for schizophrenic disorders were even above average. This finding suggests that the CIDI, although originally designed for use in epidemiological surveys, may be useful and reliable in clinical samples as well. A major limitation concerning clinical applicability refers to the long duration of the interview. First interviews ranged from 40 to 200 minutes, with an average of 102 minutes. More detailed analysis, however, showed that interview duration is reduced with increased interviewer experience (from an average of 113 minutes for the first set of 15 interviews per interviewer to an average of 92 minutes for the second set) making the time investment perhaps acceptable for clinical applications.

In comparison with the results reported by Robins et al. (1981), who used the DIS with lay interviewers in a test-retest design, quite similar k-values with respect to the majority of RDC lifetime diagnoses were obtained in the present study. Higher reliability emerged from the CIDI study in obsessive-compulsive disorder ($k = .60$), schizophrenic disorder ($k = .54$) and manic disorder ($k = .65$), whereas Briquet's disorder ($k = .52$), and panic disorder ($k = .51$) displayed lower values. The relatively poor reliability found in both studies for anxiety disorders suggests shortcomings in these specific areas, on the part of either the DIS/CIDI approach or the Research Diagnostic Criteria. It should be mentioned, however, that the sample used in the CIDI study was perhaps not particularly appropriate for evaluating anxiety disorders. In most cases, panic attacks and phobias were secondary to predominant disorders such as schizophrenia or depression, making it at least questionable whether our results can be generalized to "pure" anxiety disorders. (A more comprehensive discussion on the reliability of anxiety disorders is given in Wittchen & Semler [in press].)

Another yardstick against which to measure the CIDI is the SADS (Endicott & Spitzer, 1978). In comparison with the present study, Spitzer et al. (1978) found with the SADS considerably higher k-values for RDC schizoaffective disorder, depressed type ($k = .70$), and alcohol use disorder ($k = .95$), whereas differences in concordance in all other categories (some in favor of the CIDI and some in favor of the SADS), were quite small. It is not clear whether the interviews in the Spitzer et al. study were conducted only by physicians or (as in the CIDI study) by nonphysicians, which renders problematic the comparison between these two studies.

Highly structured interviews, such as the CIDI, may be expected to produce differences caused by the interviewer's professional background. In the present study differences in clinical experience were accompanied by little concordance. Greater variation was associated with mix in professional identification. Lowest agreement was obtained for the physician-physician pair, followed by the psychologist-psychologist pair, whereas the mixed pairs displayed the highest degree of concordance. Owing to the low number of interviewers involved in this study, these findings are tentative, but suggest that, apart from quality of training or amount of experience with the interview, specific interviewer variables affect the results to some degree.

As mentioned earlier, the CIDI and its major predecessor, the DIS, were developed for use in epidemiological surveys in which severe psychiatric disorders are rarely found and milder variations are more prominent than in clinical samples. In several recent publications, objections are raised about the comparability of findings from general population surveys and clinical studies (Helzer et al., 1985; Robins, 1985; Sackett, Haynes & Tugwell, 1985). It has been pointed out that the assignment of a diagnosis is more difficult the closer a given patient's symptomatology comes to the cut-off point of diagnostic definition. This may suggest that agreement in terms of reliability or validity of a diagnostic procedure should be better in clinical samples than in population samples. In addition, it has been suggested that psychiatric symptoms assessed in the general population differ considerably with respect to their structure and quality in comparison with clinical samples. Thus, the interpretation of the findings reported in this study has to be restricted to the use in clinical samples. Although there is much evidence that the CIDI is a reliable interview in clinical settings, a similar statement cannot be made for its use in population samples until further investigations have demonstrated comparable reliability in epidemiological surveys.

As for the generalizability of the results obtained in this study, another fact must be considered. Owing to the low number of interviewers and the above-mentioned sensitivity of the CIDI to individual interviewers, it seems important to control for individual interviewers' influence on the total results. One way to do this is to ensure equal distribution of all relevant variables, that is, by having all interviewers do the same number of first and second interviews and paying attention to proper rotation of interviewer pairing and equal distribution of male and female patients among the interviewers. Another way would be to involve a large number of interviewers (see, for example, Spitzer et al., 1979) in order to stabilize the judgments. However, because of cost, organizational effort, and training demands, such a procedure is unlikely to be used much. More realistically, appraisal of the reliability of a diagnostic procedure can be based on a series of individual studies aimed at covering the whole range of reliability aspects, under comparable methodological conditions. A first step has been reported in this chapter assessing the reliability of the CIDI. Further investigations may verify and extend the results reported here.

ACKNOWLEDGMENTS

This research was funded by the German Research Foundation (DFG). The study was done in close collaboration with the members of the task force on instrument development established in the framework of the joint WHO/ADAMHA project on diagnosis and classification. Part of the reliability analysis was done under an NIMH contract.

REFERENCES

American Psychiatric Association. 1980. *Diagnostic and Statistical Manual of Mental Disorders*. 3rd ed. (DSM-III). Washington D.C.

Andreasen, N. C., Grove, W. M., Shapiro, R. W., Keller, M. B., Hirschfeld, M. R. A., and McDonald, S. P. 1981. Reliability of lifetime diagnoses. A multicenter collaborative perspective. *Arch. Gen. Psychiat.* 38: 400–405.

Ash, P. 1949. The reliability of psychiatric diagnoses. *J. Abnorm. Soc. Psychol.* 44: 272.

Beck, A. T., Ward, H., Mendelson, M., Mock, J. E., and Erbaugh, J. K. 1962. Reliability of psychiatric diagnosis: II. A study of consistency of clinical judgments and ratings. *Amer. J. Pychiat.* 119: 351–357.

Bishop, Y. M. M., Fienberg, S. E., and Holland, P. W. 1975. *Discrete Multivariate Analysis: Theory and Practice.* Cambridge, Massachusetts: MIT Press.

Blashfield, R. K. 1984. The classification of psychopathology. *Neo-Kraepelinian and Quantitative Approaches.* New York: Plenum Press.

Boisen, A. T. 1938. Types of dementia praecox: a study in psychiatric classification. *Psychiatry* 1: 233–236.

Boyd, J. H., Robins, L. N., Holzer C. E., III., VonKorff, M., Jordan, K. B., and Escobar, J. I. 1985. Making diagnosis from DIS data. In *Epidemiologic Field Methods in Psychiatry. The NIMH Epidemiologic Catchment Area Program*, ed. W. W. Eaton and L. G. Kessler, pp. 209–231. Orlando, Fla.: Academic Press.

Burnam, M. A., Karno, M., Hough, R. L., Escobar, J. I., and Forsythe, A. B. 1983. The Spanish Diagnostic Interview Schedule. Reliability and comparison with clinical diagnoses. *Arch. Gen. Psychiat.* 40: 1189–1196.

Cohen, J. 1960. A coefficient of agreement on nominal scales. *Educ. Psychol. Measure.* 20: 37–46.

Cooper, J. E., Kendell, R. E., Gurland, B. J., Sharpe, L., Copeland, J. R. M., and Simon, R. 1972. *Psychiatric Diagnoses in New York and London.* London: Oxford University Press.

Eaton, W., Regier, D., Locke, B., and Taube, C. 1981. The Epidemiological Catchment Area program. *Publ. Health Rep.* 96: 319–325.

Emerson, J. D., and Strenio, J. 1983. Boxplots and batch comparison. In *Understanding Robust and Exploratory Data Analysis.* ed. D. C. Hoaglin, F. Mosteller, and J. W. Tukey, pp. 58–96. New York: Wiley & Sons.

Endicott, J., and Spitzer, R. L. 1978. A diagnostic interview. The Schedule for Affective Disorders and Schizophrenia. *Arch. Gen. Psychiat.* 35: 837–844.

Feighner, J. P., Robins, E., Guze, S. B., Woodruff, R. A., Winokur, G., and Muñoz, R. 1972. Diagnostic criteria for use in psychiatric research. *Arch. Gen. Psychiat.* 26: 57–63.

Foulds, G. A. 1955. The reliability and the validity of psychological diagnoses. *J. Ment. Sci.* 101: 851–862.

Helzer, J. E., Clayton, P. J., Pambakian, R., Reich, T., Woodruff, R. A., Jr., and Reveley, M. A. 1977. Reliability of psychiatric diagnosis. II. The test/retest reliability of diagnostic classification. *Arch. Gen. Psychiat.* 34: 136–141.

Helzer, J. E., Robins, L. N., McEvoy, L. T., Spitznagel, E. L., Stoltzman, R. K., Farmer, A., and Brockington, I. F. 1985. A comparison of clinical and Diagnostic Interview Schedule diagnoses. Physician reexamination of lay-interviewed cases in the general population. *Arch. Gen. Psychiat.* 42: 657–666.

Hunt, W. A., Wittson, C. L., and Hunt, E. B. 1953. A theoretical and practical analysis of the diagnostic process. In *Current Problems in Psychiatric Diagnosis*, ed. P. Hoch and J. Zubin. New York: Grune & Stratton.

Katz, M. M., Cole, J. O., and Lowry, H. A. 1969. Studies of the diagnostic process: The influence of symptom perception, past experience, and ethnic background on diagnostic decisions. *Amer. J. Psychiat.* 125: 937–947.

Kendell, R. E., Cooper, J. E., Gourlay, A. J., Copeland, J. R. M., Sharpe, L., and Gurland, B. J. 1971. Diagnostic criteria of American and British psychiatrists. *Arch. Gen. Psychiat.* 25: 123–130.

Kreitmann, N. 1961. The reliability of psychiatric diagnosis. *J. Ment. Sci.* 107: 876–886.

Masserman, J. H., and Carmichael, H. T. 1938. Diagnosis and prognosis in psychiatry: with a follow-up of the results of short-term general hospital therapy of psychiatric cases. *J. Ment. Sci.* 534: 893–946.

Norris, V. 1959. *Mental Illness in London*. Maudsley Monograph no. 6. London: Chapman & Hall Ltd.

Robins, L. N. 1985. Epidemiology: Reflections on testing the validity of psychiatric interviews. *Arch. Gen. Psychiat.* 42: 918–924.

Robins, L. N., Helzer, J. E., Croughan, J., and Ratcliff, K. S. 1981. National Institute of Mental Health. Diagnostic Interview Schedule. Its history, characteristics and validity. *Arch. Gen. Psychiat.* 38: 381–389.

Sackett, D. L., Haynes, R. B., and Tugwell, P. 1985. *Clinical Epidemiology: A Basic Science for Clinical Medicine*. Boston: Little, Brown.

Sandifer, M. G., Hordern, A., Timbury, G. C., and Green L. M. 1968. Psychiatric diagnosis: A comparative study in North Carolina, London and Glasgow. *Brit. J. Psychiat.* 114: 1–9.

Sandifer, M. G., Pettus, G., and Quade, D. 1964. A study of psychiatric diagnosis. *J. Nerv. Ment. Dis.* 139: 350–356.

Schmidt, H. O., and Fonda, C. P. 1956. The reliability of psychiatric diagnosis: A new look. *J. Abnorm. Soc. Psychol.* 52: 262–267.

Semler, G., and Wittchen, H.-U. 1983. Das Diagnostic Interview Schedule. Erste Ergebnisse zur Reliabilität und differentiellen Validität der deutschen Fassung. In *Gemeindepsychologische Perspektiven*, ed. D. Kommer and B. Röhrle, pp. 109–117. Köln.

Spitzer, R. L., Endicott, J., and Robins, E. 1978. Research Diagnostic Criteria. Rationale and reliability. *Arch. Gen. Psychiat.* 35: 773–782.

Spitzer, R. L., and Fleiss, J. L. 1974. A re-analysis of the reliability of psychiatric diagnosis. *Brit. J. Psychiat.* 125: 341–347.

Spitzer, R. L., Forman, J. B. W., and Nee, J. 1979. DSM-III field trials: I. Initial interrater diagnostic reliability. *Amer. J. Psychiat.* 136: 815–817.

Spitznagel, E. L., and Helzer, J. E. 1985. A proposed solution to the base rate problem in the kappa statistic. *Arch. Gen. Psychiat.* 42: 725–728.

Tukey, J. W. 1977. *Exploratory Data Analysis*. Reading, Mass.: Addison-Wesley.

Ward, C. H., Beck, A. T., Mendelson, M., Mock, J. E., and Erbaugh, J. K. 1962. The psychiatric nomenclature: Reasons for diagnostic disagreement. *Arch. Gen. Psychiat.* 7: 198–205.

Wing, J. K., Cooper, J. E., and Sartorius, N. 1974. *The Description and Classification of Psychiatric Symptoms: An Instruction Manual for the PSE and CATEGO Program*. Cambridge: Cambridge University Press.

Wing, J. K., Nixon, J. M., Mann, S. A., and Leff, J. P. 1977. Reliability of the PSE (ninth edition) used in a population survey. *Psychol. Med.* 7: 505–516.

Wittchen, H.-U. and Semler, G. In press. Diagnostic reliability of anxiety disorders. In *Panic and Phobias: Empirical Evidence of Theoretical Models and Longterm Effects of Behavioral Treatments*, ed. I. Hand and H.-U. Wittchen. Berlin: Springer.

World Health Organization. 1973. *The International Pilot Study of Schizophrenia*. Vol. 1. Geneva.

Yule, G. U. 1912. On the methods of measuring association between two attributes. *J. Roy. Statist. Soc.* 75: 581–642.

Zubin, J. 1967. Classification of the behavior disorders. *Ann. Rev. Psychol.* 18: 373–401.

21 Experience with the semistructured Initial Evaluation Form in Peru and the United States

DANTE E. WARTHON, CECILIA SOGI, JUAN E.
MEZZICH, IGNACIO LÓPEZ-MERINO, AND
JORGE CASTRO (Peru)

INTRODUCTION

Along with concern for improved diagnostic formulations to enhance both clinical care and clinical research, the need for patient evaluation procedures that are reasonably rigorous as well as clinically valid has become increasingly apparent. As part of this concern, there has been noticeable interest in "structuring" the diagnostic interview, that is, controlling some of its sources of undesirable variability. In fact, a number of observations and studies (Climent, Plutchik & Estrada, 1975; Greist, van Cura, & Kneppreth, 1973; Helzer, 1981; Kiernan, McCreadie & Flanagan, 1976; Saghir, 1971; Weitzel, Morgan & Guyden, 1973) have documented that structured interviews tend to yield more reliable and comprehensive information than the traditional free-format interview. Furthermore, a variety of well-recognized interview procedures have been published, including the Present State Examination (PSE) (Wing, Cooper & Sartorius, 1974), the instrument developed by the Association for Methodology and Documentation in Psychiatry (AMDP system) (Scharfetter, 1972); the Schedule for Affective Disorders and Schizophrenia (SADS) (Endicott & Spitzer, 1978); the Diagnostic Interview Schedule (DIS) (Robins et al., 1981); the Composite International Diagnostic Interview (CIDI) (Robins, 1985); and the Structured Clinical Interview for Diagnosis (SCID) (Spitzer, 1985).

However, some researchers and clinicians (e.g., Spitzer et al., 1982; Ganguli & Saul, 1982) have noted that the best-known structured interviews, because they are too highly structured, tend to interfere with the establishment of an appropriate relationship with the interviewee, which is critical in a clinical setting, and also restrict the possibilities of probing and thereby undermine the validity of the data to be obtained. These problems point out both the need for semistructured approaches and the complexity of the issues involved. Consideration of the fundamental types of interviews may have a clarifying value here.

Richardson, Dohrenwend, and Klein (1965) conceptually analyzed a diversity of interviewing tasks and the personal characteristics and behaviors of interviewers, and concluded that interviews can first be classified into standardized and non-standardized.

The standardized interview is aimed at obtaining the same classes of information

235

from each respondent, requires the advanced specification of all items of information sought, and involves formalized (if not quantifiable) data. This type of interview is in turn classified into scheduled and nonscheduled.

The scheduled standardized interview is characterized by the determination in advance of the wording and sequence of the questions involved.

The nonscheduled standardized interview involves the participation of a thoroughly trained interviewer in order to vary the wording and sequence of the questions as needed for maximal effectiveness with individual respondents. This type of interview assumes, first, that no unique wording of sequence will suffice for all respondents and that such wording and sequence should be adjusted when the respondent shows discomfort or resistance. Further, it assumes that carefully trained interviewers can tailor the questions and the sequence so that equivalence of meaning is obtained for all respondents.

The nonstandardized interview does not conform to the above requirements and it is typically used for the exploration and development of concepts and the detailed description of new phenomena.

In addition to structural issues related to the interview process, other key factors must be considered in the development of adequate psychiatric evaluation procedures. These include (1) the phenomenological approach in the sense of an empathetic and sensitive attitude toward the patient (Carpenter, Strauss & Bartko, 1981); (2) nonsymptomalogical aspects of the clinical condition, such as family history, personal and social history, and adaptive functioning, (Hesselbrock et al., 1982); (3) all sources of available information (Brockington & Meltzer, 1982; Spitzer, 1983); and (4) the inclusion of narrative statements in addition to structured elements (Brockington & Meltzer, 1982). Also note that the most highly structured diagnostic instruments tend to cover only a limited number of diagnostic categories (Ganguli & Saul, 1982; Robins & Helzer, 1982).

The above considerations point out the need for semistructured evaluation approaches responsive to these issues. The Initial Evaluation Form described below represents a contribution in this area.

THE DEVELOPMENT OF THE INITIAL
EVALUATION FORM

The Initial Evaluation Form (IEF) was originally developed at the Western Psychiatric Institute and Clinic of the University of Pittsburgh (Mezzich et al., 1981) and was then implemented as the first component of that institution's computerized clinical information system (Mezzich, Dow & Coffman, 1981). More recently, the instrument was revised, along with a manual for its use (Mezzich et al., 1986).

The IEF, in reference to the previously described typology of Richardson et al. (1965), is a flexibly scheduled standardized procedure; that is, it occupies an intermediate position between nonscheduled and fully scheduled standardized interviews. The IEF approach differs, on the one hand, from traditional free-format interviews in that most aspects of the information to be obtained are specified and defined, and it contains some guidelines for conducting the interview. On the other hand, it differs from rigidly structured interviews in that it makes use of the skills of well-trained clinicians to decide on the wording, probing, and sequence of the questions.

The procedure also fosters a phenomenological attitude, in the sense of "being with the patient," which seems to be important to help elucidate deep-seated psychopathological experiences. In the words of Jaspers (1963), psychopathology description requires intimate awareness of the inner world of patients, that is, becoming familiar with the patient's subjective experience through both language-oriented, cognitive processes and empathetic communication. Carpenter, Strauss, and Bartko (1981) point out that the scientific foundation of psychiatry is clinical observation, and that the failure of clinical research methods to achieve phenomenological soundness not only leaves the field inadequately informed but is misleading as to the complex nature of disease and treatment. Therefore, the patient-clinician relationship should be considered every bit as important as the gathering of data necessary to formulate diagnosis.

Another important feature of the IEF approach is its use of all available sources of information, not only the patient himself, but also relatives and associates, past clinical records, school and legal reports, and so on. The clinician is then expected to exercise professional judgment in weighing the consistency and credibility of the information obtained from various sources in order to make evaluative statements that will be as sound as possible.

The basic format of the IEF involves narrative and structured components which complement each other. The narrative component allows for flexibility in describing the particularities of the patient's condition in natural language, while the standardized component ensures that key informational items are systematically covered. The standardized component specifies the list of items to be considered and through instructions presented on the form and in its manual, provides item definitions and related guidelines.

The side-by-side layout of the narrative and structured components of the various sections of the IEF implements their mutually complementary nature and facilitates their completion. Laska (1974), upon conducting a critical review of clinical information systems, found that those involving completely separate narrative and structured forms require a significant amount of duplicate clinical reporting and may, paradoxically, lead to incomplete documentation.

Another important feature of the IEF is that it leads to a full DSM-III (American Psychiatric Association, 1980) diagnostic formulation, including all its categories and axes. Because of the broadness of the IEF symptom inventory, it is also possible to make diagnoses according to ICD-9 (World Health Organization, 1977) and other standard diagnostic systems.

SECTIONS OF THE INITIAL EVALUATION FORM

The sections of the IEF cover most of the clinical aspects that are usually considered important for presenting a concise but reasonably comprehensive

Table 21.1. *Format of the initial evaluation form (IEF), 1982 version*

Narrative component	Structured component
	Demographic information
	Financial/insurance information
Reasons for referral and evaluation	
History of present illness	Psychiatric history markers
History of other psychiatric disorders	
Mental status observations	Symptom inventory
	Cognitive functioning inventory
Family history	Family history markers
Personal and social history and current social support system and assets	Personal and social history and social support markers
Medical history and examination	Checklist of current physical problems and presence/absence of positive examination findings
Narrative assessment summary, problem list and recommendations, plans for family members	Confidence in the information obtained Diagnostic summary and disposition
Evaluators' signatures	Evaluators' codes and signature dates

Note: A supplemental DSM-III Diagnostic Criteria Checklist plan documents the fulfillment of criteria and subcriteria for Axes I and II diagnoses made.

description of the patient's condition and for supporting disposition and initial management decisions.

These sections (see Table 21.1) encompass psychiatric history and examination, family, personal, social and general medical histories, diagnostic summary, and disposition – all of which are organized around narrative and structured components.

Aspects of the standardized Symptom Inventory, the Personal and Social History and the Diagnostic Summary are presented next to illustrate representative features of the IEF.

The purpose of the *Symptom Inventory* (Figure 21.1) is to provide a general mapping of the patient's psychopathology. It includes 64 general items plus 22 supplementary symptoms for children and adolescents. This evaluation covers three time frames: the "past", "the current episode," and "during the interview." With respect to the "current episode," each symptom is rated as "absent," "mild," "moderate," or "severe" according to its frequency and intensity.

The purpose of the *Personal and Social History* (Figure 21.2) is to provide highlights of the biography of the patient relevant to clinical understanding and care. The structured component concentrates on problems and deficits, and the corresponding narrative clarifies any noted abnormalities and de-

SYMPTOM INVENTORY (continuation)

	NEVER PRESENT	PAST	CURRENT EPISODE	DURING INTERVIEW
		N=Absent Y=Present ?=Unknown	N=Absent 1=Mild 2=Moderate 3=Severe ?=Unknown	Y=Observed or reported as present
46. SUSPICIOUSNESS feelings that everything is not as it should be; inappropriate interpretiveness, hyper-vigilance, guardedness	□	N Y ?	N 1 2 3 ?	Y
47. SOMATIC PREOCCUPATION hypochondriasis	□	N Y ?	N 1 2 3 ?	Y
48. SUICIDAL INDICATORS death wishes, suicide ideas or attempts	□	N Y ?	N 1 2 3 ?	Y
49. HOMICIDAL IDEATION	□	N Y ?	N 1 2 3 ?	Y
50. HOMICIDAL BEHAVIOR	□	N Y ?	N 1 2 3 ?	Y
51. OBSESSIONS AND COMPULSIONS repetitive, intrusive thoughts or behavior experienced against conscious resistance	□	N Y ?	N 1 2 3 ?	Y
52. DEPERSONALIZATION experiencing self and surroundings as unreal	□	N Y ?	N 1 2 3 ?	Y
53. SCHNEIDERIAN SYMPTOMS voices arguing or commenting on one's actions or speaking thoughts aloud; somatic passivity; thought withdrawal, insertion or broadcasting; "made" feelings, impulses, or acts; primary delusional perception	□	N Y ?	N 1 2 3 ?	Y

Figure 21.1. Aspect of the IEF symptom inventory

scribes key indicators of the patient's history and his personal, family, and social resources.

The *Diagnostic Summary* (Figure 21.3) is a multiaxial formulation covering all five axes of DSM-III plus a sixth one on current functioning (occupational role, with family, and with other individuals and groups). For each typological axis (I, clinical psychiatric syndromes; II, personality and specific developmental disorders; and III, physical disorders), the format provides slots for a main formulation of diagnostic terms and codes, as well as for alternatives to be ruled out.

For Axis IV (psychosocial stressors), slots are provided for listing up to four stressors in decreasing order of importance; then their overall severity is marked on a 7-point scale.

Similarly, for Axis V (highest level of adaptive functioning in the past year) and Axis VI (current functioning), the appropriate ratings are marked on the linear scales presented on the format.

The IEF manual, as well as the back of the diagnostic page of the IEF, provides detailed instructions for rating Axes IV, V, VI, which are in line with, but are more specific than, those included in DSM-III.

PERSONAL AND SOCIAL HISTORY (*Developmental, educational, marital, sexual, military, occupational, and legal history. Current family structure and social support system* [availability of confidant, group and community support]. *Assets* [talents, adaptive means of coping, motivation for treatment, etc.] *useful for treatment planning.*)

	NO	YES	NOT KNOWN
	N	Y	?
1. Perinatal problems	N	Y	?
2. Developmental delays	N	Y	?
3. Broken family or serious family problems while growing up	N	Y	?
4. Academic difficulties at school	N	Y	?
5. Behavioral, discipline and social problems at school	N	Y	?
6. Difficulties during military service or less than "honorable" discharge	N	Y	?
7. Considerable past periods of unemployment or poor work performance	N	Y	?
8. History of marital disharmony or divorce	N	Y	?
9. Arrests with convictions	N	Y	?
10. Lack of confidant	N	Y	?
11. Lack of supportive interpersonal and community resources	N	Y	?

Figure 21.2. Personal and social history section of the IEF

DIAGNOSTIC SUMMARY

I. Clinical psychiatric syndromes *(Instructions and codes on back of pages 6 and 7)*

Main Formulation: Codes   Alternatives to be ruled out   Codes

1.
2.
3.
4.

II. Personality and specific developmental disorders *(Instructions and codes on back of pages 6 and 7)*

Main Formulation: Codes   Alternatives to be ruled out: Codes

1.
2.

III. Physical Disorders *(Instructions on back of page 7)*

Main Formulation: Codes   Alternatives to be ruled out: Codes

1.
2.
3.
4.

IV. Psychosocial stressors *(Instructions on back of this page)*

A. Ranked list:
1.
2.
3.
4.

B. Overall stressor severity:

1	2	3	4	5	6	7	0
None	Minimal	Mild	Moderate	Severe	Extreme	Catastrophic	Unspecified

V. Highest level of adaptive functioning during the past year *(Instructions on back of this page)*

1	2	3	4	5	6	7	0
Superior	Very Good	Good	Fair	Poor	Very Poor	Grossly Impaired	Unspecified

VI. Current functioning: *(Instructions on back of this page)*

	Superior	Very Good	Good	Adequate	Slightly Impaired	Moderately Impaired	Markedly Impaired	Unspecified
A. Occupational	1			2	3	4	5	0
B. With family	1			2	3	4	5	0
C. With other indiv. & groups	1			2	3	4	5	0

Figure 21.3. IEF diagnostic summary

THE IEF'S SPANISH TRANSLATION AND ADAPTATION FOR USE IN PERU

The 1980 version of the IEF was translated and adapted by three bilingual psychiatrists (I. Lopez Merino, K. Tejada, and A. Castillo) at the Instituto Nacional de Salud Mental "Honorio Delgado-Hideyo Noguchi" of Lima, Peru (Peruvian National Institute of Mental Health, NIMH).

The translation and adaptation of the 1982 version were even more formalized and included the preparation of a draft by two bilingual psychiatrists (Cecilia Sogi and Dante Warthon) at the above-mentioned institution. This draft was then critically reviewed by an international panel of bilingual psychopathologists (J. Castro, I. Lopez-Merino, J. Mariategui, A. C. Mezzich, J. E. Mezzich, A. Perales, and H. Tovar). Their suggestions were collated, on the basis of which a new draft was prepared and reviewed again by the panel. A final version was prepared using the new set of corrections and suggestions.

The adaptation of the IEF for use in Peru involved the following modifications: (1) use of appropriate Spanish sounds for the assessment of articulation speech problems, (2) specification of special education for mental retardation as a treatment modality, among psychiatric history markers, (3) elimination of "honorable discharge" from the appraisal of military service history, and (4) adjustments in the disposition section to reflect legal regulations for mental-health care in Peru.

EVALUATION OF THE IEF

The evaluation of the interrater reliability of the IEF was conducted at the Peruvian NIMH on the basis of 24 general psychiatric patients assessed by two attending psychiatrists (DW, CS), and at the University of Pittsburgh on the basis of 42 general psychiatric patients evaluated by two teams each composed of a psychiatric nurse and a faculty psychiatrist. These types of evaluator arrangements are the typical ones used routinely at the corresponding institutions. In each case, the two evaluating teams jointly interviewed the patient but completed the IEF independently from each other.

To illustrate the findings obtained, Table 21.2 presents the intraclass correlation coefficients measuring the reliability for the IEF symptom inventory, divided into sections. The overall reliability coefficient was 0.78 in Lima and 0.57 in Pittsburgh.

The interrater reliability of the various axes contained in the IEF diagnostic summary are presented in Table 21.3. The reliability of the psychiatric syndrome's axis was 0.80 in Lima and 0.60 in Pittsburgh. In both settings, substantial and very similar reliability values were obtained for the adaptive functioning axes, and the lowest reliability, among all axes, was obtained for overall stressor severity. These findings probably reflect different levels of conceptual clarity and scale specificity among these quantitative axes.

There was a tendency for reliability findings to be higher in Lima than in

Table 21.2. *Interrater reliability of the IEF symptom inventory*

Sections	Lima (N = 24) r	Pittsburgh (N = 42) r
Vegetative, substance related and characterological	0.95	0.56
General appearance and behavior	0.71	0.55
Speech and thought patterns	0.84	0.59
Mood and affect	0.80	0.64
Thought content and perception	0.76	0.67
Cognitive functioning	0.64	0.42

Note: r = intraclass correlation coefficient.

Table 21.3. *Interrater reliability of the IEF diagnostic formulation*

Axes	Lima (N = 24)	Pittsburgh (N = 42)
I. Clinical syndromes (k)	0.80	0.60
II. Personality disorders (k)	1.00	0.61
III. Physical disorders (k)	0.92	0.66
IV. A. Specific psychosocial stressors (k)	0.68	0.55
B. Overall stressor severity (r)	0.65	0.32
V. Highest functioning in the past year (r)	0.73	0.72
VI. Current functioning (r)	0.74	0.72

Note: k = Kappa; r = intraclass correlation coefficient.

Pittsburgh. This may reflect the different types of evaluators involved in the two settings, that is, two separate psychiatrists in Lima and two nurse-psychiatrist teams in Pittsburgh, as well as the fact that the two psychiatrists performing the evaluations in Lima were familiar with the IEF procedure, as they were instrumental in translating and adapting it.

The second evaluative study involved the assessment of the quality of the IEF as perceived by panels composed of most of the clinicians using the IEF at the Peruvian NIMH and at the University of Pittsburgh. The clinicians appraised the first version of the IEF in terms of four variables (format organization, clarity of items, accuracy of portrayal of the patient's condition, and feasibility and ease of use) each measured on a 4-point scale (very good, fairly good, rather poor, and very poor) (see Table 21.4). Across the items, 71–100 percent of the ratings were at one of the two highest levels, with the large majority of the ratings being at the "very good" level.

Additional information on the suitability and usefulness of the IEF was ob-

Table 21.4. *Clinicians' perceptions of IEF quality*

Survey variables	Very good and fairly good levels[a]	
	Lima (%)	Pittsburgh (%)
Format organization	79	98
Clarity of items	71	100
Portrayal of patient's condition	93	99
Feasibility and ease of use	100	89

[a]Two highest levels on 4-point scale.

tained through studies conducted by quality review boards at both institutions upon inspecting representative samples of routinely completed IEFs. They found that the vast majority of sections and items of the IEF were completed satisfactorily. Across cases and IEF sections, the overall average of satisfactory completion was judged to be 89 percent in Lima and 78 percent in Pittsburgh. With respect to the diagnostic documentation value of the IEF, it was found that in 94 percent of the cases in Lima and 91 percent in Pittsburgh, there was adequate clinical information recorded in the body of the form to satisfy the criteria required in the DSM-III manual for the diagnoses made.

TRAINING AND IMPLEMENTATION

The training of clinical evaluators for proper psychiatric evaluations along the lines of the IEF represents an ongoing program at both institutions, as it involves an orientation to new groups of evaluators as well as refresher activities. The manual is a key element of this training program. The program typically involves the following components: (1) Didactic review of diagnostic evaluation topics and of the approach and sections of the IEF; (2) demonstration of interviewing techniques by senior clinicians; (3) individual practice with live patients and videotaped interviews, followed by group discussions of the ratings made; (4) monitoring of all completed IEFs by administrative clinicians who then provide feedback to the clinical evaluators as needed; and (5) periodic peer reviews and group discussions of sampled IEFs.

The IEF is currently used to articulate the assessment of all new patients presenting for care at both the Peruvian NIMH and the University of Pittsburgh. In Lima, the evaluations are conducted fully by either an attending or a resident psychiatrist, while in Pittsburgh they are carried out by a team composed of a primary evaluator (typically a specially trained nurse, a psychiatric resident or a psychology intern) and a supervising faculty psychiatrist.

All IEFs generated in the clinical operation are checked for completion and clarity of coding by medical records clerks. A growing data base is being con-

Table 21.5. *Most frequent current symptoms*

Frequent symptoms	Lima (%; N = 103)	Pittsburgh (%; N = 174)
Hyposomnia	81	74
Appetite decreased	76	66
Depressed mood	67	80★
General anxiety	64	62
Social withdrawal	61	65
Weight decreased	60	46★
Poor concentration	53	72★★
Suicidal indicators	39	60★★
Low self-esteem	28	60★★★

Note: Difference statistically significant at $p < 0.05$(★); < 0.01 (★★); < 0.001 (★★★).

tinuously developed, which, by the end of 1986, amounted to over 15,000 unduplicated patients seen since 1980 at WPIC in Pittsburgh, and to the 6,000 unduplicated patients seen since 1982 at the Peruvian NIMH.

UTILITY OF THE IEF INFORMATION

The information obtained with the IEF can be used to enhance patient care, to answer clinical-epidemiological research questions including those related to diagnosis and classification, and to facilitate administrative operations and planning.

To illustrate some of the informational findings that can be obtained from IEF data bases, results from analyses conducted on two groups of quasi-randomly selected general psychiatric patients, 103 in Lima and 174 in Pittsburgh, will be presented next. In regards to sex distribution, females amounted to 61 percent in Lima and 64 percent in Pittsburgh. The age distribution of the Peruvian group included 47 percent for ages 18 to 29 and only 7 percent for ages 60 and older, while the corresponding figures in the U.S. group were 31 percent and 20 percent, which grossly reflect the different age distributions in the two cities.

Table 21.5 shows the most frequent current symptoms in the two patient samples. Reflecting considerable cross-national similarity in this regard, hyposomnia and depressed mood were among the top symptoms in both samples. On the other hand, low self-esteem, suicidal indicators, poor concentration, and depressed mood (all psychic symptoms) were significantly more frequent in the Pittsburgh sample, while decreased weight (a somatic sign) was significantly more frequent in Lima.

Table 21.6 displays the frequencies of the DSM-III Axis I diagnoses in the

Table 21.6. *Distribution of patients by clinical psychiatric syndromes (DSM-III Axis I, listed as primary, secondary, tertiary, and quaternary diagnoses)*

DSM-III Axis I Clinical psychiatric syndromes	Lima (%; N = 103)	Pittsburgh (%; N = 174)
Organic mental disorder	4	6
Alcohol use disorder	9	15
Other substance abuse	4	7
Schizophrenic disorders	17	6*
Other psychotic disorders	8	2
Bipolar disorder	4	6
Major depression, single episode	16	17
Major depression, recurrent	11	21*
Dysthymic disorder	11	11
Phobic disorders	3	0
Anxiety states	11	4*
Somatoform disorders	2	2
Psychosexual disorders	4	0*
Adjustment disorders	10	6
Other psychiatric disorders	3	14
Deferred or no diagnosis	3	8

*Difference statistically significant at $p < 0.05$.

Lima and Pittsburgh samples. Despite the relatively small samples, most broad categories in Axis I were covered. Schizophrenia, anxiety, and psychosexual disorders were significantly more frequent in Lima, whereas recurrent major depression was more frequent in Pittsburgh.

Finally, Table 21.7 presents a comparative distribution of broad categories of psychosocial stress. Stressors were identified much more frequently in the Pittsburgh sample, and here the most frequent and differential stressors were those related to work, love and marriage, and financial problems.

SUMMARY

The IEF is a semistructured psychiatric evaluation procedure that involves a standardized and flexibly scheduled interview, allows a phenomenological attitude in the evaluator, covers several key aspects of the clinical condition, uses all sources of information available, and has a recording format that contains structured and narrative components complementing each other. It yields a multiaxial formulation covering all diagnostic categories and axes of DSM-III.

Adequate levels of reliability, clinician acceptability, informational utility, and full implementation in comprehensive institutions in Lima and Pittsburgh have been documented for this instrument.

Table 21.7. *Broad categories of psychosocial stress*

Broad categories	Lima (%; N = 103)	Pittsburgh (%; N = 174)
Health	28	26
Love and marriage	23	36*
Parental	10	16
Other familial relationship	12	13
Housing/environmental	9	16
Work	8	30***
School	8	6
Financial	7	16*
Bereavement	7	14
Others	11	30***
No stressors	29	8***

Note: Difference statistically significant at $p < 0.05$ (*); $p < 0.01$ (**); $p < 0.001$ (***).

As a semistructured procedure, the IEF is inappropriate for a number of purposes (e.g., community surveys conducted by laymen or investigations of certain specific syndromes in laboratory settings). However, given its applicability in general patient care settings and broad informational coverage, the IEF appears to be a promising instrument for the naturalistic study of diagnostic systems and related processes in a real clinical context.

REFERENCES

American Psychiatric Association. 1980. *Diagnostic and Statistical Manual of Mental Disorders*. 3rd ed. (DSM-III). Washington, D.C.

Brockington, I. F., and Meltzer, H. Y. 1982. Documenting an episode of psychiatric illness: need for multiple information sources, multiple raters, and narrative. *Schizophrenia Bulletin* 8: 485–492.

Carpenter, W. T., Strauss, J. S., and Bartko, J. J. 1981. Beyond diagnosis: the phenomenology of schizophrenia. *American Journal of Psychiatry* 138: 948–953.

Climent, C. E., Plutchik, R., Estrada, H., Gaviria, L. F., and Arevalo, W. 1975. A comparison of traditional and symptom-checklist-based histories. *American Journal of Psychiatry* 132: 450–453.

Endicott, J., and Spitzer, R. L. 1978. A diagnostic interview: the schedule for Affective Disorders and Schizophrenia. *Archives of General Psychiatry* 35: 837–844.

Ganguli, M., and Saul, M. C. 1982. Diagnostic Interview Schedule (Letter to the Editor). *Archives of General Psychiatry* 39: 1442–1444.

Greist, J. H., van Cura, L. J., and Kneppreth, N. P. 1973. A computer interview for emergency room patients. *Computer Biomedical Research* 6: 254–265.

Helzer, J. E. 1981. The use of a structured diagnostic interview for routine psychiatric evaluation. *Journal of Nervous and Mental Disease* 169: 45–49.

Hesselbrock, V., Stabenau, J., Hesselbrock, M., Mirkin, P., and Meyer, R. 1982. A comparison of two interview schedules. The Schedule for Affective Disorders and Schizophrenia – life time and the National Institute of Mental Health Diagnostic Interview Schedule. *Archives of General Psychiatry* 39: 674–677.

Jaspers, K. 1963. *General Psychopathology*. Transl. J. Hoening and M. W. Hamilton Chicago: University of Chicago Press.

Kiernan, W. E. S., McCreadie, R. G., and Flanagan, W. L. 1976. Trainee's competence in psychiatric case writing. *British Journal of Psychiatry* 129: 107–172.

Laska, M. L. 1974. The multi-state information system, in *Progress in Mental Health Information Systems*, ed. J. L. Crawford, D.W. Morgan, and D.T. Gianturc. Cambridge, Mass.: Ballinger.

Mezzich, J. E., Dow, J. T., and Coffman, G. A. 1981. Developing an efficient clinical information system for a comprehensive psychiatric institute. I. Principles, design and organization. *Behavior Research Methods and Instrumentation* 13: 459–463.

Mezzich, J. E., Dow, J. T., Rich, C. L., Costello, A. J., and Himmelhoch, J. M. 1981. Developing an efficient clinical information system for a comprehensive psychiatric institute. II. Initial Evaluation Form. *Behavior Research Methods and Instrumentation* 13: 464–478.

Mezzich, J. E., Ganguli, R, Munetz, J. R., Zettler-Segal, M., and Dow, J. T. 1986. Computerized initial and discharge evaluations in *Clinical Care and Information Systems in Psychiatry*, ed. J. E. Mezzich. Washington, D.C.: American Psychiatric Press.

Richardson, S. A., Dohrenwend, B. S., and Klein, D. 1965. *Interviewing: Its Forms and Function*. New York: Basic Books.

Robins, L. N. 1985. Composite International Diagnostic Review. Paper presented at the 138th Annual Meeting of the American Psychiatric Association, Dallas, May 21.

Robins, L. N., and Helzer, J. E. 1982. Diagnostic Interview Schedule, Letters to the Editor. *Archives of General Psychiatry* 39: 1443–1445.

Robins, L. N., Helzer, J. E., Croughan, J. L., and Ratcliff, K. 1981. The NIMH Diagnostic Interview Schedule: its history, characteristics and validity, in *What Is a case?: The problem of definition in psychiatric community surveys*, ed. J. K. Wing, P. Bobbington, and L. N. Robins. London: Grant McIntyre.

Saghir, M. T. 1971. A comparison of some aspects of structured and unstructured psychiatric interviews. *American Journal of Psychiatry* 128: 180–184.

Scharfetter, C. 1972. *Das AMDP-System. Manual zur Dokumentation Psychiatrischer Befunde*. 2nd ed. Berlin: Springer.

Spitzer, R. L. 1983. Psychiatric diagnosis: Are clinicians still necessary? *Comprehensive Psychiatry* 24: 399–411.

Spitzer, R. L. 1985. Structured Clinical Interview for Diagnosis. Paper presented at the 138th Annual Meeting of the American Psychiatric Association, Dallas, May 21.

Spitzer, R. L., Skodol, A. E., Williams, J. B, Gibbon, M., and Kass, F. 1982. Supervising intake diagnosis: A psychiatric "Rashomon." *Archives of General Psychiatry* 39: 1299–1305.

Weitzel, W. D., Morgan, D. W., Guyden, T. E., and Robinson, J. A. 1973. Toward a more efficient mental status examination. *Archives of General Psychiatry* 28: 215–218.

Wing, J. K., Cooper, J. E., and Sartorius, N. 1974. *Measurement and Classification of Psychiatric Symptoms: An Instruction Manual for the PSE and CATEGO Program.* Cambridge: Cambridge University Press.

World Health Organization. 1977. *Manual of the Ninth Revision of the International Classification of Diseases (ICD–9).* Geneva.

PART IV

Current nosological issues and prospects

22 A review of the usage of diagnostic systems in national admission statistics

LETTEN SAUGSTAD (Norway)

AN EMPIRICAL INVESTIGATION

The chapter on mental disease in the eighth revision of the International Classification of Diseases (ICD-8) (World Health Organization, 1967) was implemented internationally about 1970. One of the main reasons for the earlier reluctance to accept international standards had been the prevailing national discrepancies in diagnostic practice. In Norway and Denmark, where the Kraepelinian nosology was traditional, a need was felt for a third category of functional psychoses ("reactive" or "psychogenic" psychosis) in addition to schizophrenia and manic-depressive (affective) disorder. As shown in Table 22.1, more than 42 percent of first admissions to Norwegian psychiatric hospitals were given this diagnosis in 1965, and in Denmark 39 percent of first admissions in 1965–6 were so classified. In France, an intermediate category was introduced in the past century. Such a diagnosis, particularly in its acute form (*bouffée délirante*), has been much used (Pichot, 1982). In other countries such as Sweden, the United States, the Soviet Union, and the United Kingdom, psychiatrists have felt no need for such categories, because they employed either an extremely wide concept of schizophrenia (USA, USSR) or of affective disorder (UK). In Sweden, the intermediate category of functional psychoses is probably included in the nonpsychotic categories, which (in 1962–4) comprised more than 60 percent of first admissions.

The World Health Organization proposed a change in diagnostic practice in ICD-8 by reserving the three-digit category 298 for the intermediate (other) functional psychoses. It was expected to reduce the international discrepancy through a narrowing of the concepts of schizophrenia and affective disorder. ICD-8 also introduced three new subgroups of schizophrenia that by definition had a favorable prognosis (295.4, 295.5, 295.7), thereby engendering a change in the concept of schizophrenia as a disorder with an inevitably unfavorable outcome. This fundamental change in attitude was probably an important reason why the general reluctance was overcome and the ICD-8 was internationally accepted. Admittedly, the disagreement between experts prevailed in the classification test of 12 atypical psychoses presented at the second WHO seminar on diagnosis, classification, and statistics in psychiatry held in Oslo in 1966 (Astrup & Odegård, 1970). The Norwegian psychiatrist Odegård diagnosed 9

253

Table 22.1. *Proportion of first admissions by diagnosis before 1970 (both sexes combined)*

ICD-8 Diagnoses	Denmark (1965–6)	Sweden (1962–4)	Poland (1969)	Norway (1965)	United States (1969)
295	5.4	13.9	16.7	19.0	46.1
296	15.2	15.1	5.6	10.4	8.5
297, 298, 299	39.3[a]	9.6	37.3[b]	42.2	10.7
300, 306–8	40.1	61.4	40.4	28.4	34.7[c]
Total admissions	4,179	15,870	35,185	4,272	194,543

Note: Diagnostic codes: 295: schizophrenia; 296: major affective disorders; 297: paranoid states; 298: other psychoses; 299: unspecified psychosis; 300: neuroses; 306: special symptoms; 307: transient situational disturbances; 308: behavior disorders of childhood and adolescence.
[a]Includes 306–8.
[b]Includes organic and symptomatic psychoses and involutional melancholia.
[c]26.3 percent was nonpsychotic depression (300.4).

of the 12 cases as intermediate (reactive) psychoses, and the Danish representative Strömgren diagnosed 7 of the 12 cases in this way. The representatives from the United States and the Soviet Union did not use this diagnosis at all but preferred the diagnosis of schizophrenia in 8 and 10 cases, respectively. The representative from the United Kingdom classified 8 of the cases as affective disorder. Another important reason why the ICD-8 was internationally accepted was that uniformity in diagnostic practice became essential after the introduction of psychotropic drugs in the 1950s. If clinical psychiatrists wanted to profit from one another's experience, they had to speak the same diagnostic language.

International communication about psychiatric conditions rests on a classification that is internationally accepted and practiced in such a way that the official statistics are comparable. Information on first admissions to psychiatric hospitals with a breakdown by ICD code was available only from seven WHO member countries after 1970: Norway, Denmark, England, France, Poland, Australia (Province of Victoria), and the United States. The functional psychoses were divided in three groups: schizophrenia (295), affective disorder (296), and the "intermediate" psychoses (297, 298, 299). A proportion of nonpsychotic conditions (300, 306–8) was also included, while the following diagnoses were left out of the analysis: organic and symptomatic psychoses (290–4) and alcoholism and drug addiction (301, 303–4) (Saugstad & Odegård, 1983).

As seen from the admission statistics for the mid–1970s in Table 22.2, the proportion of intermediate psychoses ranged from 8.3 percent in Australia and 11.8 percent in the United States to 36.8 percent in Denmark, where admissions classified as schizophrenia amounted to 7.4 percent, compared with 11.5 percent in England and Wales and 46.6 percent in the United States. Affective disorder

Table 22.2. *Proportion of first admissions by diagnosis after 1970 (both sexes combined)*

ICD-8 Diagnosis	Denmark (1974–5)	England[a] (1976)	Norway (1972–4)	France[b] (1974)	Poland[c] (1976)	Australia[d] (1972–5)	USA[e] (1975)
295	7.4	11.5	12.8	14.5	18.0	29.7	46.6
296	25.5	42.5	6.4	17.0	12.2	15.7	37.1
297, 298, 299	36.8	13.4	28.1	23.3	29.7	8.3	11.8
300, 306–8	30.3	32.6	52.7	45.2	41.1	46.3	4.5
Total admissions	4,173	56,080	5,274	77,700	44,849	11,350	53,217

Note: For diagnostic codes see Table 22.1.

[a]295 includes 297, and "depressive disorder not elsewhere specified" is included with 296.

[b]298 also includes nonpsychotic depressions (300.4).

[c]297, 298, 299 also include 290–4, and involutional melancholia.

[d]Victoria.

[e]296 includes 298.0 and 300.4, while 297, 298, 299 include 310–5, 302, 305, 306, and 316–9. The information is from a sample survey conducted by the National Institute of Mental Health (Department of Health and Human Services).

was diagnosed in only 6.3 percent of the admissions in Norway, compared with 3.71 percent of those in the United States and 42.5 percent in England and Wales, where "depressions not elsewhere classified" were included in this category. The proportion of nonpsychotic admissions ranged from less than 5 percent (USA) to more than 50 percent (Norway). The discrepancy in diagnostic distribution is, therefore, more or less the same as it was before the introduction of the ICD-8 (Table 22.1). The new intermediate category (298) had no success in the United States, where admissions labeled as schizophrenia remained around 46 percent. Neither was there an increased use of the 298 diagnosis in England and Wales, despite an even further decrease in the use of the diagnoses of schizophrenia and paranoid psychosis after 1970. A reduction in the use of the intermediate category (298) was observed in Denmark, Poland, and Norway, accompanied by a rise in the use of the diagnoses of schizophrenia and affective disorder in Denmark and Poland. In Norway there was a continuous decline in the use of these diagnoses, as less than 5 percent of first admissions were given one of these diagnoses in 1978 (Saugstad & Odegård, 1980). In particular, the new subgroups of schizophrenia (295.4, 295.5, 295.7) were used in only 1.2 percent, and nonpsychotic diagnoses at admission now predominate in this country (52.7 percent). A wide concept of affective disorder (including depressions not elsewhere classified) persists in England and Wales (42.5 percent), where an additional one-third of first admissions were classified as nonpsychotic depressions (300.4). This preference for depressions as the least stigmatizing mental disorder goes back to Aubrey Lewis's (1934) influential paper establishing a concept of affective disorder that includes those depressive psychoses classified as "reactive" or "psychogenic" in Norway and Denmark, and probably also cases that in the United States would have been diagnosed as schizophrenia or schizoaffective psychosis (Kantor & Glassman, 1977). The persistent predominance of a wide concept of psychophrenia in the United States (46.6 percent of first admissions) indicates that the social stigma attached to the term "psychosis," and particularly to schizophrenia, is of less importance in that country. In contrast to Norway, there is a veritable flight from the Kraepelinian disease entities, as well as from the term "psychosis."

A narrowing of the concept of schizophrenia that accompanied the high frequency of social remissions in the 1960s led to a predominance of admission with a diagnosis of intermediate (reactive) psychosis (Table 22.1). After 1970, the use of psychotropic drugs further accelerated the narrowing of the concept of schizophrenia to a disease with a necessarily unfavorable outcome (some 5 percent of admissions) concomitantly with a decline in admissions classified as "reactive" psychosis. The present predominance of nonpsychotic admissions to Norwegian psychiatric hospitals may be a result of the inability to eliminate the social stigma attached to the term "psychosis." Psychiatrists in Norway prefer a diagnosis that traditionally implies a favorable outcome, and nonpsychotic depression (300.4) is the preferred diagnosis in around 20 percent (Saugstad & Odegård, 1980).

The present fundamental differences in the diagnostic distribution observed in these seven countries with similar nosological concepts cannot be explained satisfactorily as variation in psychiatric morbidity. They must result from persistent national differences in diagnostic practice. The general reluctance to adhere to international diagnostic standards, which was seemingly overcome when the ICD-8 was universally accepted, is now evident in these national differences, as well as in the restricted official use of ICD-8. During the last 10 years or so, additional problems have been created through the development of a multitude of new national and local diagnostic and classificatory systems. For example, the Research Diagnostic Criteria (Spitzer, Endicott & Robins, 1978) has been used in the United States while CATEGO and the Index of Definition (ID) (Wing, Cooper & Sartorius, 1974) have been developed in Britain. Specific operational criteria as well as multiaxial systems (Mezzich, 1979) have been proposed in several countries. The replacement of ICD-8 by a national classification, DSM-III (American Psychiatric Association, 1980), further aggravated this situation.

It was hoped that the wide acceptance of ICD-8 would result in its effective official use. As we have seen, information was available only from seven WHO member countries, and of these only two countries, Norway and Denmark, strictly adhered to the ICD-codes. In the remaining countries various codes are grouped together, such as 295 and 297 (schizophrenia and paranoid psychosis), 296 and 311 (affective disorder and "depressive disorder not elsewhere classified"), as well as 298 and 290–4 (other psychosis and organic and symptomatic psychoses). Neither the concept of other psychosis (298) nor the three new subgroups of schizophrenia (295.4, 295.5, 295.7) were widely accepted.

The most striking finding in the present investigation is, however, the complete lack of information from any developing country regarding the use of ICD-8 or ICD-9. The developing countries contain about three-fourths of the world's population. They have limited economic resources, and very few psychiatrists. Mental health has a low priority in those countries. They are mostly forced to use nonpsychiatric service personnel. These developing countries accepted chapter V (mental disorder) in the ICD-8 together with the other parts of ICD-8, probably more as a necessary evil than as a clinically useful instrument. They have already exposed shortcomings in the ICD, and stated that it must become more truly international by paying adequate attention to the type of mental disorders encountered in countries culturally different from those of Western Europe or the United States. It should be remembered that the reason why ICD-7 was not internationally accepted was that it was too Anglo-Saxon, whereas the ICD-8 is more "European," with its incorporation of French and Scandinavian diagnostic concepts.

The present investigation clearly illustrates the problems encountered in international cooperation. To judge from Norwegian experience, possibly the ICD-8 is already too complicated for international statistical usage. More than 30 percent of hospitalized psychotics in 1977–8 were classified as "unspecific" (fourth digit 9). There was, in reality, nonusage of the fourth digit (Saugstad & Odegård, 1980), whether because of a lack of clinical information or doubt in clinical diagnosis. This was also the case in England and Wales, where the most frequently used diagnosis was the unspecific "depressive disorder not elsewhere classified" (about one-third of admissions). It has, however, already been shown how the proportion of these cases could be reduced to only 1 percent through furnishing clinical psychiatrists with a WHO glossary and instructing them in its use (Zigmond & Sims, 1983). Even in our psychiatrically "developed" countries, diagnostic (clinical) practice can, therefore, be considered improved.

ISSUES IN THE DEVELOPMENT OF ICD-10

Revision of the International Statistical Classification of Diseases, Injuries and Causes of Death, or ICD, takes place regularly in order to resolve some of the differences associated with the previous revision, to adapt it to current practice, and to keep up with scientific advancement. The tenth revision (ICD-10) is already in preparation, and it seems reasonable to comment on some of the suggested changes related to the present investigation. Psychiatry was the first branch of medicine to publish official morbidity statistics, which in Norway date back to the middle of the nineteenth century, with separate recording of first admissions and readmissions by diagnoses since 1916. The psychiatric classification had to meet particular requirements stemming from its being part of a comprehensive classification of diseases. In fact, the mental disorder section or chapter V was the last chapter to gain international acceptance. As we have observed, however, very few countries use the ICD in a way that could make comparable their official admission statistics by diagnosis. There was a frequency analysis by ICD codes in only two countries, while the remaining countries used various combinations of diagnoses, such as affective disorder with "depressive disorder not elsewhere classified," and schizophrenia with paranoid psychosis.

The ICD is a statistical classification which means that only a limited number of categories are used to describe the whole range of mental disorder. A certain further reduction in the number of categories seems advisable as it could facilitate the usage of ICD-10 in official statistics. Under the heading F30–39 (affective mood disorders) where the distinction between a depressive neurosis and depressive psychosis has been abandoned, seven different categories of depressive disorder are included. This seems to be an adaptation to current practices in the United Kingdom, and in the United States. To a certain extent, it is also in agreement with the fact that mood stability is a fundamental personality trait with a normal distribution. What is considered within or outside normal variation is, therefore, arbitrary and related to sociocultural conditions. With this in mind, it would have been helpful to have all depressive disorders included under adjustment disorder within the class of mood disorders. Instead, several are listed as F40–49 (neurotic, stress-related, and somatization disorders). More important, and contrary to the statement that the distinction between neurotic and psychotic depressions has been abandoned, three different categories of depressive psychoses are classified in chapter F20–29 (schizophrenia and other psychotic disorders) as acute psychotic episode (depressive type), schizoaffective disorder (depressive type), and reactive (psychogenic) psychoses (depressive type). It remains to be seen whether these last categories will be used to a great extent. Another question is where to place anxiety with underlying depression. As mentioned earlier, we have seen the development of specific diagnostic criteria for patient evaluation during the last 10 years or so. The ICD-10 will eventually include, in addition to the basic glossary, a number of documents, such as one containing precise diagnostic criteria. There is, however, a disturbing lack of consensus regarding diagnosis between the present British and American systems, as has been verified by Dean and coworkers (1983) in their Edinburgh community sample. There was agreement about diagnostic labeling in only 16.7 percent of cases of anxiety and 56 percent of cases of depression. The often difficult clinical task of deciding whether depression or anxiety predominates, and their similarities in treatment, suggest that the transfer of neurotic depression should have been accompanied by a similar relocation of anxiety as a mood disorder.

The present general reluctance to diagnose schizophrenia and the failure of its three new subgroups with a favorable outcome (acute, latent, and schizoaffective) to gain acceptance suggest that a narrow concept of schizophrenia now predominates. There is, however, probably no particular change in incidence despite the observed decline in the proportion of first-admission patients classified as schizophrenics. The increasing prevalence may be due to the accumulation of chronic cases. The expansion of schizophrenia coding from one to four three-character codes (paranoid, residual, schizoaffective, and other types) therefore comes as a surprise. So far, no biological or genetic marker has been identified defending further subclassification. In Norway, during 1977–8, the most frequently used schizophrenic subtypes were paranoid (33.6 percent) and unspecific (20 percent), whereas only 7 percent of the patients were diagnosed as schizoaffective and 1 percent as residual (Saugstad & Odegård, 1980).

The most striking finding in the present investigation of the usage of ICD-8 was the complete lack of information from developing countries. The totally new feature in ICD-10 with its reservation of a particular three-character code for acute psychotic episode is particularly welcome. It is seen as an adaptation to the clinical psychiatric picture frequently seen in developing countries. It is hoped that ICD-10 will be widely used and will reduce the reluctance to use the international classification. It is extremely important for the WHO to succeed in this task, since the majority of the world population resides in these countries.

It is further planned that Chapter V will consist of a family of classifications that includes the presently discussed core classification with its basic glossary and instructions designed to meet the needs of morbidity, and mortality classification and statistical reporting, and in addition a number of adaptations, extensions, and associated classifications, as well as documents for special purposes. Chapter V is, therefore, complicated and it may already have "complicated" itself out of ICD-10. With more than 70 percent of the world population residing in developing countries and having only one or two psychiatrists per million persons, classification cannot be operated by clinical psychiatrists. An international classification should, therefore, be simple enough to be used by nonpsychiatric medical personnel; it must seem clinically useful and relevant to their psychiatric experience and be bias-free. The number of categories should be limited to a minimum, since we will have classifications available for research and for local and national purposes.

The proposed expansion of ICD-10 to cover a total of 100 three-character codes with the further possibility of a large number of fourth-digit codes creates a formidable task for its future users. With such an abundance of categories to choose from and a variety of additional documents, the ICD-10 core classification of mental disorders (chapter V) may be too complicated for international statistical usage. The frequent argument that ICD-10 will be more satisfactory and scientifically superior to ICD-8 and ICD-9 usually is made on the basis of its prospective use of operational criteria and definitions. Diagnostic concepts are posed as more reliable and valid because they are amenable to translation into operational diagnostic criteria. This may not be true. According to Kendell (1982), the development of various sets of operational criteria seems to have decreased international agreement in psychiatry. Furthermore, there is an alarming lack of consensus between the predominant British and American systems (Saugstad & Odegård, 1983, 1985).

The ongoing cooperation between the WHO and the American Psychiatric Association to facilitate the convergence between ICD-10 and DSM-IV suggests that ICD-10 will become more Americanized than any of its predecessors. This may deter the developing countries from using ICD-10, as they have tended to react negatively to the "Western" orientation of previous ICDs. International communication in psychiatry has been made more difficult by the replacement in the United States in 1980 of the ICD by the national DSM-III classification system. A few years after its implementation, DSM-III is already being revised, perhaps because of the limited empirical justification of its 200 categories of mental disorder, and the often arbitrary nature of their definitions. There is the risk that a multitude of new national and local diagnostic classification systems will be developed, using different operational criteria and sometimes disregarding the fundamentals of psychopathology. This would create a confusing situation in psychiatric classification, reminiscent of the conditions described by Dr. P. Renaudin, the director of the asylum at Meurthe in France in 1856:

It is thus essential to understand the significance of words, i.e. the elements of a rational classification and the value of the signs reflecting the observational method. It is evident that this understanding does not exist any longer; we must be seriously concerned about indefinitely postponing a future stage, or it may reestablish itself. After having fought victoriously against administrative and judicial prejudice, which excluded certain cases from the picture of mental derangement, after medical-legal expertise has won true victories which honor science and humanity, we see anarchy dividing our ranks and pressing us to loose the fruits of our predecessors' labors.

How can we prevent such a situation? It may be possible to simplify the proposed ICD-10 by pushing it away from becoming a nomenclature (in which a unique code is assigned to every mental condition that can be specifically described) and focusing, instead, on simple and fairly general categories relevant to a truly core classification.

How can we limit the number of three-character codes? Perhaps by eliminating some aspects of the proposed classification that psychiatrists in the developing countries find unsatisfactory, and by preserving some continuity with previous ICD revisions. The forced distinction between organic and so-called functional or nonorganic conditions should be abandoned, as it can be assumed that all mental disorders have, to some extent, an organic basis. It is only a matter of time and research for etiological factors or causes to be identified. The classification should, therefore, be based solely on the clinical syndrome presented by the individual patient, and the fourth digit reserved for etiological factors. Instead of following the suggestion that "all the mental disorders attributable to demonstrable organic causes (with the exception of those due to substance use) are grouped together, regardless of whether their predominant manifestations are psychotic or nonpsychotic," patients with similar clinical symptoms should be grouped together, irrespective of cause. Psychiatric disease entities differ from those in general medicine because a variety of different etiological factors may give rise to the same mental disorder which may be considered a nonspecific response of the patient's personality. On the other hand, the same etiological factor may lead to different disease entities in different individuals. Thus, to stimulate acuity in clinical observation and further research on causation, it is important to base the classification on the clinical symptoms only.

In addition to the two problems mentioned above, we have the arbitrary definition of what is abnormal regarding mood disorders and their relations to social and cultural factors. As a first step, all mood disorders should be grouped together in one major class.

We found questionable the inclusion of personality, adjustment, somatoform, and psychosomatic disorders in the core classification, since their identity as mental disorders is problematic. Perhaps they should be included only if they result in hospital admission or social disadvantage (inability to work requiring an invalid pension, etc.) (Saugstad, 1986). There is an element of psychiatric propaganda in considering all reactions and personality conditions as mental disorders. It is also discriminating. Not all patients with somatic problems are recorded specifically in official health statistics.

One may consider as an example of possible ways to operate with a small number of three-character codes the Egyptian psychiatric classification system (DMP–1). (See Chapter 5.) It is based on several classifications such as ICD-8, DSM-II, and the INSERM French classification with additional influence from Anglo-Saxon and Soviet psychiatry. It contains 16 major classes of mental disorder, with cross-references to the international classification. Even an instrument such as the Composite International Diagnostic Interview (CIDI) (see

Chapter 19), which is aimed at producing diagnoses according to various classification systems, operates with 43 categories instead of the 200 DSM-III and the 100 currently proposed for ICD-10.

REFERENCES

American Psychiatric Association. 1980. *Diagnostic and Statistical Manual of Mental Disorders*. 3rd ed. (DSM-III). Washington, D.C.

Astrup, C., and Odegård, O. 1970. Continued experiments in psychiatric diagnosis. *Acta Psychiatrica Scandinavica* 46: 180–210.

Dean, C., Surtees, P. G., and Sashidharan, S. P. 1983. Comparison of research diagnostic systems in an Edinburgh community sample. *British Journal of Psychiatry* 142: 247–256.

Kantor, S. J., and Glassman, A. H. 1977. Delusional Depressions. Natural History and Response to Treatment. *British Journal of Psychiatry* 131: 351–360.

Kendell, R. E. 1982. The choice of diagnostic criteria for biological research. *Archives of General Psychiatry* 39: 1334–1339.

Lewis, A. J. 1934. Melancholia: Clinical survey of depressive states. *Journal of Mental Science* 80: 277–378.

Mezzich, J. E. 1979. Patterns and issues in multiaxial psychiatric diagnosis. *Psychological Medicine* 9: 125–137.

Pichot, P. 1982. The diagnosis and classification of mental disorders in French-speaking countries: background, current views, and comparisons with nomenclatures. *Psychological Medicine* 12: 475–492.

Renaudin, P. 1856. Observations sur les recherches statistiques relative a l'alienation mentale. *Annales Medico-Psychologiques* 2: 339–360.

Saugstad, L. 1986. The advantage of a register which goes back to 1916. The National Norwegian Case Register. In *Psychiatric Case Registers*, ed. R. Giel, S. ten Horn, and G. Gulbinat. Amsterdam: Elsevier.

Saugstad, L., and Odegård O. 1980. Ingen internasjonal tilnaerming etter 10 ar med den internasjonale diagnoseliste ICD–8. *Nord. Psyk. Tidsk.* 34: 455–464.

Saugstad, L., and Odegård, O. 1983. Persistent discrepancy in international diagnostic practice since 1970. *Acta Psychiatrica Scandinavica* 68: 501–510.

Saugstad, L., and Odegård, O. 1985. In defence of International Classification. *Psychological Medicine* 15: 1–2.

Saugstad, L., and Odegård, O. 1986. Chorea Huntington in Norway. *Psychological Medicine* 16: 39–48.

Saugstad, L., and Odegård, O. In press. Inbreeding and functional psychosis (schizophrenia). *Clinical Genetics*.

Spitzer, R. L., Endicott, J., and Robins, E. 1978. Research diagnostic criteria. *Archives of General Psychiatry* 35: 773–782.

Wing J. K., Cooper, J. E., Sartorius, N. 1974. *Measurement and Classification of Psychiatric Symptoms*. Cambridge: Cambridge University Press.

World Health Organization. 1967. *Manual of the International Classification of Diseases*. 8th rev. ed. (ICD-8). Geneva.

Zigmond, A. S., and Sims, A. C. 1983. The effect of the use of the International Classification of Diseases, Ninth Revision, upon hospital in-patient diagnoses. *British Journal of Psychiatry* 142: 409–413.

23 *The revision of DSM-III*

Process and changes

ROBERT L. SPITZER AND
JANET B. W. WILLIAMS (USA)

INTRODUCTION

DSM-III was published in February of 1980. Shortly thereafter a Committee to Evaluate DSM-III was appointed by the American Psychiatric Association (APA). This committee was charged with reviewing both the impact of DSM-III and the problems related to its use. In 1983 that committee recommended to the APA Board of Trustees that a new group be formed to begin work on a revision of DSM-III, and in May of that year the Work Group to Revise DSM-III was constituted with the senior author as its chair. Ultimately, the Work Group has numbered, in addition to the two authors of this chapter, eleven persons: Drs. Dennis Cantwell, Allen Frances, Ken Kendler, Gerald Klerman, David Kupfer, Roger Peele, Judith Rapoport, Darrel Regier, Bruce Rounsaville, George Vaillant, and Lyman Wynne. The mandate of the Work Group was to act as a steering committee and guide the clarification of ambiguities and inconsistencies in the classification, diagnostic criteria, and text, and to make changes in the text and criteria based on new data that had become available since the publication of DSM-III. Further, the Work Group had to maintain consistency with ICD–9-CM, the Clinical Modification of the ICD that is used in the United States.

No sooner had the Work Group begun its project than people began to ask if a revision was really necessary, seemingly so soon after DSM-III had come into use. The view of the APA and the Work Group was that a revision, to be published in 1987, was timely because of the explosion of research studies carried out on DSM-III categories that had suggested numerous revisions that should be made. Any changes, however, had to be well thought out and based on careful consideration.

THE PROCESS OF REVISION

Basically, there have been four phases to our work. The first phase, which began in May 1983 and lasted about six months, was an "outreach" phase. During this time, the Work Group assembled a list of people whom we thought could make contributions to the revision. This list of more than two

263

Table 23.1. *DSM-III-R Advisory Committees*

Infancy, Childhood, and Adolescence (General)
Pervasive Developmental Disorders
Specific Developmental Disorders
Attention Deficit, Conduct, and Oppositional Disorders
Stereotyped Movement Disorders
Substance Use Disorders
Substance-induced (nonalcohol) Organic Mental Disorders
Sleep Disorders
Eating Disorders
Impulse Control Disorders
Psychotic Disorders
Mood (Affective) Disorders
Dysthymic Disorder
Melancholia
Anxiety Disorders
Post-traumatic Stress Disorder
Somatoform, Organic Mental Disorders, and 316
Dissociative Disorders
Gender Identity Disorders
Psychosexual Dysfunctions
Paraphilias
Factitious Disorder
Premenstrual Dysphoric Disorder
Personality Disorders
Defense Mechanisms
Multiaxial System
Cross-cultural Issues

hundred persons was gleaned from our work on DSM-III, from the journal literature, and from other professional contacts. Most of the people were in the United States, although many were from outside the country. We notified these people of the plan for the revision and invited them to submit suggestions; many of them then became members of the various Advisory Committees.

The advisory-committee phase began in early 1984. Table 23.1 presents a list of the various Advisory Committees. To date, we have had more than 30 Advisory Committee meetings, and each meeting has included from 4 to more than 30 persons. Frequently, after a meeting of a full Advisory Committee, smaller subgroups of the committee have been assembled to work out various specific problems not fully resolved at the initial meeting.

On several occasions it has been impossible to resolve certain issues at Advisory Committee meetings. One instance of this took place after an Advisory Committee meeting on attention deficit, conduct, and oppositional disorders, when, after several attempts, the committee was unable to reach a consensus about the revised criteria. The committee did agree to conduct a field trial in 10 different child evaluation centers, where provisional revised criteria were subsequently tried out. The results of this field trial ensured that the final proposed revisions were based on empirical data.

The third phase of the revision involved the submission of proposed changes in the classification and criteria to the APA Board of Trustees and Assembly of District Branches, as well as to the panels of experts assembled in the first place. For the three months of this third phase, we responded to criticisms of the proposed criteria and suggestions for further revisions. A complete draft of the proposed changes was also made available to the field, to facilitate more review and evaluation of our work.

In the final, one-year, phase of our work we revised the text of DSM-III. Changes in the text often follow changes in the criteria, so the revised criteria had to be established in order for this final phase to proceed. The completed document was submitted to the Board of Trustees and Assembly in late 1986, for publication in 1987. Since the publication of ICD-10 is expected in 1993, the timing of DSM-III-R is approximately midway between DSM-III itself in 1980 and DSM-IV in 1993.

CHANGES

The major changes in DSM-III-R fall into two categories: those that affect the entire classification, and those that involve revisions in individual categories or diagnostic classes.

Changes affecting the entire classification

In both the DSM-III and DSM-III-R classifications, each major diagnostic class includes a residual category for disorders that are best classified within that class of disorders, but that do not meet the diagnostic criteria for any of the specific disorders within that class. The term "not otherwise specified" (NOS) replaces the term "atypical" that was used in DSM-III for each of these residual categories. Thus, for example, the terms "atypical psychosis" and "atypical depression" are replaced in the revision by "psychotic disorder NOS" and "depressive disorder NOS." The reason for this change is that many have complained that the use in DSM-III of the term "atypical" is, in itself, an atypical use of the term. In addition, this change brings DSM-III-R more in line with ICD-9-CM, which uses the term NOS. It solves another problem by clearing up the confusion that has existed with the use of the term "atypical depression." Dr. Donald Klein and his associates, as well as other investigators, have long used the term to identify a particular type of depression that is characterized by a particular constellation of symptoms and that appears to be responsive to monoamine oxidase inhibitors (Liebowitz et al., 1984).

Another new convention that affects the overall classification is the provision that enables clinicians to indicate the current severity of each mental disorder as either mild, moderate, severe, in partial remission (or residual state), or in complete remission. "Mild," "moderate," and "severe" should be used to indicate the severity of a current disorder at the time of the evaluation when all of the diagnostic criteria are met. The distinction among these three indications of severity should take into account the number and intensity of the signs and symptoms of the disorder, and any resultant impairment in functioning. For some of the disorders, specific criteria for these differing severities are provided.

Revisions in the multiaxial system of DSM-III have been among the most difficult about which to reach consensus, undoubtedly because of the lack of empirical research on multiaxial classification since the publication of DSM-III (Williams, 1985). However, Axes I and II have been reorganized, and Axes IV and V revised. Axes I and II comprise the entire classification of mental disorders. In DSM-III Axis II included the personality disorders and specific developmental disorders, and Axis I included all of the other mental disorders. In DSM-III-R, Axis II includes the personality disorders and all of the developmental disorders, which are defined as mental retardation, and the pervasive and specific developmental disorders. The disorders on Axis II, then, are those that generally have an onset in childhood or adolescence and usually persist in a stable form (without periods of remission or exacerbation) into adult life. With only a few exceptions (e.g., the gender identity disorders and paraphilias), these features are not characteristic of the Axis I disorders. The Axis I–Axis II distinction in evaluating children emphasizes the need to consider disorders involving the development of cognitive, social, and motor skills. For adults, as in DSM-III, the separation between Axis I and Axis II ensures that consideration is given to the possible presence of personality disorders that may be overlooked when attention is directed to a usually more florid Axis I disorder.

A list of defense mechanisms and their definitions are added to the Glossary of Technical Terms in DSM-III-R. Axis II, then, can be used to indicate specific personality traits that don't meet the criteria for a personality disorder (as in DSM-III), or habitual use of particular defense mechanisms.

The revision of Axis IV, severity of psychosocial stressors, has been especially problematic, since many believe it lacks clinical utility, but no one has proposed a satisfactory solution. However, one improvement is being made by suggesting that clinicians note the specific relevant psychosocial stressors, and further specify them as either "predominantly acute events" (with a duration of less than six months) or "predominantly enduring circumstances" (that have lasted longer than six months). Examples of predominantly acute events are death of a loved one, an accident, or beginning a new school or job. Examples of predominantly enduring circumstances include chronic marital or parental discord, and persistent and harsh parental discipline. This distinction may be important in formulating a treatment plan that includes attempts to remove the psychosocial stressor(s) or to help the individual cope with it. Furthermore, there is evidence that predominantly enduring psychosocial stressors are more likely to predispose children to develop psychopathology than predominantly acute events (Rutter & Shaffer, 1980).

In DSM-III Axis V was a rating scale for indicating an individual's highest level of adaptive functioning during the past year. Adaptive functioning was defined as including social and occupational functioning, and, in individuals functioning at a high level, also their use of leisure time. This scale was criticized as being too limited in not measuring overall severity of illness, and of questionable prognostic validity (Rutter & Shaffer, 1980). Therefore, Axis V in DSM-III-R permits a clinician to indicate his or her overall judgment of an individual's psychological, social and occupational functioning on a continuum of mental health-illness. A new scale called the Global Assessment of Functioning Scale is presented in Table 23.2. It was derived from the Global Assessment Scale (Endicott et al., 1976) and the Children's Global Assessment Scale (Shaffer et al., 1983). Ratings are made both for the individual's current level of functioning, and for the highest level during the past year. Ratings of current functioning will generally reflect the current need for treatment or care, and have been shown to have some predictive power (Mezzich et al., 1984).

Revisions in the diagnostic classes and categories

The revised classification of mental disorders is presented in the appendix to this chapter. Following is a brief overview of the major changes affecting the categories themselves:

Turning first to the childhood disorders, we see that the DSM-III categories of infantile autism and childhood onset pervasive developmental disorder have been combined into a single category of autistic disorder. Those two disorders in DSM-III were distinguished merely on the basis of the age at onset's being before or after 30 months. Our Advisory Committee did not believe this was a meaningful distinction. This change also represents a general trend within the revision to avoid including age at onset in the diagnostic criteria unless it is strongly supported by data. For autistic disorders, we suggest that the age at onset be noted by the clinician as either infantile (before three years), in childhood, or unknown.

Next among the childhood disorders, notice that attention deficit–hyperactivity, oppositional-defiant, and conduct disorders have been grouped together as disruptive behavior disorders, since these three categories tend to be highly intercorrelated and represent a significant differential diagnostic problem. Another issue is the extent to which attention deficit–hyperactivity disorder and conduct disorder actually represent two distinct diagnostic entities.

Note that the DSM-III category of attention deficit disorder without hyperactivity has been relegated to residual status in DSM-III-R as undifferentiated attention deficit disorders, given the revised criteria for attention deficit–hyperactivity disorder. Schizoid disorder of childhood or adolescence has been deleted, since a defect in the capacity to form social relationships appears to be observable only in the presence of psychopathological signs suggesting a pervasive developmental disorder.

The class of psychoactive substance–induced organic mental disorders lists

Table 23.2. *Global Assessment of Functioning Scale (GAFS)*

Consider psychological, social, and occupational functioning on a hypothetical continuum of mental health-illness. Do not include impairment in functioning owing to physical (or environmental) limitations.

Code

81–90   Absent or minimal symptoms (e.g., mild anxiety before an exam, an occasional argument with family member), good functioning in all areas, interested and involved in a wide range of activities, socially effective, generally satisfied with life, no more than everyday problems or concerns.

71–80   If symptoms are present, they are transient and expectable reactions to psychosocial stressors (e.g., difficulty concentrating after family argument); no more than slight impairment in social, occupational, or school functioning (e.g., temporarily falling behind in school work).

61–70   Some mild symptoms (e.g., depressed mood and mild insomnia, occasional truancy, or theft within the household) OR some difficulty in social, occupational, or school functioning, but generally functioning pretty well, has some meaningful interpersonal relationships.

51–60   Moderate symptoms (e.g., few friends and conflicts with peers, flat affect and circumstantial speech, occasional panic attacks) OR moderate difficulty in social, occupational, or school functioning.

41–50   Serious symptoms (e.g., no friends, unable to keep a job, suicidal ideation, severe obsessional rituals, frequent shoplifting) OR any serious impairment in social, occupational, or school functioning.

31–40   Some impairment in reality testing or communication (e.g., speech is at times illogical, obscure, or irrelevant) OR major impairment in several areas, such as work or school, family relations, judgment, thinking, or mood (e.g., depressed man avoids friends, neglects family, and is unable to work; child frequently beats up younger children, is defiant at home, and is failing at school).

21–30   Behavior is considerably influenced by delusions or hallucinations OR serious impairment in communication or judgment (e.g., sometimes incoherent, acts grossly inappropriately, suicidal preoccupation) OR inability to function in almost all areas (e.g., stays in bed all day; no job, home, or friends).

11–20   Some danger of hurting self or others (e.g., suicide attempts without clear expectation of death, frequently violent, manic excitement) OR occasionally fails to maintain minimal personal hygiene (e.g., smears feces) OR gross impairment in communication (e.g., largely incoherent or mute).

1–10   Persistent danger of severely hurting self or others (e.g., recurrent violence) OR persistent inability to maintain minimal personal hygiene OR serious suicidal act with clear expectation of death.

Note: Use intermediate codes when appropriate, e.g., 45, 68, 72.

several specific substance-induced disorders not recognized in DSM-III, such as posthallucinogen perception disorder. The distinction between substance abuse and dependence has been minimized. What used to be called abuse will now be included to large extent in a broader concept of behavioral dependence.

DSM-III emphasized a distinction between abuse and dependence based on physiologic tolerance or withdrawal. The Advisory Committee believed that this distinction is often a difficult one to make and that the real issue is the extent to which involvement with a drug tends to dominate an individual's life. By making this change, we are again moving closer to the current ICD–10 proposal that includes the concept of behavioral dependence on drugs.

Next in the DSM-III-R classification appear the sleep and arousal disorders. The appendix in DSM-III includes a classification of sleep disorders that was prepared by two major sleep disorder associations. This was considered for inclusion within the classification of mental disorders during the development of DSM-III, but was finally judged too complicated for general clinical use. It contains many categories, such as rapid time zone change ("jet lag") syndrome, that make sense from a sleep pathology point of view, but do not represent clinically significant mental disorders. For the revision of DSM-III, we have developed a classification that is much simpler, more clinically oriented, and that is by and large limited to the major chronic sleep disorders.

As for schizophrenic disorders, the major change has been a modification of the A criterion to make it simpler and take into account changes in the criteria for delusional (paranoid) disorders. The B criterion has also been revised to take into account onset in childhood and to avoid the term "deterioration," which suggests that recovery never occurs. The requirement that the illness begin before age 45 has been eliminated, partly on the basis of conceptual arguments made by Kendell and others (Kendell, 1983). In addition, several studies have not supported the validity of this DSM-III criterion; that is, they have found that course and familial prevalence did not change significantly if one used age at onset to distinguish the groups (Gold, 1984). DSM-III-R, however, recommends that age at onset be noted if it is after 45 (late adult life), so that this issue can be studied further.

The category for paranoid disorders is defined very narrowly in DSM-III by the requirement of either persecutory delusions or delusions of jealousy. In DSM-III-R the concept is expanded to bring it more in line with Kraepelinian tradition, by including other monosymptomatic delusions such as somatic delusions and erotomania. The name of paranoid disorders has been changed to the more nosologically descriptive term "delusional (paranoid) disorders," suggested by Winokur (1977) and Kendler (1980), since the term "paranoid" in English suggests only suspiciousness.

The residual class of psychotic disorders not elsewhere classified will still include categories for schizophreniform disorder, schizoaffective disorder, and brief reactive psychosis. The inclusion criterion for schizophreniform disorder has been revised to cover features that are generally associated with good prognosis so that as few cases as possible will eventually go on in time to meet the criteria for schizophrenia. The minimal duration criterion has been eliminated so that the diagnosis could even be made within the first week or two of the disturbance, provided the illness does not meet the criteria for brief reactive psychosis.

As is well known, schizoaffective disorder is the only specific category in DSM-III that does not have formally specified diagnostic criteria. In the revision, we have included criteria that have been taken from the examples of the category that were given in the text of DSM-III. There is some research evidence suggesting that schizoaffective disorder, depressed, has an outcome closer to that of schizophrenia and that schizoaffective disorder, bipolar, is closer to affective disorder (Brockington, Kendell & Wainwright, 1980; Brockington, Wainwright & Kendell, 1980) so there is a provision in DSM-III-R for making that distinction.

Brief reactive psychosis is a category that required several changes. For one, its maximum duration in DSM-III is two weeks, yet there is much clinical experience indicating that this is often too short a period for a short-lived reactive psychosis. There seems to be a consensus that a duration of four weeks will handle the vast majority of cases. In addition, there will be acknowledgment that the stressors may be cumulative and must be viewed in the context of the individual's subculture. This differs from DSM-III, in which the stressor had to be one that would be markedly stressful for almost anyone.

Note that in the revised classification the term "affective disorders" has been changed to "mood disorders." This latter term had been considered during the development of DSM-III, but was not adopted at that time because of the long tradition of referring to such disorders as affective disorders. However, the term is now being proposed again with the recognition that the the term affective disorder actually translates in many languages into "mood," and that "mood" is a more precise term. Within the mood disorders, the classification has been reorganized to group the bipolar disorders (bipolar disorder and cyclothymia) together, and the depressive disorders (major depression and dysthymia) together.

Within the anxiety disorders, there are two major changes. First, in DSM-III-R the category of panic disorder is given more prominence, and has two subtypes: with agoraphobia, and without agoraphobia. The meaning of agoraphobia will be broadened to include any degree of significant phobic avoidance, in keeping with the more traditional use of the term. Thus, this category will subsume DSM-III cases of agoraphobia with panic attacks. In addition, the DSM-III category of agoraphobia without panic attacks will be retained as agoraphobia without history of panic attacks, and again, the definition of agoraphobia will be broadened.

There was much discussion among the Work Group and Advisory Committee members about the placement in the classification of obsessive compulsive disorder. At one point, the Advisory Committee voted to remove the category from the anxiety disorders and give it status as a diagnostic class in its own right. On further reflection, however, the arguments in favor of retaining it as an anxiety disorder appeared stronger, and the Committee reversed its decision. The committee also considered the placement of post-traumatic stress disorder (PTSD), giving thought to its placement within the dissociative disorders because of the dissociation involved in reexperiencing the traumatic event in memory, dreams, and real life. In time, however, this too was rethought, and PTSD will remain an anxiety disorder.

Within the somatoform disorders, we have included a new category called undifferentiated somatoform disorder. A similar category is included in recent ICD-10 proposals. Although we are not entirely happy with the actual name of the category, we believe the concept, that is, chronic multiple physical complaints that are apparently of psychological origin yet do not meet the criteria for somatization disorder or any other somatoform disorder, is an important one, particularly in developing countries. Also new to the classification in this class is a category for body dysmorphic disorder, more commonly known in the literature as dysmorphophobia. This condition, in which an individual has a nondelusional preoccupation with some deformity in their physical appearance that is out of proportion to any actual physical abnormality that may exist, was included in DSM-III as an example of atypical somatoform disorder.

The psychosexual disorders of DSM-III are divided in DSM-III-R into gender, identity disorders, and sexual disorders, in order to better reflect the language of experts in these areas. The sexual dysfunctions are now to be specified as "psychogenic only" or "psychogenic and biogenic." If biogenic only, these conditions are coded in Axis III.

Recently there has been considerable interest and research in the complicated and controversial area of premenstrual syndromes (Haskett et al., 1980; Hamilton et al., 1984). We assembled an advisory committee of experts working in that area, who drafted diagnostic criteria. In order to narrow the boundaries of the syndrome to those that would define a disorder, the criteria require a clustering of the symptoms, a disappearance of the symptoms shortly after the onset of menses, and impairment in social or occupational functioning. This controversial category, with the name of periluteal dysphoric disorder, is listed in the appendix of DSM-III-R to facilitate field evaluations.

Finally, the personality disorders. One of the most fundamental changes in this class is the adoption of a consistent format for all of the diagnostic criteria. The new format is polythetic; that is, it lists an index of items for each disorder and requires a certain number of those items for the diagnosis. With this format, two different individuals may qualify for the same personality disorder diagnosis even though there may be relatively little overlapping of their symptoms. We believe that with this change in criteria format, the reliability of the personality disorder diagnoses will increase, since with a polythetic model it is not necessary to have agreement on each and every item of the criteria that are met. We believe that this approach is also more consistent with the way clinicians tend to think about personality, that is, comparing individuals to a characteristic prototype.

A category called self-defeating personality disorder has been listed for field evaluation in the appendix of DSM-III-R. This category is similar to the traditional concept of masochistic personality disorder, but because in the DSM-III-R definition of the category there is no assumption that people enjoy the suffering they subject themselves to, "self-defeating personality disorder" is a more precise term. A category for sadistic personality disorder has also been added to the appendix for individuals who have a pervasive pattern of cruel, demeaning, and aggressive behavior. It may be that this category will be important in forensic psychiatry, for example, in the court-mandated evaluation of individuals accused of spouse or child abuse.

We believe the various changes described here will make the manual more useful to clinicians and researchers. Clinical experience and empirical data with DSM-III-R should be helpful for a future revision of the manual.

APPENDIX. DSM-III-R CLASSIFICATION: AXES I AND II CATEGORIES AND CODES

All official DSM-III-R codes are included in ICD-9-CM. Codes followed by a * are used for more than one DSM-III-R diagnosis or subtype in order to maintain compatibility with ICD-9-CM.

A long dash following a diagnostic term indicates the need for a fifth digit subtype or other qualifying term.

The term *specify* following the name of some diagnostic categories indicates qualifying terms that clinicians may wish to add in parentheses after the name of the disorder.

NOS = Not Otherwise Specified

The current severity of a disorder may be specified after the diagnosis as:

mild
moderate   } currently meets diagnostic criteria
severe

in partial remission
(or residual state)
in complete remission

DISORDERS USUALLY FIRST EVIDENT IN INFANCY, CHILDHOOD, OR ADOLESCENCE

DEVELOPMENTAL DISORDERS
Note: These are coded on Axis II.

Mental Retardation
317.00   Mild mental retardation
318.00   Moderate mental retardation
318.10   Severe mental retardation
318.20   Profound mental retardation
319.00   Unspecified mental retardation

Pervasive Developmental Disorders
299.00   Autistic disorder
299.80   Pervasive developmental disorder
          NOS

Specific Developmental Disorders
    Academic skills disorders
315.10   Developmental arithmetic disorder
315.80   Developmental expressive writing disorder
315.00   Developmental reading disorder

    Language and speech disorders
315.39   Developmental articulation disorder
315.31* Developmental expressive language disorder
315.31* Developmental receptive language disorder

    Motor skills disorder
315.40   Developmental coordination disorder

315.90* Specific developmental disorder
       NOS

Other Developmental Disorders
315.90* Developmental disorder NOS

Disruptive Behavior Disorders
314.01   Attention-deficit hyperactivity disorder

    Conduct disorder
312.20   Group type
312.00   Solitary aggressive type
312.90   Undifferentiated type

313.81   Oppositional defiant disorder

Anxiety Disorders of Childhood or Adolescence
309.21   Separation anxiety disorder
313.21   Avoidant disorder of childhood or adolescence
313.00   Overanxious disorder

Eating Disorders
307.10   Anorexia nervosa
307.51   Bulimia nervosa
307.52   Pica
307.53   Rumination disorder of infancy
307.50   Eating disorder NOS

Gender Identity Disorders
302.60   Gender identity disorder of childhood
302.50   Transsexualism
       Specify sexual history: asexual, homosexual, heterosexual, unspecified
302.85* Gender identity disorder of adolescence or adulthood, nontranssexual type
       Specify sexual history: asexual, homosexual, heterosexual, unspecified

302.85* Gender identity disorder NOS

Tic Disorders
307.23   Tourette's disorder
307.22   Chronic motor or vocal tic disorder
307.21   Transient tic disorder
          Specify: single episode, recurrent
307.20   Tic disorder NOS

Disorders of Elimination
307.70   Functional encopresis (*Specify* primary or secondary type)
307.60   Functional enuresis (*Specify* primary or secondary type, nocturnal/diurnal)

Speech Disorders Not Elsewhere Classified
307.00*   Cluttering
307.00*   Stuttering

Other Disorders of Infancy, Childhood, or Adolescence
313.23   Elective mutism
313.82   Identity disorder
313.89   Reactive attachment disorder of infancy or early childhood
307.30   Stereotypy/habit disorder
314.00   Undifferentiated attention deficit disorder

ORGANIC MENTAL DISORDERS

Dementias Arising in the Senium and Presenium
          Primary degenerative dementia of the Alzheimer type, senile onset,
290.30   With delirium
290.20   With delusions
290.21   With depression
290.00*   Uncomplicated
          (Note: code 331.00 Alzheimer's Disease on Axis III)

Code in fifth digit:
1 = with delirium, 2 = with delusions, 3 = with depression, 0* = uncomplicated.
290.1x   Primary degenerative dementia of the Alzheimer type, presenile onset, _____
          (Note: code 331.00 Alzheimer's Disease on Axis III)
290.4x   Multi-infarct dementia, _____

290.00*   Senile dementia NOS
              Specify etiology on Axis III if known
290.10*   Presenile dementia NOS
              Specify etiology on Axis III if known (e.g., Pick's disease, Jakob-Creutzfeldt
              disease)

Psychoactive Substance-Induced Organic Mental Disorders

Alcohol
303.00   Intoxication
291.40   Idiosyncratic intoxication
291.80   Uncomplicated alcohol withdrawal
291.00   Withdrawal delirium
291.10   Amnestic disorder
291.30   Hallucinosis
291.20   Dementia associated with alcoholism

Amphetamine or similarly acting sympathomimetic
305.70*   Intoxication
292.00*   Withdrawal
292.81*   Delirium
292.11*   Delusional disorder

Caffeine
305.90*   Intoxication

Cannabis
305.20*   Intoxication
292.11*   Delusional disorder

Cocaine
305.60*   Intoxication
292.00*   Withdrawal
292.81*   Delirium
292.11*   Delusional disorder

Hallucinogen
305.30*   Hallucinosis
292.11*   Delusional disorder
292.84*   Mood disorder
292.90*   Posthallucinogen perception disorder

Inhalant
305.90*   Intoxication

Nicotine
292.00*   Withdrawal

Opioid
305.50*   Intoxication
292.00*   Withdrawal

Phencyclidine (PCP) or similarly acting arylcyclohexylamine
305.90*   Intoxication
292.81*   Delirium
292.11*   Delusional disorder
292.84*   Mood disorder

292.90*   Organic mental disorder NOS

Sedative, hypnotic, or anxiolytic
305.40*   Intoxication
292.00*   Uncomplicated sedative, hypnotic, or anxiolytic withdrawal
292.00*   Withdrawal delirium
292.83*   Amnestic disorder

Other drug or unspecified psychoactive substance
305.90*   Intoxication
292.00*   Withdrawal
292.81*   Delirium
292.82*   Dementia
292.83*   Amnestic disorder
292.11*   Delusional disorder
292.12   Hallucinosis
292.84*   Mood disorder
292.89*   Anxiety disorder
292.89*   Personality
292.90*   Organic mental disorder NOS

Organic Mental Disorders associated with Axis III physical disorders or conditions, or whose etiology is unknown

293.00   Delirium
294.10   Dementia
294.00   Amnestic disorder
293.81   Organic delusional disorder
293.82   Organic hallucinosis
293.83   Organic mood disorder
             Specify: manic, depressed, mixed
294.80*   Organic anxiety disorder
310.10   Organic personality disorder
             Specify if explosive type
294.80*   Organic mental disorder NOS

PSYCHOACTIVE SUBSTANCE USE DISORDERS

Alcohol
303.90   Dependence
305.00   Abuse

Amphetamine or similarly acting sympathomimetic
304.40   Dependence
305.70*   Abuse

Cannabis
304.30   Dependence

305.20*   Abuse

Cocaine
304.20   Dependence
305.60*   Abuse

Hallucinogen
304.50*   Dependence
305.30*   Abuse

Inhalant
304.60   Dependence
305.90*   Abuse

Nicotine
305.10   Dependence

Opioid
304.00   Dependence
305.50*   Abuse

Phencyclidine (PCP) or similarly acting arylcyclohexylamine
304.50*   Dependence
305.90*   Abuse

Sedative, hypnotic, or anxiolytic
304.10   Dependence
305.40*   Abuse

304.90* Polysubstance dependence

304.90* Psychoactive substance dependence NOS
305.90* Psychoactive substance abuse NOS

SCHIZOPHRENIA
Code in fifth digit: 1 = subchronic, 2 = chronic, 3 = subchronic with acute exacerbation, 4 = chronic with acute exacerbation, 5 = in remission, 0 = unspecified.

Schizophrenia,
295.2x   Catatonic, _____
295.1x   Disorganized, _____
295.3x   Paranoid, _____
                Specify if stable type
295.9x   Undifferentiated, _____
295.6x   Residual, _____
            Specify if late onset

DELUSIONAL (PARANOID) DISORDER
297.10   Delusional (Paranoid) disorder

Specify type: Erotomaniac
Grandiose
Jealous
Persecutory
Somatic
Other

PSYCHOTIC DISORDERS NOT ELSEWHERE CLASSIFIED
298.80   Brief reactive psychosis
295.40   Schizophreniform disorder
    Specify: without good prognostic features, with good prognostic features
295.70   Schizoaffective disorder
    Specify: bipolar type, depressive type
297.30   Induced psychotic disorder
298.90   Psychotic disorder NOS (Atypical psychosis)

MOOD DISORDERS
Code current state of Major Depression and Bipolar Disorder in fifth digit:
1 = mild
2 = moderate
3 = severe but without psychotic features
4 = with psychotic features (*specify* mood-congruent or mood-incongruent)
5 = in partial remission
6 = in full remission
0 = unspecified

For major depressive episodes, *specify* if chronic and *specify* if melancholic type.

For Bipolar Disorder, Bipolar Disorder NOS, Recurrent Major Depression, and Depressive Disorder NOS, *specify* if seasonal pattern.

Bipolar Disorders
    Bipolar disorder,
296.6x   mixed, _____
296.4x   manic, _____
296.5x   depressed, _____
301.13   Cyclothymia
296.70   Bipolar disorder NOS

Depressive Disorders
    Major Depression,
296.2x   single episode, _____
296.3x   recurrent, _____

300.40   Dysthymia (or Depressive neurosis)
        Specify: primary or secondary
        Specify: early or late onset
311.00   Depressive disorder NOS

ANXIETY DISORDERS (or Anxiety and phobic neuroses)
        Panic disorder,
300.21   with agoraphobia (*Specify* current severity of agoraphobic avoidance and panic attacks)
300.01   without agoraphobia (*Specify* current severity of panic attacks)
300.22   Agoraphobia without history of panic disorder
        Specify with or without limited symptom attacks
300.23   Social phobia
        Specify if generalized type
300.29   Simple phobia
300.30   Obsessive compulsive disorder (or Obsessive compulsive neurosis)
309.89   Post-traumatic stress disorder
        Specify if delayed onset
300.02   Generalized anxiety disorder
300.00   Anxiety disorder NOS

SOMATOFORM DISORDERS
300.70*   Body dysmorphic disorder
300.11   Conversion disorder (or Hysterical neurosis, conversion type)
        Specify: single episode, recurrent
300.70*   Hypochondriasis (or Hypochondriacal neurosis)
300.81   Somatization disorder
307.80   Somatoform pain disorder
300.70*   Undifferentiated somatoform disorder
300.70*   Somatoform disorder NOS

DISSOCIATIVE DISORDERS (or Hysterical neuroses, dissociative type)
300.14   Multiple personality disorder
300.13   Psychogenic fugue
300.12   Psychogenic amnesia
300.60   Depersonalization disorder (or Depersonalization neurosis)
300.15   Dissociative disorder NOS

SEXUAL DISORDERS
Paraphilias
302.40   Exhibitionism
302.81   Fetishism
302.90*   Frotteurism
302.20   Pedophilia
        Specify: same sex, opposite sex, same and opposite sex
        Specify if limited to incest
        Specify: exclusive or nonexclusive type

302.83   Sexual masochism
302.84   Sexual sadism
302.30   Transvestic fetishism
302.82   Voyeurism
302.90*   Paraphilia NOS

Sexual Dysfunctions
Specify: psychogenic only, psychogenic and biogenic (Note: If biogenic only, code on
Axis III);
Specify: lifelong or acquired;
Specify: generalized or situational

      Sexual desire disorders
302.71   Hypoactive sexual desire disorder
302.79   Sexual aversion disorder

      Sexual arousal disorders
302.72*   Female sexual arousal disorder
302.72*   Male erectile disorder

      Orgasm disorders
302.73   Inhibited female orgasm
302.74   Inhibited male orgasm
302.75   Premature ejaculation

      Sexual pain disorders
302.76   Dyspareunia
306.51   Vaginismus

302.70   Sexual dysfunction NOS

Other Sexual Disorders
302.89*   Sexual disorder NOS

SLEEP DISORDERS
Dyssomnias
      Insomnia disorder
307.42*   Related to another mental disorder (nonorganic)
780.50*   Related to known organic factor
307.42*   Primary insomnia

      Hypersomnia disorder
307.44   Related to another mental disorder (nonorganic)
780.50*   Related to a known organic factor
780.54   Primary hypersomnia

307.45* Sleep-wake schedule disorder
   Specify: advanced or delayed phase type, disorganized type, frequently changing type

   Other dyssomnias
307.40* Dyssomnia NOS

Parasomnias
307.47   Dream anxiety disorder (Nightmare disorder)
307.46* Sleep terror disorder
307.46* Sleepwalking disorder
307.40* Parasomnia NOS

FACTITIOUS DISORDERS
         Factitious disorder,
301.51   with physical symptoms
300.16   with psychological symptoms
300.19   Factitious disorder NOS

IMPULSE CONTROL DISORDERS NOT ELSEWHERE CLASSIFIED
312.34   Intermittent explosive disorder
312.32   Kleptomania
312.31   Pathological gambling
312.33   Pyromania
312.39* Trichotillomania
312.39* Impulse control disorder NOS

ADJUSTMENT DISORDER
         Adjustment disorder,
309.24   With anxious mood
309.00   With depressed mood
309.30   With disturbance of conduct
309.40   With mixed disturbance of emotions and conduct
309.28   With mixed emotional features
309.82   With physical complaints
309.83   With withdrawal
309.23   With work (or academic) inhibition
309.90   Adjustment disorder NOS

PSYCHOLOGICAL FACTORS AFFECTING PHYSICAL CONDITION
316.00   Psychological factors affecting physical condition
            Specify physical condition on Axis III

PERSONALITY DISORDERS
Note: These are coded on Axis II.

Cluster A
301.00   Paranoid
301.20   Schizoid
301.22   Schizotypal
Cluster B
301.70   Antisocial
301.83   Borderline
301.50   Histrionic
301.81   Narcissistic
Cluster C
301.82   Avoidant
301.60   Dependent
301.40   Obsessive compulsive
301.84   Passive aggressive

301.90   Personality disorder NOS

V CODES FOR CONDITIONS NOT ATTRIBUTABLE TO A MENTAL DISORDER THAT ARE A FOCUS OF ATTENTION OR TREATMENT

V62.30   Academic problem
V71.01   Adult antisocial behavior
V40.00   Borderline intellectual functioning (Note: This is coded on Axis II.)
V71.02   Childhood or adolescent antisocial behavior
V65.20   Malingering
V61.10   Marital problem
V15.81   Noncompliance with medical treatment
V62.20   Occupational problem
V61.20   Parent–child problem
V62.81   Other interpersonal problem
V61.80   Other specified family circumstances
V62.89   Phase of life problem or other life circumstance problem
V62.82   Uncomplicated bereavement

ADDITIONAL CODES

300.90   Unspecified mental disorder (nonpsychotic)
V71.09*   No diagnosis or condition on Axis I
799.90*   Diagnosis or condition deferred on Axis I

V71.09*   No diagnosis or condition on Axis II
799.90*   Diagnosis or condition deferred on Axis II

REFERENCES

Brockington, I. F., Kendell, R. E., and Wainwright, S. 1980. Depressed patients with schizophrenic or paranoid symptoms. *Psychological Medicine* 10: 665–675.

Brockington, I. F., Wainwright, S., and Kendell, R.E. 1980. Manic patients with schizophrenic or paranoid symptoms. *Psychological Medicine* 10: 73–83.

Endicott, J., Spitzer, R. L., Fleiss, J. L., and Cohen, J. 1976. The Global Assessment Scale: A procedure for measuring overall severity of psychiatric disturbance. *Archives of General Psychiatry* 33: 766–771.

Gold, D. D. 1984. Late age of onset schizophrenia: Present but unaccounted for. *Comprehensive Psychiatry* 25: 225–237.

Hamilton, J. A., Parry B. L., Alagna, S., Blumenthal, S., and Herz, E. 1984. Premenstrual mood changes: A guide to evaluation and treatment. *Psychiatric Annals* 14:426–435.

Haskett, R. F., Steiner, M., Usmun, J. N., and Carroll, B. J. 1980. Severe premenstrual tension: Delineation of the syndrome. *Biological Psychiatry* 15: 121–139.

Kendell, R. E. 1983. A major advance in psychiatric nosology. In *International Perspectives on DSM-III*, ed. R. L. Spitzer, J. B. W. Williams, and A. E. Skodol, pp. 55–68. Washington, D.C.: American Psychiatric Press.

Kendler, K. S. 1980. The nosological validity of paranoia (simple delusional disorder): A review. *Archives of General Psychiatry* 37: 699–706.

Liebowitz, M. R., Quitkin, F. M., Stewart, J. W., McGrath, P. J., Harrison, W., Rabkin, J., Tricamo, E., Markowitz, J. S., and Klein, D. F. 1984. Phenelzine v imipramine in atypical depression. *Archives of General Psychiatry* 41: 669–677.

Mezzich, J. E., Evanczuk, K. J., Mathias, R. J., and Coffman, G. A. 1984. Admission decisions and multiaxial diagnosis. *Archives of General Psychiatry* 41: 1001–1004.

Rutter, M., and Shaffer, D. 1980. DSM-III: A step forward or back in terms of the classification of child psychiatric disorders? *Journal of the American Academy of Child Psychiatry* 19: 371–394.

Shaffer, D., Gould, M. S., Brasic, J., Ambrosini, P., Fisher, P., Bird, H., and Aluwahlia, S. 1983. Children's Global Assessment Scale (CGAS). *Archives of General Psychiatry* 40: 1228–1231.

Williams, J. B. W. 1985. The multiaxial system of DSM-III: Where did it come from and where should it go? II. Empirical studies, innovations, and recommendations. *Archives of General Psychiatry* 42: 181–186.

Winokur, G. 1977. Delusional disorder (paranoia). *Comprehensive Psychiatry* 18: 511–521.

24 The diagnostic process and classification in child psychiatry

Issues and prospects

DONALD J. COHEN, JAMES F. LECKMAN, AND
FRED R. VOLKMAR (USA)

SCOPE OF MENTAL DISORDER IN CHILDHOOD

We no longer think of childhood as a carefree, innocent phase of life. Yet, even physicians and psychiatrists may be surprised by the findings in epidemiological studies of the abundance of mental suffering and illness that afflict children. Various surveys have revealed that 7 percent or more of all 10- and 11-year-old children have clinically significant psychiatric maladjustment. For children with physical illnesses the percentage is almost double, and fully one-third of children with brain disorders, including mental retardation, are likely to have psychiatric illness as well (Lapouse & Monk, 1959; Rutter & Graham, 1968; Earls, 1980; Links, 1983; Gould & Shaffer, 1985). The range of estimates of psychiatric disorder (6–30 percent) in different studies may result from differences in methods for ascertainment, environmental factors, social differences, or other problems in methodology. Furthermore, little information is available concerning the prevalence of specific disorders in different population subgroups. In spite of the scarcity of data, it is clear that mental disorders in childhood are common and of importance for mental-health planners as well as clinicians.

Some childhood disorders are likely to remit with maturation; others may continue for decades and into adulthood or predispose individuals to other forms of mental disorder as adults. Regardless of their temporal course, mental disorders of childhood are sources of pain and suffering for the child and its family and limit the fulfillment of a child's potential. The most serious disorders, such as autism and serious attentional and conduct disorders, are persistent and expensive. For example, the care of an autistic child in a residential program may cost from $30,000 to $90,000 a year in the United States; with a normal life expectancy, treatment for one child may run to well over $1,500,000. The social cost of conduct disorder leading to antisocial behavior may be harder to define, but the burdens on society of crime and drug abuse are obvious. For developing nations as well as for technologically advanced countries, mental illness in childhood, then, presents major concerns for social planning, allocation of health resources, educational priorities, and optimal development of human resources.

284

To understand fully the extent and nature of childhood mental disorders, to chart aspects of natural history, and to plan rational mental-health and special educational services requires much more information about what constitutes mental disorder than is currently available, as well as valid and reliable methods for measurement (Mechanic, 1970). In this context, diagnosis and classification of mental disorders are fundamental to further knowledge; in turn, empirical studies may generate more refined nosologies and criteria.

THE FUNCTIONS OF DIAGNOSIS

Diagnoses function in many different types of clinical contexts and "language games" (Wittgenstein, 1958). When a clinician or educator talks with a family about a child, or discusses a child's problems with the child himself, he may use diagnostic terms to summarize his observations, relate the findings to general bodies of knowledge, suggest pathways to treatment, offer a sense of natural history, or provide consolation. Often, the "diagnostic" summary session is the start of the treatment process or may constitute the treatment (e.g., reassurance that the difficulties are transient or part of normal development).

Diagnoses are also used among professionals to convey similar sets of information about etiology, course, and treatment response. The diagnostic precision in this type of discourse may differ greatly from patient-doctor discussions. Among researchers, diagnoses are basic to clinical research: They organize the clinical problems under investigation and suggest rational hypotheses for study (e.g., the association of types of presentations of the "same" disorder or different disorders). Each type of researcher, however, may need diagnoses of different forms. For example, in epidemiological studies it may be most relevant to have very reliable classifications simply of the presence or absence of maladjustment and severity of impairment; in biological research, fine-grained distinctions based on genetic, natural history, current symptoms, and other data may be needed to subgroup patients who are diagnostically otherwise similar (e.g., overanxious children with and without family histories of anxiety disorder).

Whereas laymen may accept a psychiatric diagnosis as a term for a "real thing," it is obvious among professionals that there are complex epistemological questions concerning the ontological status of a diagnosis or classification. The fact that diagnoses function within so many different communicative contexts is an indication that the diagnostic concepts are likely to be flexible. The flexibility also relates to changing models of the mind and of mental disorder. Additional flexibility arises from changes in scientific orientation as to what are the best ways of categorizing different types of troubles (e.g., from the perspective of internal distress or impairment in functioning), additional knowledge, and availability of resources for intervention (e.g., whether a patient is described as mentally retarded or as psychotic, when a range of symptoms substantiating both may be present).

The provision of diagnostic criteria is an attempt to conventionalize the usage of diagnostic terms. However, just as with other terms, a dictionary definition of what appears to be a simple noun is only a guide to use and suggestive of a range of meanings. Use is expected to alter with context and function; the full and appropriate "meaning" of a term is clear to those who speak the language. Thus, a psychiatric term may be given greater clarity through specifications of various types (including the provision of criteria), but its meaning will be in its use by those who speak the same clinical and psychiatric language. And this use will change with time, place and purpose.

These epistemological issues are central to all aspects of psychiatric diagnosis and may be particularly relevant to child psychiatry. In child psychiatry, mental disorders are presented not by the patient himself but by the child's community, and they are thus from the start defined within the social context of what adults conceive as normal development or functioning. Also, because child psychiatric classification has a shorter history as an area of research and study, issues which may be more obscured in relation to adult disorders are still relatively clearer in child psychiatry.

THE DIAGNOSTIC PROCESS IN CHILD PSYCHIATRY

The diagnostic process in child psychiatry is a systematic attempt to delineate meaningful clusters of symptoms and behaviors (disorders) that have importance either as targets of intervention or as they provide one with an understanding of etiological factors (Group for the Advancement of Psychiatry, 1966; Cohen, 1976). The process involves the review of information from diverse sources: discussions with the child's caregivers (parents and others) and teachers; interviews and observations of the child; formal psychological and behavioral testing; review of relevant historical and current information concerning functioning (such as school attendance and achievement records, court reports, family and peer relations, leisure-time activity); assessment of genetic and biomedical factors; and assessment of the impact of previous and current treatments. Diagnosis is more than the determination of an appropriate "label" or "coded classification." It is a continuing process of investigation and clinical understanding in which the issues concerning classification are an important aspect (Cantwell, 1980, 1985).

Empirical and conceptual issues concerning nosology in adult psychiatry are also found in child psychiatry; in addition to shared concerns (e.g., whether a disorder should be defined polythetically, i.e., by fullfillment of not all but only a subset of criteria or by whether the child exemplifies a more loosely defined "model" of the condition), some issues are specific or more salient in relation to childhood psychopathology. During the past several years, an increasing number of investigators, often using epidemiological methods, have begun to study issues concerning childhood disorders (Rutter, Shaffer & Shepherd, 1975; Achenbach & Edelbrock, 1978, 1981; Gould & Shaffer, 1985). In spite of this new work which has helped shape current nosologies (such as DSM-III), there are many fundamental empirical and conceptual problems in need of study (Rutter & Shaffer, 1980).

DIFFICULTIES IN CHILDHOOD DIAGNOSIS

Various difficulties are encountered in the process of child psychiatric diagnosis. These include fundamental questions concerning the definition of what constitutes a disorder. At an early point in answering this question, the clinician and investigator need to define some point of demarcation to distinguish normative difficulties (e.g., stranger anxiety, regression around the birth of a sibling or family move) from early or manifest disorders. Delays and deviations that may be in the normal range must be distinguished from those that are of concern, either at the moment or prognostically. Another problem concerns the definition of who the patient is. Often, family and social factors are prominent in the presentation of a child for treatment, and in the disorder itself; the question may then arise about "whose problem is it?" or to what degree is the problem "in the child" or "in his environment." This may be particularly true in relation to a child who has suffered from overt abuse or neglect but equally can be raised in relation to a child who may be showing some antisocial or depressive difficulties during parental divorce.

In defining a disorder, it is useful if one can rely upon several types of stable relations: a stable relation between a set of antecedent conditions and a particular type of disorder (etiological invariance) and a stable relation between a disorder and natural history (outcome invariance). For most conditions in child psychiatry, it is far more likely to expect variance than invariance. The same type of adverse experience or endowment may lead to several types of developmental difficulties or none at all ("invulnerable children"). On the other hand, various adverse experiences may lead to similar behavioral difficulties (producing multiple "phenocopies").

Similar "openness" is found in relation to the short- and long-term natural history of children with difficulties. With the exception of the most severe developmental disorders (e.g., autism and severe mental retardation), for most disorders of childhood there is a broad range of natural histories. Children with severe problems at one stage may become relatively or completely adapted later in life or, on the other hand, may show progressive exacerbation of their problems. The reasons for this type of openness or variability in childhood are closely related to the biological and behavioral flexibility of developing systems and the availability of alternate pathways for development and coping (Kagan, 1971). They also suggest the multiple, interacting factors (particularly environmental forces) that are so critical in buffering or exacerbating emotional difficulties in childhood.

Diagnosis in childhood is complicated by the fact that children's difficulties tend to not be discrete, especially early in childhood. Multiple areas of functioning may be affected – including emotional, behavioral, and physiological processes, with varying emphases – and these may respond in tandem or progressively to intervention. An initial clinical presentation may be more polymorphous in character, with elements then emerging as the predominant areas of dysfunction.

Finally, all of these difficulties raise questions about the relation between what are simply clusters of symptoms (e.g., overactivity and inattentiveness) and what is a "disorder" (attention deficit disorder), and on what grounds this distinction can be made. This is particularly acute in relation to symptoms which are of very high frequency. For example, a well-done epidemiological survey of childhood symptomatology using the Achenbach Child Behavior Checklist in Holland (Verhulst, Berden & Sanders-Woudstra, 1985) found that more than 40 percent of all six-year-old boys were rated as sometimes or often ("somewhat or sometimes true" or "very true or often true") having the following: talks too much, temper tantrums, teases a lot, unusually loud, stubborn, argues a lot, bragging, can't concentrate, hyperactive, demands attention, disobedient at home, easily jealous, fighting. Many other symptoms were rated almost as highly. Given such high rates, one could arbitrarily create any number of diagnostic subgroups (e.g., bragging with and without hyperactivity). How can one define what is a "valid" and what is an "arbitrary" subgroup or disorder? (For a review of studies and a model epidemiological study, see Verhulst, Akkerhuis & Althaus, 1985; Verhulst, Berden & Sanders-Woudstra, 1985.)

MODELS OF DIAGNOSIS

At present, various models of diagnosis are used in child psychiatry, and each has its specific values and limitations. Some models work better for specific disorders.

The *developmental model* is characterized by the study of the unfolding of fundamental processes (such as socialization, language development, the regulation of self-esteem) (Zigler & Glick, 1986). In this model of diagnosis, the emphasis is on the ways in which underlying processes are expressed differently through the course of maturation, on whether systems emerge synchronously or with dysharmony across systems, and on the development of increasingly complex behavioral and mental structures (e.g., metacognitive processes, internalized sense of morality, desire for peer acceptance). Psychosocial and constitutional factors are conceptualized as complementary, and the diagnostic processes focus on defining how and why development in one or more areas has been delayed, distorted, or derailed. Anna Freud's (1965) concept of using developmental lines in understanding psychopathology is an example of a developmental model. In this model, multiple processes may interact in a specific developmental line (e.g. the line leading from dependency to bodily self-care).

The *process model* of diagnosis is related to the developmental, in the search for underlying or organizing processes, but it is less concerned with historical change than with mechanisms of functioning. This approach may be analogized to physiological models in general medical diagnosis in which surface manifestations of dysfunction are correlated with underlying biological processes (such as high blood pressure to autonomic control of periperhal vascular resistance). A recent example of this approach tries to understand developmental disorders in relation to hemispheric lateralization (Tanguay, 1984). The diagnostic process utilizing this model attempts to explicate spheres of functioning which are most impaired, and to trace the impact of the underlying dysfunction on other areas (e.g., how disturbances in anxiety regulation may lead to personality difficulties, or how attentional problems may affect thinking). Typical disorders may be clustered together under dimensions that "cut across" phenotypic expression (such as disorders primarily of arousal or anxiety, mood or self esteem, or development).

The *dimensional model* of diagnosis is characterized by the search for broad spheres of behavior that are closely related phenomenologically and in terms of etiology and prognosis. In child psychiatry, some have recently attempted to delineate dimensions based on current behavioral symptoms (Achenbach & Edelbrock, 1981); using factor analytic methods, symptoms have been grouped into two broad broad dimensions of symptomatology: disruptive/acting out/externalizing, on one hand, and emotionally upset/internalizing, on the other. Within these broad dimensions, children with various types of disorders and with tremendous differences in impairment are categorized together. Other dimensions can be derived from different types of data (e.g., results of psychological and cognitive testing).

The *categorical model* in childhood, as in adulthood, assumes that there are discrete disorders of mental illness that can be explicated on the basis of factors such as current and past symptoms, etiology, natural history, treatment response, or a combination of such factors. In DSM-III, as an example of a simplified categorical approach, categories are defined almost exclusively on the basis of current symptoms (behavioral problems or items), with little or no regard for context (developmental phase, social situation, "meaning of the symptoms to child or family," treatment response, salient etiological factors, etc.). This model of diagnosis is sometimes referred to as the "medical model," wherein a "strep throat" is the same bacterial infection regardless of the age, social situation, or feelings of the patient; the assumption of stability of etiological factors, presentation, and outcome are most clear in this model. It should be noted, however, that most medical diagnoses, especially in more advanced fields of medicine, do not rely solely (or sometimes even to a large degree) on symptoms and signs; historical and contextual factors are considered and there is extensive use of observation and testing and the application of understanding of underlying processes.

The *clinical formulation model* is the approach used in the actual practice of child psychiatry, and is a mixture of the developmental, process, dimensional, and categorical models. In this model, the child's difficulties are seen in the context of his or her endowment, family and personal history, and psychosocial status. In addition to delineating current symptoms and signs, the diagnostic process focuses on defining areas of competence, the child's and family's mode of adaptation to the underlying difficulties, and severity of impairment in different spheres of internal and behavioral development. The process attends to the different areas in which the child functions – at home, in school, with peers, in broader society, while alone – and recognizes the various skills and weaknesses that may emerge differentially in these areas of functioning. This differentiation of "dysfunction" is used in assessing the nature of the disorder (e.g., why children may reserve their worst behavior for those they love the most, or keep their feelings mostly to themselves). Thus, disagreement among observers (parent, teacher, child) about the child's difficulties may be expected to provide useful information.

The result of this approach to diagnosis is thus a portrait or, more precisely, a historic panorama; the clinical formulation is an attempt to vividly depict interactions between biological and psychosocial factors and the unfolding fabric of family life as the child's problems shape and are shaped by his experiences within his family, school and community. This formulation includes the child's increasingly complex sense of self and his or her attempts, conscious or unconscious, to adapt to his or her own emotional difficulties and the difficulties of his situation, as well as the changing patterns of dysfunction (within the child and those who are charged with caring for, or responding to, him or her). In this model of diagnosis, there is attention to forces that may have preceded the child's birth and issues concerning his or her future; the child's biological and psychological functioning; the roles the child plays in the family and outside; the resources of family and community life, including the limitations and potentialities for fostering autonomy and development; modes of adaptation to deficits or trauma; and the like.

In the clinical approach, the formulation will highlight the most impressive difficulties in specific developmental lines, dimensions of difficulty, and the presence of disorders that can be defined categorically. All of these statements are placed in context. Perhaps it is specifically in relation to contextualization (historical, social, personal-dynamic) that this approach most differs from the categorical approach of DSM-III.

The clinical model is closely associated with the broad sense of "clinical understanding" in which the specific facts about a child and family and their community are integrated through the application of relevant theory; it is associated, as well, with the use of such knowledge to be of service to the child and those around him. This model includes the importance of recognizing specific, categorical diagnoses that may be present and the focus of treatment (e.g., diagnosing manic-depressive disorder that may be responsive to medication) as well as the social and communal context in which the child lives and which may bring him for treatment or make such treatment ineffective (e.g., chronic economic disadvantage and lack of vocational opportunities as a determinant of the child's mode of adaptation or sense of anger/despair).

MULTIAXIAL SYSTEMS AND MODELS OF DIAGNOSIS

The emphasis of DSM-III on multiaxial classification is an outcome of the recognition of the limitation of categorical diagnosis, as such, and, more specifically, the limitations of categorical diagnosis relying solely on current signs and symptoms. Issues concerning specific problems in the establishment of diagnostic criteria for disorders are beyond this discussion. It should be noted, however, that there are unsolved difficulties of considerable importance in relation to even the most common symptoms (and disorders) of childhood, such as hyperactivity with and without conduct difficulties. These problems concern fundamental epistemological questions, including what shall be taken to constitute a disorder or, more precisely, for what purposes should a range of specific difficulties and level of impairment in specific areas be counted as a disorder? To what degree is suffering (and whose suffering?) to be considered? To what extent is psychiatric diagnosis ahistorical and to what degree must it consider the individual and broader history of the person being diagnosed? When should areas of disturbance (e.g., inattentiveness) be left to the understanding of the clinician to assess in a particular situation and when should specific behavioral items (e.g., jumps up to run around at mealtime) be required for diagnosis?

There is also epistemological tension between diagnosis for different purposes – for epidemiological research, for biomedical and other investigation, for planning services, and for delivering clinical care. For some purposes, children conveniently and usefully may be broadly grouped on the basis of the troubles they cause or are likely to cause society or the types of intervention that are both available and of proved benefit. For other purposes, finely graded distinctions among children who are quite similar in their difficulties are needed. For example, a therapist requires a rich understanding of individuality and of specific community and family resources; an investigator may need to make distinctions among patients in a category on the basis of severity or etiology that are not needed for survey purposes (e.g., the hepatologist must distinguish the multiple varieties of jaundice, whereas the epidemiologist for some purposes need only determine who has jaundice and whether they have sought treatment). To what degree can a system of classification serve all such purposes, and when can overgeneralization of a system derived from one set of data or from one purpose (e.g., epidemiology) be dangerous for the progress of functioning in another area?

At the present time, classification systems appear to be driven by the desire to perform efficient epidemiological studies. Diagnoses may be reduced to counting the presence of a certain number of symptoms which can be ascertained with reliability using survey techniques. The range of epistemological assumptions underlying this approach requires further study. For example, the groupings of symptoms into dimensions or categories as derived from such work may not be the same which would be derived from different populations or different methods. Some "disorders" may be diagnosed with unbelievable frequency (if based on very commonly reported symptoms) because of lack of consideration of other factors (e.g., impairment or actual performance), whereas uncommon disorders (such as autism) may fail to emerge at all. Other issues need to be clarified where this approach deviates from the clinical formulation model, for example, the changing manifestations of an underlying disorder in the course of development or in different contexts, the presence of multiple phenocopies.

A major contribution of DSM-III to formal classification is the provision of

Axis IV (psychosocial stress) and Axis V (adaptive functioning). However, neither of these axes has gained wide acceptance within child psychiatric practice because of problems in their operational definition. For childhood, psychosocial stress must be defined more broadly than the types of acute events prominent in adult psychiatric studies; instead, cumulative, process stressors and the presence of factors that enhance or burden development require explication. These broader factors include the provision of continuity of supportive caregiving at important phases of development, adequacy of education, quality of relations with caregivers, and the like.

Adaptive functioning has been more emphasized within child psychiatry than adult psychiatry, but the scales provided in DSM-III are inadequate for conveying the spheres of adaptation in childhood; they tend, therefore, to cluster the most seriously disturbed children within a small range. Instead of such global assessment, child psychiatric diagnosis requires finely differentiated assessment of adaptation in major developmental areas (language and communication, socialization, emotional regulation, self-care). Well-standardized scales such as the Revised Vineland Adaptive Behavior Scales are available for this purpose (Sparrow, Balla & Ciccheti, 1985). In addition to the assessment of adaptive functioning, it is often critical in child psychiatric practice and research to have careful determinations of an individual's intellectual abilities. For the diagnosis of mental retardation, the clinician must assess both adaptive functioning and intelligence; this two-factor approach provides information of central importance for all developmental disorders and for children who are having difficulties in school or with academic achievement (regardless of specific diagnosis). Since adaptation and intelligence are important prognostically for the futures of virtually all children, their careful evaluation within a system of classification and diagnosis seems worthy of specific recognition, perhaps through coding on the same axis (Axis V).

Finally, DSM-III does not provide for a sense of how severe any problem or diagnosis is or, when a child has multiple areas of difficulty, how they relate to one another and which are most contributory to the level of the child's impairment in different areas of his life. Assessment of severity of a disorder and level of impairment, however, are critical to thinking about the need for treatment and designing treatment strategies.

The clinical formulation model of diagnosis in child psychiatry in some ways can be seen to move from Axis V to Axis I. The clinician begins with a discussion of the child's functioning in various developmental areas – the child's adaptive functioning relative to children of the same age and cognitive abilities as well as the areas of greatest impairment, and their relations to each other (Axis V). From this, the clinician describes the child's social context, the stresses that have been experienced during the course of development, and factors that have been and currently are facilitating his or her maturation (Axis IV). These environmental factors are related to the presence of any biomedical problems (Axis III), which are specifically related to the persistent developmental or personality difficulties presented by the child (Axis II) or the emergent, more immediate difficulties he is experiencing (Axis I).

FUTURE WORK ON NOSOLOGY IN CHILD PSYCHIATRY

The diagnostic process within child psychiatry involves the utilization of methodologies of various types, and with different emphases than in adult psychiatry. By and large, in the practice of adult psychiatry, the primary informant is the patient himself or herself, and the major (and often sole) source of data is the patient's self-report. Rarely is this the case in child psychiatry. Just as in clinical work, research studies in classification in child psychiatry require the utilization of multiple sources of information, including structured interviews with parents, children, and other informants; rating scales completed by the parents and teachers, and sometimes the child; structured measures for determining adaptive functioning; formal observational methods; psychological and psychometric testing; and a gamut of biomedical approaches (neuromaturational and neurological examination, imaging techniques, electrophysiological measures, neurochemical studies, etc.). Each of these formal methods provides useful information that may be complementary. What is reported by the child about his or her inner life and experiences may enrich the reports of parents, and these descriptions are further broadened by the accounts of teachers, child-care workers, social service agencies, and so on. In turn, the very richness of sources of information may be overwhelming in the number of "subtypes" that may emerge (hyperactive children with and without signs of neuromaturational delay, for example) and when there are important discrepancies in the reports from different informants.

Advances in studies of classification and nosology in child psychiatry are likely to come not from ignoring these challenges but from increasingly addressing them. The goals of this work include the satisfaction of the criteria for what categories should be included in a medical classification. As explicated by Rutter and Shaffer (1980), the five major criteria for inclusion of a category are: that the syndrome is identifiable; that the diagnosis can be made reliably; that the disorder is handicapping and warrants clinical concern; that the syndrome differs from others in terms of etiology, course, treatment response; and that it is either sufficiently common or severe as to require specific coding. In reviewing the current status of childhood nosology and future prospects, it would appear that the following areas of study will help to address the current challenges to a rational classification system and provide suitable categories for communication with patients, among clinicians, for mental-health planners, and for investigators:

1. Studies of relatively limited areas of disorder are needed. Instead of trying to undertake research projects aimed at defining an entire classification system, projects should focus on domains of dysfunction. These domains may be defined

differently for different purposes, consistent with the alternate models of diagnosis. In this work, research should make use of current diagnostic groups as hypotheses for further investigation. It should be appreciated that the kinds of data and studies which will help illuminate one area of developmental disorder (e.g., the developmental language disorders) may not be useful with another (e.g., conduct disorders), and that the models of diagnosis in one area should not necessarily constrain the other.

2. There needs to be continued development of valid and reliable methods of assessment of the various domains that are considered in child psychiatric diagnosis. Overemphasis on one type of approach (e.g., symptom and sign checklists) can distort the diagnostic system. In this process, there can be no single "gold standard" against which all other information is tested; rather, information from various methods must be integrated in various ways by individuals trained in developmental psychopathology in order to achieve convergent validity. For the time being, this process of multimodal approach to validation or diagnostic triangulation seems more reasonable than an assumption that one method (e.g., an interview with the child and/or parent, etc.) conveys the "truth."

3. The benefits and disadvantages of different research approaches must be more fully appreciated. The careful study of clinical populations is critical to defining new subgroups or disorders in which surface features (symptoms) are related to underlying processes and developmental history. Disorders such as Tourette's syndrome would be as unlikely to "emerge" from surveys of childhood disorders as would inborn errors of metabolism such as PKU from collecting the urine samples of a thousand children and subjecting the metabolites in them to factor analysis. On the other side, without detailed knowledge of community prevalence and the spectrum of a disorder that may not appear in a clinic, generalizations from clinic data can be hazardous in trying to understand the nature of the disorder or approaches to treatment and prevention. For example, only through epidemiological methods can we fully understand the relation between severe Tourette's disorder and milder manifestations and the full spectrum of tic disorders.

4. Studies of classification cannot be separated from other forms of clinical investigation aimed at elucidating basic mechanisms of developmental psychopathology, understanding natural history, or attempting amelioration through treatment. Classification is needed for such research to progress but, in turn, must be shaped by results of such work.

5. In studies of classification in child psychiatry, multiple domains (in addition to current symptoms and signs as reported by parent or child) must be considered. Especially important are the data of real life (school attendance, academic achievement, use of leisure time, social and cultural achievements, police record, etc.) as well as findings from psychological and behavioral testing. It is to be expected that there will not be full agreement across domains of information about a child, even when very similar methods are applied (e.g., the use of formal, structured interviews). The child, parents, teachers, and others may see

the "same" child and his difficulties from different angles; also, the child may be quite different when being seen by different individuals or in different contexts. These different perspectives are useful for understanding a child (as they would be for an adult patient, whose employer, spouse, and neighbors we rarely or ever have the opportunity of hearing from), although they make the work of the researcher more difficult.

6. The use of "best estimate" techniques in diagnosis can help in integrating information from various types of informants and methods, but major aspects of the epistemology of "best estimate diagnosis" require further study and have not been formally assessed (e.g., the role of expert knowledge base of the individual doing the diagnosis, whether a personal interview by the expert would add to his or her understanding, etc.). Although it would be helpful if formal decision algorithms could be constructed to lead from current symptoms to final diagnosis, this should be seen as a long-term goal. An attempt to force available data from a limited domain (present symptoms) into a formal decision-making model is likely to distort the natural hierarchies, interrelations, and modifying factors which need to be considered in forming a diagnosis. For example, it remains unclear when an individual receives five or six diagnoses by a categorical approach (DSM-III), how these should be organized into a coherent picture of the individual and his difficulties for purposes of treatment or research. At this stage of our knowledge, it is important to retain as much information as possible in diagnostic estimates and to make use of the subclassification of the estimates themselves as "possible," "probable," or "definite" based on the level of confidence associated with the full set of available data.

7. Natural history studies of various types (follow-up studies, case control studies, high-risk studies) can provide important information about underlying factors that lead to persistent disorder and changing manifestations of a diathesis. In this type of work, categorical diagnosis is embedded in the developmental model, and the range of facilitating and disturbing influences on development can be examined. By understanding these modifying influences, one can better understand the essential features of a diagnostic category.

8. With further elucidation of genetic markers (or the actual gene[s]) for a disorder, it will be possible to do genetic case-control studies in which children from the same family with and without the relevant gene can be studied prospectively to determine the precursor behavioral problems and the emergent difficulties as well as the factors that modify the expression of a genetic vulnerability. These studies will lead toward newer forms of classification based on biological markers. Similarly, behavioral findings (e.g., attentional disorder, dysfunctions of specific social or communicative competence) could serve in classification schemes if they are robustly related to vulnerability, natural history of psychiatric disorder, specific types of deficit, or the like.

The diagnostic process and systems of classification build upon the entire range of knowledge concerning normal development and the multiple, interactive forces that can impair these processes. The diagnostic process is also shaped by various types of concerns for children and families (clinical, social,

and even political) and by the sensitivity of the clinicians and clinical investigators to various factors. In turn, rational and useful classification of disorders,
like the classification of other natural phenomena, is essential for advancing our
understanding of basic social, psychological, and biological mechanisms. Debate
is likely to continue among professionals accustomed to their own models and
domains of data, about whose perspective provides the least obstructed view of
reality. And such debate may be informative, in turn, about the range of social,
historical, psychological, and medical factors that do impinge on children.

A complex and interesting dialectic process is thus likely to develop over the
coming years, between advances in the developmental biological and behavioral
sciences, clinical expertise and concern, and advances in achieving broadly
accepted and helpful classification schemes. In this dialectic, classification
schemes (such as DSM-III) provide hypotheses for potential refutation or refinement, while new data are incorporated into nosological sophistication. It is
in this context that we describe in Chapter 10 of this volume the hypotheses
suggested by DSM-III concerning pervasive developmental disorders, studies
that have derived from these hypotheses, and new approaches to classification.

ACKNOWLEDGMENTS

We wish to thank Dr. Gwen Zahner for her discussions concerning
classification as well as our collaborators in studies of classification, including
Dr. Rhea Paul and Dr. Bennett Shaywitz. This research was supported by
NICHD grant 03008, Mental Health Clinical Research Center MH 30929, The
Children's Clinical Research Center RR00125, the John Merck Fund, the W. T.
Grant Foundation, Leonard Berger, and the MacArthur Foundation.

REFERENCES

Achenbach, T., and Edelbrock, C. 1978. The classification of child psychopathology:
A review and analysis of empirical efforts. *Psychological Bulletin* 85: 1275–1301.
Achenbach, T., and Edelbrock, C. 1981. Behavioral Problems and Competencies Re-
ported by Parents of Normal and Disturbed Children Aged 4 through 16. Mono-
graphs of the Society for Research in Child Development. Vol. 46. Serial 188.
Cantwell, D. P. 1980. The diagnostic process and diagnostic classification in child psy-
chiatry – DSM-III. *Journal of American Academy of Child Psychiatry* 19: 345–355.
Cantwell, D. P. 1980. The diagnostic process and diagnostic classification in child psy-
chiatry – DSM-III. *Journal of American Academy of Child Psychiatry* 19: 345–355.
Cantwell, D. P. 1985. Classification. In *Psychiatry*, vol. 2, ed. R. Michels and J. Cavenar,
Chap. 19. Philadelphia: J.B. Lippincott.
Cohen, D. J. 1976. The diagnostic process in child psychiatry. *Psychiatric Annals* 6: 29–
56.
Earls, F. 1980. Prevalence of behavior problems in 3-year old children: A cross-national
replication. *Archives of General Psychiatry* 37: 1153–1157.
Freud, A. 1965. *Normality and Pathology in Childhood: Assessments of Development.* New
York: International Universities Press.
Gould, M., and Shaffer, D. 1985. Epidemiology and Child Psychiatry. In *Psychiatry*,
ed. R. Michels and J. Cavenar, Chap. 11. Philadelphia: J. B. Lippincott.

Group for the Advancement of Psychiatry. 1966. Psychopathological Disorders in Childhood. GAP Report No. 62.

Kagan, J. 1971. *Change and Continuities in Infancy*. New York: Wiley.

Lapouse, R., and Monk, M. 1959. Fears and worries in a representative sample of children. *American Journal of Orthopsychiatry* 24: 803–818.

Links, P. S. 1983. Community surveys of the prevalence of childhood psychiatric disorders: A review. *Child Development* 54: 531–548.

Mechanic, D. 1970. Problems and prospects of psychiatric epidemiology. In *Psychiatric Epidemiology*, ed. E. H. Hare and J. K. Wing. London: Oxford University Press.

Rutter, M., and Graham, P. 1968. The reliability and validity of the psychiatric assessment of the child: I. Interview with the child. *British Journal of Psychiatry* 114: 563–579.

Rutter, M., and Shaffer, D. 1980. DSM-III: a step forward or back in terms of the classification of child psychiatric disorders? *Journal of American Academy of Child Psychiatry* 19: 371–394.

Rutter, M., Shaffer, D., and Shepherd, M. 1975. *A Multiaxial Classification of Child Psychiatric Disorders*. Geneva: World Health Organization.

Sparrow, W., Balla, D., and Ciccheti, D. 1985. *Vineland Adaptive Behavior Scales*. Circle Pines, Minn.: American Guidance Service.

Tanguay, P. 1984. Toward a new classification of serious psychopathology in childhood. *Journal of American Academy of Child Psychiatry* 23: 373–384.

Verhulst, F., Akkerhuis, G., and Althaus, M. 1985. Mental health in Dutch children: I. A cross-cultural comparison. *Acta Psychiatrica Scandinavia*. Supp. no. 323. vol. 72.

Verhulst, F., Berden, G., and Sanders-Woudstra, J. 1985. Mental health in Dutch children: II. The prevalence of psychiatric disorder and relationship between measures. *Acta Psychiatrica Scandinavica*. Supp. no. 324. vol. 72.

Wittgenstein, L. 1958. *Philosophical Investigations*. Oxford: Basil Blackwell.

Zigler, E., and Glick, M. 1986. *A Developmental Approach to Psychopathology*. New York: Wiley.

25 Structural methodology for designing diagnostic systems

JUAN E. MEZZICH (USA and Peru)

The concept of diagnosis in medicine in general, and psychiatry in particular, is an intricate one. Although traditional, narrower views focus on the identification of a disease entity, more encompassing and dynamic notions of diagnosis are gaining interest. The latter emphasize the role of diagnosis within the process of clinical reasoning and decision making (Whitbeck, 1981) and may lead to complex informational statements. Thus, a diagnostic system, which in this chapter means the set of concepts and rules underlying a diagnostic formulation, should be flexibly structured.

In addressing the design of a diagnostic system, it would be useful to point out first that such a system is supposed to be a parsimonious model of reality, a summarized representation of the world of the ill and illness. It should attempt to reflect the patient's condition as faithfully as possible, although we know that it will never be able to furnish a full account. The widely accepted purposes of a diagnosis are to enhance professional communication, treatment decisions, prognosis, public-health policies, and theoretical understanding. Methodologically, a diagnostic system is expected to be (1) as accurate as possible (in this sense, attempting to identify precisely the condition of the patient through careful data gathering and differential diagnosis processes), (2) reasonably thorough (providing a penetrating and comprehensive picture of the morbid condition and its context), and (3) codified (formalized in such a way as to allow efficient appraisal, storage, and retrieval of the information it contains).

The construction of such a summarized model of reality requires decisions and steps in regard to the various aspects of its structure. One fundamental issue has to do with how psychopathological information is scaled. Should it be categorical, consisting of a catalog of syndromes, or should it be quantitative, indicating, for example, the standing of an individual on a psychotic dimension? Another important question concerns the categorization approach used for defining morbid entities. Should it be the traditional, classical model or the so-called prototypical approach? Also critical are the ways in which diagnostic entities are organized, grouped, and hierarchically interconnected. What principles should be used to vertebrate a classification of disorders? What dominant relations are appropriate between syndromes (the formulation of one syndrome

298

excluding the formulation of another when the manifestations of both overlap chronologically)? The final questions refer to the scope and architecture of the diagnostic formulation: Should multiple diagnoses be allowed? Should the whole formulation be uniaxial or multiaxial? In the latter case, what would be the most appropriate types and number of diagnostic axes?

A brief review of the various issues enumerated above constitute the thrust of this chapter.

SCALING OF PSYCHOPATHOLOGY

Virtually all psychopathology descriptive systems of wide use to date have been categorical. Perhaps this reflects the deep need for naming that human beings have exhibited since the dawn of mankind. Raven, Berlin, and Breedlove (1971) have proposed that the development of the human mind has been closely related to the perception of discontinuities in nature. It indeed appears that people's functioning and survival have depended on their ability to recognize and communicate similarities and differences among objects and events. The preference noted for categorical descriptions of psychopathology also reflects long-standing clinical traditions, from the first version of the International Classification of Diseases in 1893 to its current ninth revision (World Health Organization, 1978).

However, in recent years we are seeing a renewed interest in exploring dimensional approaches, particularly in psychopathological areas that are perceived as inchoate and blending with normality, such as personality problems. Here it is worth mentioning two developments. One is the consideration, for psychiatric assessment, of a profile of dimensional constructs underlying personality conditions. According to this, the personality of a patient would be described in terms of a profile of highs, mediums, or lows, along dimensions such as paranoid, obsessive-compulsive, and dependent. Also of interest is the so-called personality circumplex. This is a development originally proposed by Wiggins (1982) to try to organize interpersonal aspects of personality functioning in terms of a circle that is vertebrated by two main considerations, dominance or control vertically, and gregariousness horizontally, and has a number of intermediate points. This model has been recently expanded in terms of the richness of its dimensions by Kiesler (1983). Within this construct it is possible to place many current concepts of personality disorders. For example, as shown in Figure 25.1, dependent personality disorder may be placed in the lower right quadrant of the circle, reflecting the notion that individuals with this personality disorder tend to be submissive and agreeable (Widiger and Frances, 1985). How to incorporate concepts and procedures like these in an efficient, usable diagnostic system remains to be seen. But at least they represent a direction that may be worth exploring, particularly in traditionally challenging areas such as personality conditions.

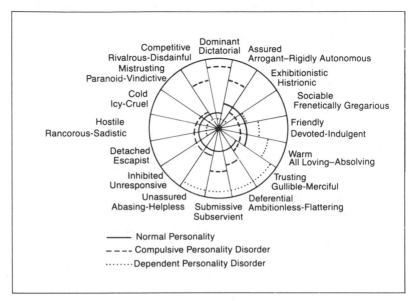

Figure 25.1. Personality circumplex for a normal case, a dependent personality disorder, and a compulsive personality disorder (from Widiger & Frances, 1985)

CATEGORICAL DEFINITION AND ASSIGNMENT

There are two issues of paramount importance concerning how syndromes or diagnostic entities are defined. One refers to the level of definitional specificity and the other to the categorization model used to conceptualize the structure of a diagnostic group.

Level of definitional specificity refers to the degree of clarity, precision, explicitness, or operationality of the presentation of a diagnostic entity and the rules governing the adjudication of a diagnostic category to individuals under evaluation. Degree of specificity oscillates from the rather general and connotative diagnostic definitions offered in ICD-9 (World Health Organization, 1978) to the formalized and denotative criteria contained in DSM-III (American Psychiatric Association, 1980). Both levels of specificity could be represented under the same diagnostic system. For example, as explicated in the essays by Jablensky (Chapter 30) and Cooper (Chapter 28) in this volume, current proposals for ICD-10 call for the use of less strict clinical guidelines for patient-care purposes and more demanding criteria for research work.

With respect to the conceptualization of diagnostic entities and groups, two models of categorization are to be considered: the classical and the prototypical. On the one hand, the classical approach assumes homogeneous categorical groups, having distinct boundaries, and defined by singly necessary and jointly sufficient features. On the other hand, the prototypical model, epistemologically discussed by Wittgenstein (1953), is based on the notion of prototypes representing categorical entities. It considers that categorical groups are heterogeneous in membership, have overlapping boundaries, and are characterized by features correlated with group membership, but not singly necessary and jointly sufficient for such characterization. When one looks at the hierarchical organization of categories, the classical model assumes perfect nesting of a broad category's features in its subsets. For example, if a high-order category named anxiety disorders includes under it conditions such as panic disorder, obsessive-compulsive disorder, and generalized anxiety disorder, these conditions according to the classical model should share in full the defining features of the head category. No such perfect nesting is required by the prototypical approach.

The classical model appears to hold well when applied to theoretical objects such as geometric figures. For example, the concept of a triangle requires the existence of both three sides and three angles, and the presence of these two features in a geometrical figure makes it a triangle. On the other hand, the prototypical model appears to be applicable in most natural areas, including diagnosticians' cognitive processes (Cantor et al., 1980). Concerning scientific classification, the classical model represents a deterministic approach while the prototypical model corresponds to a probabilistic approach.

The implications of the prototypical model in psychopathology include, first, the acceptance of multiple diagnoses for describing a patient's condition. Second, it favors polythetic as opposed to nomothetic diagnostic criteria, as subjects would need to have only a subset of a list of features of a diagnostic category to qualify for it. Also, it allows weighing the importance of various diagnostic criteria to characterize a given disorder. Finally, as noted by Widiger and Frances (1985), it makes it plausible to measure the typicality of a given case, for example by determining the proportion of criteria of major depression met by a given patient.

SYNDROME GROUPING AND HIERARCHICAL ORGANIZATION

This section examines how specific disorders or syndromes are arranged or organized within a whole classification. First, consider the classificatory principles vertebrating a classification of mental disorders. Two major perspectives are etiology and phenomenology. As Stengel (1959) noted in his review of classification systems used in various parts of the world, these two viewpoints have traditionally been used in various combinations to articulate most psychiatric classifications. Within the etiological perspective, the predominant summarizing factors appear to be the biological and the psychosocial, although not always with the same weight. From the phenomenological standpoint, there are two main views. One emphasizes the use of higher order concepts such as psychosis and neurosis. These may be taken here as major classificatory principles, not necessarily on the basis of their controversial etiological connotations but, alternatively, with focus on their descriptive roles. The other phenomenological view, which has been gaining interest, emphasizes more discrete symptomatological configurations such as affective, anxiety, paranoid, and somatoform disorders.

The second organizational issue refers to hierarchical arrangements. One of these corresponds to the various layers of psychiatric classes, from broad categories (such as schizophrenia), to symptomatological types (such as paranoid schizophrenia), to decimal digit coding subtypes that may refer to severity or course of illness (such as subacute paranoid schizophrenia). Another important arrangement concerns dominant relations between disorders. These are expressed through exclusionary elements in the diagnostic criteria or definition of a disorder, which may preclude the use of that diagnostic category if its manifestations overlap to a large extent with manifestations of a more encompassing or prior condition considered more important. These rules may simplify the diagnostic formulation by limiting multiple diagnoses, but they may lead to ignore syndromes which may be suitable targets of therapeutic intervention.

To illustrate some of the previous issues, we may consider the case of a patient with a depressive condition. If clear-cut organic factors are identified as pertinent, the diagnosis may be directed to an affective type of organic mental disorder. If no such factor is elucidated, the diagnosis may be oriented toward a phenomenological formulation, for example, manic-depressive disorder versus depressive neurosis, and then, perhaps, specification of episodicity or severity subtypes. The presence of strong psychosocial stressors precipitating psychopathology may conceivably influence the selection of a diagnosis, such as adjustment disorder, particularly if the clinical manifestations of depression are rather inchoate.

THE ARCHITECTURE OF A DIAGNOSTIC FORMULATION

In considering the scope and structure of diagnostic formulations, the first dilemma is the contrast between uniaxial and multiaxial approaches. The traditional uniaxial model is characterized by the intent to synthetize what is important in a morbid state through a simple categorical statement (e.g., paranoid schizophrenia). The multiaxial approach involves the systematic assessment and display of the patient's condition in terms of several of its key aspects such as psychopathological syndromes, impairment in social roles, and biological and psychosocial contributing factors. It represents an analytic endeavor to disentangle the critical elements of a clinical case, while attempting to present a comprehensive picture of it by ensuring that systematic attention is paid to all such elements (Mezzich, 1985).

The structure of multiaxial systems encompasses two key aspects: number and type of axes. In considering the most appropriate number of axes for a multiaxial system suitable for general clinical work, two prominent sources of elements of judgment are available. One is published experience, as represented by a review of 15 multiaxial systems originating in Brazil, the Federal Republic of Germany, France, the German Democratic Republic, Japan, Norway, Poland, Sweden, the United Kingdom, and the United States, which revealed that the modal number of axes included was five (Mezzich, 1985). Another source is a recent international consultation on multiaxial diagnosis sponsored by the World Psychiatric Association (Mezzich, Fabrega & Mezzich, 1985). Here again, five was the largest number of axes that a majority of the 175 expert diagnosticians responding from 52 countries considered feasible for regular patient care. Also pertinent is the number of statements or diagnoses allowed in each axis. This varies across multiaxial systems, from only one diagnosis in the pentaxial system for children and adolescents developed by Rutter and colleagues (1975) to several diagnoses permitted or encouraged in systems such as DSM-III (American Psychiatric Association, 1980) and the Swedish schema (von Knorring, Perris & Jacobsson, 1978).

Regarding types of axes, both the review of published multiaxial systems and the international consultation of multiaxial diagnosis mentioned above yield similar lists of highly endorsed axes. These include the following:

1. Psychiatric syndromes
2. Personality disorders
3. Physical disorders
4. Course of illness (duration, episodicity, etc.)
5. Psychosocial stressors
6. Adaptive functioning
7. Psychopathological severity
8. Specific developmental disorders
9. IQ/mental retardation
10. Etiology specified by clinician.

In light of limitations in the number of axes feasible for clinical work, this list of important axial possibilities is too long. Attempts to reorganize and shorten it could involve the following steps: First, axes with considerable conceptual similarity may be merged. For example, personality disorders, specific developmental disorders and mental retardation may be grouped together in an axis on stable behavioral handicaps. Second, potential axes that may be considered qualifiers of psychiatric syndromes may be housed within this axis and specified through additional digits in the psychiatric syndrome code. Obviously, this applies to illness course, psychopathological severity, and etiology.

These steps lead to the delineation of a schema with five axes, which is outlined in Table 25.1. Axis I corresponds to Psychiatric Syndromes, where each syndrome is further characterized in terms of symptomatological severity, course (duration, episodicity), and etiological formulation, through an extended coding arrangement. Axis II refers to a complement of psychiatric conditions, namely, stable behavioral handicaps, including personality problems, IQ/mental retardation, and specific developmental disorders. Although Axes I and II house all psychopathological disorders, the remaining three axes deal with factors contributing to psychopathology or reflecting its consequences. Axis III lists concomitant physical disorders, which may either have a causative role in

Table 25.1. *A consolidated multiaxial diagnostic scheme*

I. Psychiatric syndrome   •   + severity + course + etiology

II. Stable behavior handicaps: personality conditions, mental retardation, and developmental disorders
III. Physical disorders
IV. Psychosocial stressors/situations
V. Adaptive functioning

psychopathology or need to be considered for comprehensive treatment planning. Axis IV specifies psychosocial stressors or abnormal psychosocial situations that may be descriptive of a problematic environment. Finally, Axis V deals with adaptive functioning, covering areas such as self-management, occupational performance, and interpersonal functioning with family and others.

Other structural issues in multiaxial models include the scaling of the axes, which may be typological (e.g., psychiatric syndromes), dimensional (e.g., level of adaptive functioning), or both (e.g., psychosocial stressors assessed in terms of type of stressors as well as regarding their overall severity). Also worth considering is the possibility of specifying interaxial etiological connections, for example, by using a "dagger" to flag a stressor and an "asterisk" to flag a psychiatric syndrome, to indicate that the latter was influenced by the former.

SUMMARY

We have noted that the task of designing a diagnostic system requires decisions and developments in several structural areas: scaling of psychopathology, defining syndromes, hierarchically organizing the whole classification, and setting up the architecture of the diagnostic formulation. These tasks involve work along several methodological perspectives, including analysis of systematically gathered data and the development of consensus (intranationally and internationally) across experts and the various types of professionals using diagnostic systems.

REFERENCES

American Psychiatric Association. 1980. *Diagnostic and Statistical Manual of Mental Disorders, Third Edition (DSM-III)*. Washington, D.C.: American Psychiatric Press.
Cantor, N., Smith, E. E., French, R. D., Mezzich, J. E. 1980. Psychiatric diagnosis as prototype categorization. *Journal of Abnormal Psychology* 89: 181–193.
Kiesler, D. 1983. The 1982 interpersonal circle: A taxonomy for complementarity in human transactions. *Psychology Review* 90: 185–214.
Knorring, L. von, Perris, C., & Jacobsson, L. 1978. Multiaspects classification of mental

disorders. Experiences from clinical routine work and preliminary studies of the inter-rater reliability. *Acta Psychiatrica Scandinavica* 58: 401–412.

Mezzich, J. E. 1985. Multiaxial diagnostic systems in psychiatry. In H. I. Kaplan and B. J. Sadock, eds., *Comprehensive Textbook of Psychiatry*. 4th ed. Baltimore: Williams & Wilkins.

Mezzich, J. E., Fabrega, H., Mezzich, A. C. 1985. An international consultation on multiaxial diagnosis. In P. Pichot, P. Berner, R. Wolfe, and K. Thau, eds., *Psychiatry: The State of the Art*. London: Plenum.

Raven, P. H., Berlin, B., & Breedlove, D. E. 1971. The origins of taxonomy. *Science* 174: 1210–1213.

Rutter, M., Shaffer, D., & Sturge, C. 1975. *A Guide to a Multiaxial Scheme for Psychiatric Disorders in Childhood and Adolescence*. London: Institute of Psychiatry.

Stengel, E. 1959. Classification of mental disorders. *Bulletin of the World Health Organization* 21: 601–663.

Whitbeck, C. 1981. What is diagnosis? Some critical reflections. *Metamedicine* 2: 319–329.

Widiger, T. A., & Frances, A. 1985. The DSM-III personality disorders: Perspectives from psychology. *Archives of General Psychiatry* 42: 615–623.

Wiggins, J. 1982. Circumplex models of interpersonal behavior in clinical psychology. In P. Kendall, and J. Butcher, eds., *Handbook of Research Methods in Clinical Psychology*. New York: John Wiley & Sons.

Wittgenstein, L. 1953. *Philosophical Investigations*. Oxford: Blackwell Scientific Publications.

World Health Organization, 1978. *Manual of the International Classification of Diseases, Ninth Revision* (ICD-9). Geneva: World Health Organization.

26 The contribution of epidemiology to the advancement of nosology

JEFFREY H. BOYD, DARREL A. REGIER, AND JACK D. BURKE (USA)

Epidemiology may contribute to an understanding of nosology by addressing at least two issues for which its methods are particularly well suited. First, it provides a scientific approach for assessing the scope of currently defined illness in a total community population, and second, it attempts to identify illness correlates that identify groups at high risk in the community, an approach that may help to elucidate the causal chain of factors important to etiology.

Where nosology is based on putative etiological mechanisms, it is possible to test such causal hypotheses by epidemiologic approaches. In the DSM-III, however, as well as in many other psychiatric classification systems, the nosology is intended to be descriptive unless definitive etiologies are known, as with amphetamine psychosis (Peterson, 1980) or other specific substance-induced organic disorders.

Nosological systems, as well as the criteria for individual disorders, are amenable to testing with empirical data obtained from epidemiologic studies. To illustrate this, the application of epidemiologic data both to tests of the DSM-III system and to the individual criteria for agoraphobia are presented. The data were obtained from the National Institute of Mental Health Epidemiologic Catchment Area (ECA) Program, which established the scope of mental disorders in populations large enough to show how disorders in a diagnostic system were correlated, and determined how criteria for individual disorders were distributed in a community sample.

DIAGNOSTIC HIERARCHY

A diagnostic hierarchy has been embedded in all of the ICD and DSM classification systems. This hierarchy is also inherent in Kraepelin's writings, made explicit by Jaspers (1962). Such hierarchies may have several purposes including the following: (1) to identify the most important diagnosis for treatment and prognosis; (2) to identify the most parsimonious explanation; (3) to aid in the process of differential diagnosis by determining one of several possibilities for which the most compelling evidence is available; and (4) to identify "pure" cases, which seems to be the reasoning behind the St. Louis approach to "primary" and "secondary" diagnoses (Feighner et al., 1972). It is not clear

306

Table 26.1. *Relationship of panic disorder and major depression in the past month (weighted data from 3 ECA sites)*

| | | Panic disorder | |
		Present	Absent
Major depressive disorder	Present	1,613	17,167
	Absent	3,508	700,594

Odds ratio = 19. $p < .001$.

which of these various possible purposes lies behind the use of a diagnostic hierarchy in DSM-III. In DSM-III a criterion in the definition of 60 percent of the disorders states that the diagnosis cannot be made if the composite symptoms and disabilities are "due to" another disorder. We test the theory of a diagnostic hierarchy by observing that if a disorder such as panic, for example, might be "due to" a disorder such as major depression, then one would expect people who are in an episode of major depression to be more likely to have major panic attacks than people who are not depressed. Epidemiologists measure this type of association by means of an odds ratio.

Methods

The goals and methodology of the ECA program have been described in detail elsewhere (Regier et al., 1984; Eaton et al., 1984; Eaton & Kessler, 1985). We report here on 11,519 subjects interviewed in New Haven, Baltimore, St. Louis, and Durham, using the NIMH Diagnostic Interview Schedule (Robins et al., 1982; Burnam et al., 1983; Wittchen, Semler & von Zerssen, 1985; Anthony et al., 1985; Burke, 1985; Helzer et al., 1985; Klerman, 1985).

Results

Table 26.1 shows the relationship of major depressive episode and panic disorder. The odds ratio of 19 means that panic disorder occurs 19 times as often in the presence of major depression as we would expect if these two disorders were independently distributed. This lends support to the notion that major depression and panic are associated, and that therefore the two disorders might be considered to be hierarchically interrelated.

Table 26.2 shows the odds ratios for all disorders that are considered to be lower on the diagnostic hierarchy than major depression, at least as far as DSM-III is concerned. In every case there is significantly more co-occurrence of the two disorders than we would expect if the disorders were independently distributed. These data tend to confirm the diagnostic hierarchy found in DSM-III. The question arises, however, whether this relationship between disorders

Table 26.2. *Odds ratios for the co-occurrence of major affective disorder and other disorders lower on the DSM-III hierarchy*

Affective disorder	Other disorder	Odds ratio	Significance
Major depressive	Panic	19	$p < .001$
	Agoraphobia	15	$p < .001$
	Simple phobia	9	$p < .001$
	Obsessive compulsive	11	$p < .001$
Manic episode	Antisocial pesonality	7	$p < .05$

Table 26.3. *Odds ratios for the co-occurrence of major affective disorder and other disorders not hierarchically related*

Affective disorder	Other disorder	Odds ratio	Significance
Major depression	Alcohol abuse/dependence	4	$p < .001$
	Drug abuse/dependence	4	$p < .05$
	Somatization	27	$p < .001$
	Antisocial personality	5	$p < .01$
Manic episode	Alcohol abuse/dependence	15	$p < .001$
	Drug abuse/dependence	3	ns
	Obsessive compulsive	18	$p < .001$
	Phobia	13	$p < .001$
	Somatization	12	$p < .05$
	Panic	24	$p < .001$

follows the expected pattern of the diagnostic hierarchy, or whether *any* two disorders tend to be related to one another, even if they are not hierarchically related in our diagnostic system.

Table 26.3 shows the odds ratios between major affective disorders and other disorders that are not thought to have any specific hierarchic relationship to major affective disorders. In almost every case we find a significant increase in the occurrence of the other disorder in the presence of major depression. This suggests that different psychiatric disorders may tend to aggregate together, whether or not the two disorders are hierarchically related to each other.

Figure 26.1 displays the odds ratios of pairs of disorders, hierarchically related according to DSM-III, and those of nonhierarchically related pairs of disorders. There is considerable similarity between the two scattergrams, which suggests that there may not be anything special about the hierarchy in the DSM-III diagnostic system. Disorders tend to be associated with one another, that is, to be found in co-occurrence with another disorder, whether they are hierarchically related to one another or not.

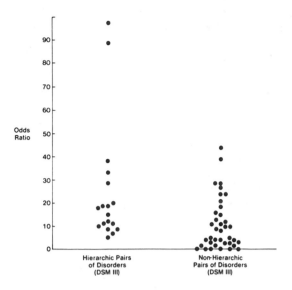

Figure 26.1. Odds ratios for pairs of disorders thought to be hierarchically related compared to odds ratios for pairs of disorders not thought to be hierarchically related

Table 26.4. *Number of co-occurring psychiatric disorders: observed versus expected*

Number of disorders	Number of subjects	
	Observed	Expected
0	10,060	9,676
1	1,150	1,722
2	215	117
3 or more	94	4
Total	11,519	11,519

Note: Chi-square = 2,209; degrees of freedom = 3; $p < .0001$.

Table 26.4 examines the question of multiple disorders co-occurring. Most of the subjects in our sample had no disorder; 13 percent of the sample had one or more disorders. Within the group that had at least one psychiatric disorder, there are higher-than-expected numbers of subjects with two or three or more psychiatric disorders simultaneously.

In summary, we have found a general tendency for psychiatric disorders to occur in the presence of other psychiatric disorders. This is certainly consistent with ordinary clinical experience. A large proportion of patients have more than one thing wrong with them. Sturt (1981) who found a similar pattern, has pointed out that this pattern could be interpreted as consistent with a hierarchic arrangement of disorders, but almost any hierarchy would work providing the more rare disorders appeared higher in the hierarchy. It is not at all clear that the specific diagnostic hierarchy found in DSM-III or in ICD-9 has any advantage over other hierarchies that might be imposed on these diagnoses. Alternatively, one might avoid having any diagnostic hierarchy and simply note that psychiatric disorder tends to increase the chance of having almost any other psychiatric disorder (Boyd et al., 1984). Because of this research, the diagnostic hierarchy has been reconsidered for the revision of DSM-III, primarily to avoid the loss of information that occurs when a diagnostic hierarchy is employed. The order in which multiple diagnoses are listed may be used to indicate which disorders the clinician considers to be most important.

PANIC ATTACKS AND AGORAPHOBIA

In addition to studies of general nosological issues, epidemiological studies also contribute to an understanding of individual diagnostic categories. Clinical studies have demonstrated that the majority of agoraphobics have a history of having had a panic attack. Table 26.5 shows 10 studies of the relationship between panic attacks and agoraphobia in clinical populations (Roberts, 1964; Mendel & Klein, 1969; Cloninger et al., 1981; Garssen, Van Veenendaal & Bloemink, 1983; Marks et al., 1983; DiNardo et al., 1983; Torgersen, 1983; Gavey & Tuason, 1984; Thyer et al., 1985; Uhde et al., 1985). The second column tells whether or not the sample was representative of a clinical population; about half the studies are trials comparing different drugs, and for such studies the study population was usually not selected to be representative. The third column gives sample size. The fourth column shows that between 61 percent and 100 percent of the agoraphobics were found to have a history of panic attacks. If we add up all the patients in these studies, 307 out of 348, or 88 percent of them had a history of panic attacks.

Table 26.6 reviews four studies that examined the temporal relationship (Mendel & Klein, 1969; Cloninger et al., 1981; Gavey & Tuason, 1984; Uhde et al., 1985) between the onset of panic attacks and the onset of agoraphobia. The study of Mendel and Klein (1969) is difficult to interpret because it is entitled "Anxiety Attacks with Subsequent Agoraphobia"; yet the authors never state whether they found any cases where agoraphobia predated the panic attacks or arose simultaneously with them. In only one case, in a study by Uhde et al. (1985), agoraphobia predated the panic attacks. That one patient had a history of long-standing separation anxiety as a child. The existence of this one patient, however, demonstrates that even in patients with panic attacks and agoraphobia one cannot assume that the panic attacks necessarily caused the agoraphobia.

Table 26.7 lists three studies that examined the question of whether a central concern of agoraphobics is a persistent fear of a recurrent panic attack. They found that between 79 percent and 100 percent of the agoraphobics reported

Table 26.5. *Studies of the percentage of agoraphobics who have had panic attacks*

Study	Representative clinical sample?	Number of agoraphobics	Percentage with panic (%)	Is the panic spontaneous?
Thyer, Parrish, Curtis, et al. (1985)	Yes	115	83	—
Uhde, Roy-Byrne, Boulenger, et al. (1985)	No	32	97	—
Garvey & Tuason (1984)	Yes	13	92	—
Garssen, Veenendaal, Bloemink (1983)	Yes	28	61[a]	—
Torgersen (1983)	No	26	69	—
DiNardo, O'Brien, Barlow, et al. (1983)	No	23	100	—
Marks, Gray, Cohen, et al. (1983)	No	45	100	Yes
Cloninger, Martin, Clayton, Guze (1981)	No	5	100	—
Mendel & Klein (1969)	Yes	25	100	—
Roberts (1964)	Yes	36	100	—

[a]Hyperventilation syndrome.

Table 26.6. *Studies of the temporal onset of panic and agoraphobia*

Study	Did the agoraphobia ever precede the panic attacks?
Uhde, Roy-Byrne, Boulenger, et al. (1985)	In 1 out of 31 cases
Gavey & Tuason (1984)	Never
Cloninger, Martin, Clayton, Guze (1981)	Never
Mendel & Klein (1969)	Presumably never

such a persistent fear (Roberts, 1964; Mendel & Klein, 1969; Garssen et al., 1983). As we inspect the clinical data in the studies listed in Tables 26.5, 26.6, and 26.7 it is clear that the results are fairly consistent from one study to another, but that the clinical data are limited. On the other hand, data from the ECA study suggest that agoraphobia without panic attacks could be more common than what is known from clinical studies.

Figure 26.2 shows the relationship of current DIS agoraphobia and a history

Table 26.7. *Studies of the fear of recurrent panic among agoraphobics*

Study	Is there a persistent fear of another panic attack?
Garssen, Veenendaal, Bloemink (1983)	Usually
Mendel & Klein (1969)	Yes
Roberts (1964)	Yes

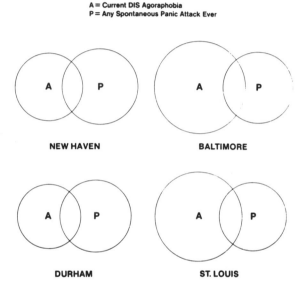

Figure 26.2. Relationship to DIS agoraphobia in the past month to any panic attacks ever

of ever having a spontaneous panic attack, as observed in the first four ECA sites. The area of the circles in this figure is proportional to the prevalence of the disorder. At all four sites the conceptual problem is the same: The majority of DIS agoraphobics do not report any spontaneous panic attacks.

At first this appears to contradict the clinical data reviewed above. We must consider, however, the issue of possible selection bias. The ECA respondents were selected to be a representative sample of community residents. In contrast, the clinical data were derived from highly selected populations. We have found that the presence of panic attacks greatly increases a person's chances of receiving mental-health treatment (Boyd, 1986). Therefore, we would expect that patients in a treatment setting would be more likely to have panic attacks than people who are not in treatment. Berkson observed in 1946 that if two disorders, in this case panic and agoraphobia, independently lead to the use of medical services

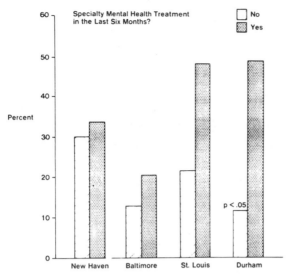

Figure 26.3. Proportion of DIS agoraphobics with a history of panic attacks at 4 ECA sites, according to treatment status in the specialty mental-health sector

then their relationship will be overestimated in studies of patient populations (Berkson, 1946).

Figure 26.3 shows frequency differences between patients with agoraphobia receiving treatment in the Specialty Mental Health Sector and those patients not receiving such treatment. The bars indicate the percentages of DIS agoraphobics who reported having had a history of panic attacks. In each ECA site we see that concomitant history of panic attacks was more frequently present in agoraphobics receiving treatment in the Specialty Mental Health Sector than in those agoraphobics not receiving such treatment. This illustrates the kind of selection bias that could result in some specialized treatment settings having an abundance of agoraphobics with panic attacks, and few agoraphobics without panic attacks.

In most cases, the growing consensus that panic attacks are the cause of agoraphobia appears to have influenced the direction of the revision of DSM-III, which now classifies much of agoraphobia as a subcategory of panic disorder. We would be wise, however, to remind ourselves that this consensus rests on studies of patient populations, and is not supported by data from the ECA studies. We must exercise caution in interpreting the ECA results because panic disorder has been difficult to assess using the DIS in clinical comparison studies (Robins et al., 1982; Burnam et al., 1983; Wittchen et al., 1985; Anthony et al., 1985; Burke, 1986; Helzer et al., 1985; Klerman, 1985).

Table 26.8 lists some of the questions we should keep in mind about the history that panic attacks cause agoraphobia. One question that needs to be asked is whether it is wise to revise our diagnostic system in advance of a

Table 26.8. *Questions relevant to the relationship between panic attacks and agoraphobia*

Question	Answer
Do most agoraphobics have a history of panic attacks?	Clinical studies 61–100% ECA studies – a minority
Are the panic attacks spontaneous?	Rarely asked
Do panic attacks predate the onset of agoraphobia?	Usually but not always; only a few studies
Do agoraphobics report an abiding fear of another attack?	Usually but not always; only 3 studies
Are agoraphobics in treatment representative of agoraphobics not in treatment relative to the proportion with panic attacks?	No

convergence of the scientific evidence or whether we would be better advised to exercise caution in such revisions, waiting for possible explanations of contradictions between studies. It should be helpful to conduct clinical follow-ups of groups of agoraphobics with and without panic attacks, using the same type of questioning used in the clinical settings. The potential for this type of follow-up now exists in all five ECA sites that can provide a more representative sample of agoraphobics than is typically found in treatment settings.

COMMENT

We have shown several examples of how epidemiologically derived data can assist in advancing our understanding of psychopathology and nosological systems. Other applications become apparent when the clinical course of disorders identified in such studies is followed longitudinally or when biological or psychosocial variables are correlated with the full clinical spectrum of a disorder. We trust that such contributions will be made with increasing frequency in the future.

ACKNOWLEDGMENTS

The Epidemiologic Catchment Area Program is a series of five epidemiologic research studies performed by independent research teams in collaboration with staff of the Division of Clinical Research, and the Division of Biometry and Applied Sciences of the National Institute of Mental Health (NIMH). The NIMH principal collaborators are Darrel A. Regier, M.D., M.P.H.; Ben Z. Locke, M.S.P.H., and Jack D. Burke, Jr., M.D., M.P.H.;

the NIMH Project Officer is William J. Huber. The principal investigators and coinvestigators from the five sites are as follows: Yale University, New Haven, CT (supported by cooperative agreement Uoi MH34224) – Jerome K. Myers, Ph.D., Myrna M. Weissman, Ph.D., and Gary Tischler, M.D.; Johns Hopkins University, Baltimore, MD (supported by cooperative agreement Uoi MH33870) – Morton Kramer, Sc.D., Sam Shapiro, Shep Kellam, Ph.D.; Washington University, St. Louis, MO (supported by cooperative agreement Uoi MH33883) – Lee N. Robins, Ph.D. and John Helzer, M.D.; Duke University, Durham, NC (supported by cooperative agreement Uoi MH35386) – Linda George, Ph.D. and Dan Blazer, M.D., Ph.D.; and University of California, Los Angeles, CA (supported by cooperative agreement Uoi MH35865) – Marvin Karno, M.D., Richard Hough, Ph.D., Javier Escobar, M.D., Audrey Burnam, Ph.D., and Dianne Timbers, Ph.D.

REFERENCES

Anthony, J. C., Folstein, M., Romanoski, A. J., VonKorff, M. R., Nestadt, G. N., Chahal, R., Merchant, A., Brown, C. H., Shapiro, S., Kramer, M., and Gruenberg, E. M. 1985. Comparison of the lay DIS and a standardized psychiatric diagnosis: Experience in Eastern Baltimore. *Archives of General Psychiatry* 42: 667–675.

Berkson, J. 1946. Limitations of the application of fourfold table analysis to hospital data. *Biometrics Bulletin* 2: 47–53.

Boyd, J. H. 1986. Panic disorder: The use of mental health services. *American Journal of Psychiatry* 143: 1569–1574.

Boyd, J. H., Burke, J. D., Gruenberg, E., Holzer, C. E., III, Rae, D. S., George, L. K., Karno, M., Stoltzman, R., McEvoy, L., and Nestadt, G. 1984. Exclusion criteria of DSM-III: A study of co-occurrence of hierarchy free syndromes. *Archives of General Psychiatry* 41: 983–989.

Burke, J. 1986. Diagnostic categorization by the Diagnostic Interview Schedule. In *The Community: Findings from Psychiatric Epidemiology*, ed. J. Barrett and R. Rose. New York City: Guilford Press.

Burnam, M. A., Karno, M., Hough, R. L., Escobar, J. I., and Forsythe, A. B. 1983. The Spanish Diagnostic Interview Schedule: Reliability and comparison with clinical diagnoses. *Archives General Psychiatry* 40: 1189–1196.

Cloninger, C. R., Martin, R. L., Clayton, P., and Guze, S. B. 1981. A blind follow-up and family study of anxiety neurosis: preliminary analysis of the St. Louis 500. In *Anxiety: New Research and Changing Concepts*, ed D. F. Klein and J. Rabkin, p. 143. New York: Raven Press.

Di Nardo, P. A., O'Brien, G. T., Barlow, D. H., Waddell, M. T., and Blanchard, E. B. 1983. *Archives of General Psychiatry* 40: 1070–1074.

Eaton, W. W., Holzer, III, C. E., VonKorff, M., Anthony, J. C., Helzer, J. E., George, L., Burnam, A., Boyd, J. H., Kessler, L. G., and Locke B. Z. 1984. The design of the Epidemiologic Catchment Area Surveys. *Archives of General Psychiatry* 41: 942–948.

Eaton, W. W., and Kessler, L. G. 1985. *Epidemiologic Field Methods in Psychiatry – the NIMH Epidemiologic Catchment Area Program*. New York: Academic Press.

Feighner, J. P., Robins, E., Guze, S. B., Woodruff, Jr., R. A., Winokur, G., and

Muñoz, R. 1972. Diagnostic criteria for use in psychiatric research. *Archives of General Psychiatry* 26: 57–63.

Garssen, B., Van Veenendaal, W., and Boemink, R. 1983. Agoraphobia and the hyperventilation syndrome. *Behavior Research Therapy* 21: 643–649.

Gavey, M. J., and Tuason, V. B. 1984. The relationship of panic disorder to agoraphobia. *Comprehensive Psychiatry* 25: 529–531.

Helzer, J. E., Robins, L. N., McEvoy, L. T., Spitznagel, E. L., Stoltzman, R. K., Farmer, A., and Brockington, I. F. 1985. A comparison of clinical and diagnostic interview schedule diagnoses. *Archives of General Psychiatry* 42: 657–666.

Jaspers, K. 1962. *General Psychopathology*. 7th ed. Trans. J. Hoenig and M. W. Hamilton, pp. 611–612. Manchester, England: Manchester University Press.

Klerman, G. L. 1985. Diagnosis of psychiatric disorders in epidemiologic field studies. *Archives of General Psychiatry* 42: 723–724.

Marks, I. M., Gray, S., Cohen, D., Hill, R., Mawson, D., Ramm, E., and Stern, R. S. 1983. Imipramine and brief therapist-aided exposure in agoraphobics having self-exposure homework. *Archives of General Psychiatry* 40: 153–162.

Mendel, J. G. C., and Klein, D. F. 1969. Anxiety attacks with subsequent agoraphobia. *Comprehensive Psychiatry* 10: 190–195.

Peterson, G. C. 1980. Organic mental disorders induced by drugs or poisons. In *Comprehensive Textbook of Psychiatry*. 3rd ed., ed. H. I. Kaplan, A. M. Freedman, and B. J. Sadock, p. 1441. Baltimore: Williams & Wilkins.

Regier, D. S., Myers, J. K., Kramer, M., Robins, N., Blazer, D. G., Hough, R. L., Eaton, W. W., and Locke, B. Z. 1984. The NIMH Epidemiologic Catchment Area Program. *Archives of General Psychiatry* 41: 934–941.

Roberts, A. H. 1964. Housebound housewives – a follow-up study of a phobic anxiety state. *British Journal of Psychiatry* 110: 191–197.

Robins, L. N., Helzer, J. E., Ratcliff, K. S., and Seyfried, W. 1982. Validity of the Diagnostic Interview Schedule, Version II: DSM-III diagnoses. *Psychological Medicine* 12: 855–870.

Sturt, E. 1981. Hierarchical patterns in the distribution of psychiatric symptoms. *Psychological Medicine* 11: 783–794.

Thyer, B. A., Parrish, R. T., Curtis, G. C., Nesse, R. M., and Cameron, O. G. 1985. Ages of onset of DSM-III anxiety disorders. *Comprehensive Psychiatry* 26: 113–122.

Torgersen, S. 1983. Genetic factors in anxiety disorders. *Archives of General Psychiatry* 40: 1085–1089.

Uhde, T. W., Roy-Byrne, P. P., Boulenger, J. P., Vittone, B. J., and Post, R. M. 1985. Phenomenology and neurobiology of panic disorder. In *Anxiety and the Anxiety Disorders*, ed. J. D. Maser and A. H. Tuma, pp. 557–576. New Jersey: Lawrence Erlbaum Associates.

Wittchen, H. U., Semler, G., and von Zerssen, D. 1985. A comparison of two diagnostic methods. *Archives of General Psychiatry* 42: 677–684.

27 Psychiatric classification issues from a sub-Saharan African perspective

FINI SCHULSINGER (Denmark)

This chapter is concerned with experiences at various levels and with certain considerations on mental health in Africa in relation to the problems and needs with regard to psychiatric classification in developing countries. The specific background for this discussion is this author's involvement, since 1981, in a Mental Health Program in Tanzania. From 1982 to 1985, a pilot phase was completed in two regions: Kilimanjaro and Morogoro. This phase has been evaluated and appraised, and it is not unlikely that the Mental Health Program will be extended throughout Tanzania before 1990.

The program was developed by the World Health Organization (WHO) in accordance with experiences from the WHO-coordinated research program on the extension of mental-health care to the primary health-care sector in a number of defined small areas in several developing countries. The Tanzania Program is the first attempt to apply these experiences on a macro level, that is, to a whole developing country. With modest support from the Danish International Development Agency (DANIDA), and a bit of luck, the Tanzanian health-care system, in a few years, may be able to offer care to all citizens who apply for help at any rural dispensary or rural health center. Such care would also comprise identification of major mental disorders, including epilepsy and alcohol and drug abuse, as well as mental retardation. At this time, 90 percent of the Tanzanian population (of which 80 percent is rural) is within 10 kilometers of such a health facility, and this proportion is steadily increasing.

One activity of the Mental Health Program is the production of regular monthly reports from all dispensaries, health centers, and hospitals. The reports include information on attendance and diagnostic distributions of mental patients. Obviously, this effort would be most useful if it were based on an appropriate classification.

MENTAL-HEALTH DIFFERENCES

One of the main issues in cross-cultural psychiatry is whether some of the psychoses seen in developing countries are specific to those countries and do not appear in the industrialized world, or whether they are just culture-related versions of the psychoses listed in ICD-9 or DSM-III. A final answer

317

may have to await the WHO-initiated and coordinated studies on acute and transient psychoses in different geographical areas.

A Dutch psychiatrist, Dr. Wilhelm Lucieer, who worked in Dar es Salaam from 1980 to 1982, once presented to this author a case history that clearly demonstrated some of the cross-cultural issues pertaining to classification. The following is a brief summary:

The patient, John, a young man of 25 residing in Dar es Salaam, met a girl at the station. She was new in town and had just left her rural family to live on her own, in personal freedom. John took her home, and they lived contentedly together. She was the most sexually attractive girl he had ever met. One day, she casually remarked that her mother had died the day before. He proposed that they should go to join the mourning. She, however, did not care to go; instead she wanted more sex, which she got.

Afterward, in the traditional way, she cleaned his penis. Immediately he felt an intense cold in the genital area and lower abdomen. He panicked, chased the girl away and rushed to his brother's room. The brother, on hearing the story, developed the same symptoms of anxiety and shriveling of the penis as John had. The brother recovered in three days, whereas John went into a stuporlike depression with feelings of being dead and of a slow disappearance of his genitals. He eventually saw and heard people preparing his burial and digging his grave.

With the help of charms and rituals by an indigenous healer, plus a little counseling and sedation from a psychiatrist, John recovered after three weeks. He felt his penis to be normal again, but he avoided dating girls.

Incidentally, he met the girl again on the street six months later, but they exchanged only a few words. Three days later he suffered severe abdominal pains and thought he would die. The brother brought him to the psychiatric department, where he was hospitalized for a few days.

He recovered quickly and began to date girls again. After intercourse with the third of these girls, he suddenly saw her as growing bigger, and he felt himself getting smaller. He realized that it was the same "djinni" who had possessed the original girl who now had taken the configuration of the present woman. After she left, he experienced a penetrating stench and heard strange noises from outside, and the next morning he found small hoof prints around the latrine. Because of the smell, he interpreted all this as evidence of a satanic orgy. He withdrew socially and became paranoid, even in relation to the psychiatrist. He recovered slowly after three weeks.

Dr. Lucieer intends to publish his interesting interpretation of this case history, in which belief in "djinnis" plays a role. They are Arab-derived spirits, supernatural and capricious, though not always malignant as Shetani is. They can be dangerously or destructively seductive when they locate themselves in a handsome woman.

The patient had left his family in North Tanzania. It belonged to a devoted Christian congregation. The case history has elements of Koro, of leaving close family life, of Christian guilt problems; and it shows psycopathology with signs of depression, hallucinations, paranoia, and withdrawal. Without help and loving care from his brother, he would not have recovered easily.

What is it that makes the difference between Western people and those in the developing countries? Is it superstition or belief in voodoo possession by "spirits"? Is it belief in ritual and magical treatment by indigenous healers?

The response to the last questions may be "yes and no." These phenomena are more openly expressed in developing countries. But magical rituals also constitute an important element of the various forms of Christian cults existing in the most developed of industrialized countries. Many people there also take all kinds of nonmedical treatments such as healing (even over the telephone), health food, amulets, herbs, homeopathic medicine, primal screams, and what not.

Why, then, are the psychiatric pictures so different between developed and developing societies, and the prognosis of severe psychosis frequently better in the latter countries? Tentatively, two very different factors may contribute to this. The first is the protection and support derived from solid traditional – almost ritual – family networks available in the rural areas of developing countries. In conjunction with this there is probably also a different attitude toward what Western psychiatrists call mental illness. The medical disease concept may be more stigmatizing than the beliefs in spirit-possession, voodoo, or interference exercised by deceased ancestors, which are conceived of as normal and non-pathological experiences.

The second factor is the much higher threshold of hospitalization observed in the developing countries. This implies that patients with an acute, dramatic, and maybe violent presentation constitute a disproportionately large amount of those cared for in developing countries by professionals trained in Western medicine. It is generally known that such cases have a much better prognosis than those with psychoses of insidious onset. If these two tentative factors were true, it is evident that the traditional Western definitions and corresponding diagnostic practices, as those, for example, used in the WHO International Pilot Study of Schizophrenia, are insufficient as clinical diagnostic and prognostic tools, not to mention research.

CAN WE DEVELOP AN IDEAL CLASSIFICATION?

Recently, Wig and his colleagues (1985) cogently discussed the problems of classification in developing countries. Their point of view was psychopathological more than logistic or operational. They outlined diagnostic classes in ICD-9, which appeared to be useless or confusing for mental health workers in the developing countries. These included the areas of chronic psychoses, acute psychoses, possibly exotic psychoses, as well as psychophysiological syndromes and the neuroses. They also pointed out that inconsistencies in conceptual framework were a major problem. The authors additionally mentioned that multiaxial classification with regard to personality, social, and cultural factors in developing countries is worthy of consideration.

Let us return to the young man in Dar es Salaam who had recurrent episodes – the first was comparable to Koro, the second was a brief, acute, psychotic episode. He eventually had one more episode and then he was well for a long time. But during outpatient contacts the psychiatrists felt that the patient was too open about himself.

It is, of course, difficult to give this patient a diagnosis other than acute psychotic episodes with schizophreniform features. This would be pertinent from a health-planning point of view. Also, the choice of therapy would be influenced by such a diagnosis. However, such a formulation would not help us to understand his disease better. Purely operational methods of classification as in DSM-III Axis I (which has considerable limitations in conceptual content) may be useful for conducting large, somewhat primitive drug assessments. Such methods may also be relevant as starting points in population-type studies. But, they do not yield data for the understanding of pathogenetic or etiological mechanisms.

The mental illness of the young man from Dar es Salaam is typical of many psychotic episodes in developing countries. They can only be understood if their social and cultural context is known, that is, the beliefs in "djinnis," the breakup from rural family to live in the metropolis, and so so. It is quite clear that multiaxial diagnoses are relevant to classification in developing countries. Transcultural psychiatry is one important avenue for the study of etiological or contributory factors in psychoses. For that reason, a transculturally oriented classificatory system, which gives adequate attention to social and cultural factors, is necessary.

A classificatory system in African and other developing regions will have to be much simpler than ICD-9 or DSM-III. The diagnoses will be made in peripheral health-care units in the rural areas, and by health workers with few years of training in health care.

The Tanzania Mental Health Program has already shown that such health workers, if properly instructed, are able to identify and treat a majority of severe mental illnesses. However, they are not scientists, an achievement that has been obtained only in few places. We may enter the era of ICD-11 or -12, or DSM-V or -VI, before a similar achievement takes place for the 75 percent of the world population who live in the rural areas of developing countries, and before there are more than a few psychiatrists available per one million inhabitants.

I propose that until this time comes, we try to develop simple classificatory systems. They must be multiaxial, covering the following areas:

1. Psychopathology
2. Personality
3. Social stressors, e.g., uprooting, poverty, deprivation
4. Physical factors, e.g., neurotoxic infections, malnutrition
5. Cultural factors, e.g., disapproval by family network, disapproval by ancestors, voodoo, spirit possessors, and djinnis

Development of such a diagnostic system may be difficult, but it will certainly be worthwhile.

REFERENCE

Wig, N. N., Setyonegoro, R. K., Shen Y.-C. and Sell, H. 1985. Problems of psychiatric diagnosis and classification in the Third World. In *Mental Disorders; Alcohol- and Drug-related Problems: International Perspectives in their Diagnosis and Classification.* Proceedings of a WHO/ADAMHA Conference. International Congress Series 669, pp. 50–60. Amsterdam: Excerpta Medica.

28   The presentation of psychiatric classifications

JOHN E. COOPER (United Kingdom)

This contribution consists largely of a plea to those responsible for preparing and presenting DSM-IV and ICD-10 to give special thought to the way in which these major classifications are presented to their potential users. The users who need special consideration are the large group of busy clinicians who are commonly required to diagnose the problems of the patients they see while performing various kinds of psychiatric services but who often have little time in which to make and record their decisions.

Although every clinician uses some form of classification even though informally and covertly, whenever they think about a psychiatric patient, the majority of clinical psychiatrists do not have a primary interest in classification as such. This means that the more a classification can be presented in a "user-friendly" manner, the more likely it is that users will find the procedure interesting and worthwhile, and the more likely that the data recorded will be reliable and accurate. The present time is particularly right for such an effort because both the major classifications noted above are in the process of development, and a good deal of international discussion and collaboration is taking place with these developments in mind.

What follows is acknowledged to be a set of ideal recommendations, not all of which are easy to put into practice. However, it is worthwhile making even ideal and somewhat optimistic suggestions in the hope that at least some of what is proposed will be reflected in the final versions of the classifications.

There is a need to deal with at least the following questions in the documents that accompany a psychiatric classification:

1. What is its main purpose, and are there any subsidiary purposes?
2. What is being classified?
3. For whom is the classification intended?
4. What type of classification is it; that is, what are the principles by which it is organized, and what is the resulting general structure?
5. How can it be best used for educational purposes, and how is it broadly related to, and different from, other classifications?

Some brief comments will be made about each of these issues, including notes on the extent to which ICD-9 (World Health Organization, 1977) and DSM-III (American Psychiatric Association, 1980) do or do not deal with them.

322

MAIN AND SUBSIDIARY PURPOSES

Almost any classification can be used for a variety of purposes, but it will always be easiest to use for the particular purpose for which it was designed. Many classifications in the literature do not contain clearly stated purposes; however both ICD-9 and DSM-III contain clear indications about theirs. ICD-9 has to be a statistical classification for the purpose of reporting international and national statistics of morbidity and mortality. Once this has been fulfilled, a variety of other uses such as a means of communication, and an educational stimulus, can be appropriately emphasized. As long as the basic statistical structure and requirements are not put at hazard, modification and additions (such as a glossary) can be introduced with these subsidiary aims in mind. DSM-III is specified as having at least 10 "goals," not presented in any obvious order of priority. The first on the list of 10 goals, however, is "clinical usefulness for making treatment and management decisions in varied clinical settings," and this purpose is also repeated elsewhere in the introductory sections of the manual. Again, a means of communication and education is high on the list, and the presence of detailed sets of criteria for most of the disorders in DSM-III also emphasizes its potential use in research.

Neither of these classifications can be criticized for not making their purposes clear, and both are well suited to their primary purpose. In contrast, both are markedly imperfect in the way in which they fulfill their subsidiary aims. These imperfections stem from the attempt to provide only one version of the classification for all purposes. However, if the same basic classifications could be presented in different ways for different purposes, with a level of detail and specific instructions deliberately designed for each purpose, the users will find them much easier to understand and use. DSM-III is particularly affected by this problem, in that the detailed diagnostic criteria it contains are at a level of detail suitable for research, and are very similar to previously published Research Diagnostic Criteria (Spitzer, Endicott & Robins, 1978). But a busy clinician may wish to make a useful and entirely appropriate "provisional" diagnosis on an admittedly incomplete set of information, and this is not allowed for in the DSM-III instructions.

The glossary of ICD-9 (World Health Organization, 1978) is not sufficiently developed to be ideal for research, simply because at the time it was drafted the use of research diagnostic criteria had not yet become widespread.

The presentation of a classification by means of separate but related documents for different purposes is discussed in more detail later in the chapter.

WHAT IS BEING CLASSIFIED?

This question needs to be answered at two levels: First, is the whole classification one of disorders, or is it one of patients? Second, what is the "unit of disorder" being used in different parts of the classification?

Disorders or patients?

Both ICD-9 and DSM-III are presented in the first instance as classifications of disorders rather than of patients, but both have given rise to problems in this respect (although of a very different sort). ICD-9 is very clearly specified as a classification of disorders, and no special provision is made or instructions provided for its transformation into a classification of patients. There are a few brief comments on this point in the accompanying "Notes for Users," and, in fact, a multiaxial system suitable for classifying patients (who may have more than one disorder) can be constructed quite easily by using the other chapters of ICD-9 and the V-codes as additional axes. However, no reports have appeared of attempts to use the ICD-9 in this way, and it is now clear that more positive statements and clearer guidance on this point would have been worthwhile.

In spite of its title *Diagnostic and Statistical Manual of Mental Disorders*, DSM-III is clearly presented in its full form as a multiaxial system for the classification of patients (see p. 8 in the manual). The five axes or aspects cover a variety of clinical and social information used in clinical assessments, although only the first two *axes* are properly developed and detailed. Axis III, "physical disorders," is left unspecified for the user to insert whatever classification he or she thinks best, Axis IV, "severity of psychosocial stresses" and Axis V, "highest level of adaptive functioning in the past year," are best described as "useful lists" rather than as developed axes or rating systems. Probably because of this uneven development of the different axes, DSM-III appears to be used far more widely as a single-axis classification of disorders than as a multiaxial classification of patients. Nevertheless, the presence of the extra axes in DSM-III is proving to be a very useful stimulus to thought, and at least brings the potential uses of multiaxial systems to the attention of its users.

Clinicians without any special interest in classification are often put off by this whole subject, by the use of terms such as "multiaxial classification," and by their first sight of the several lists or pages of ratings that are inevitably involved. They can often be reassured, however, by emphasizing the point that to use a so-called multiaxial system is to do no more than to record the familiar clinical case formulation, albeit in a compressed and coded form. A formulation contains statements about syndromes and symptoms, causes, associated physical states and social consequences; and almost all the published multiaxial systems do no more than code these familiar clinical statements in a form that can be recorded conveniently in numbers, rather than as narrative.

Diseases, syndromes, and symptoms

The patchy state of current psychiatric knowledge is reflected in the mixture of diseases, symptoms, and syndromes of which both ICD-9 and DSM-III are composed. This is acknowledged by an overall statement in the explanations which accompany both classifications, but it would be instructive and helpful to the user if both contained more detailed comments, section by section.

The psychiatric chapters of successive versions of ICD-9 have, until now, all followed a custom found in many psychiatric textbooks, by which psychiatric disorders are dealt with in the order psychoses, neuroses, personality disorders, and "the rest" (a mixed bag of syndromes and symptoms not regarded as being conceptually of the same nature as the first three). The reasons for this traditional ordering have never been stated, but presumably rest in the historical development of an extension of the responsibilities of psychiatrists as the decades of this century have passed.

Now that advances in therapy and in basic biochemical and neurophysiological research are making psychiatric classification a more lively subject, it is time for the major classifications to contain more justification of the conceptual status of the units of classification, and how they are related to each other.

FOR WHOM IS THE CLASSIFICATION INTENDED?

Three main types of users with quite different needs come immediately to mind. First, and on the largest statistical scale, are administrators, planners, and public health service doctors who need information about psychiatric services and the patients who use them. Statistics may be needed on a large scale, nationally or internationally, and on smaller scales appropriate to individual hospitals or areas. Second, clinicians and managers of individual services or units need information about their patients in order to monitor work load and developments. Even at this local or even individual level, the amount of information available and therefore, the type of classification needed, may vary widely. For instance, if services such as crisis units or emergency clinics are being studied, comparatively scanty information may be all that is available, but the need to describe and count the patients is still present. Third, research workers need quite a different level of specificity and reliability when recording their patients and the way in which they may change. Research workers usually also have ample time available for collecting detailed information, plus a more than average interest in the use of reliable classifications and ratings; they can be expected to welcome a well-developed set of diagnostic criteria and instructions. An additional important requirement is common to all users; they all need to understand the conceptual basis of the classification they are using, in spite of their very different interests and requirements.

With these points in mind, it is suggested that future versions of major classifications should be presented by means of three separate but closely related documents, namely, a set of concepts, a statistical classification for service use, and a set of research diagnostic criteria.

A set of concepts. This would be in the form of descriptions of the disease entities, syndromes, and symptoms that constitute the classification. The descriptions would be in some detail, although strict definitions would not be achieved. Conceptual similarities and differences between different disorders would be described, and notes on the history of the concepts would be included.

A statistical classification for clinical and service use. Users would need to be familiar with the set of concepts already described. This statistical classification would have a layout similar to the ICD-9 Glossary and Guide, showing clearly the nomenclature and code numbers at three- and four-digit levels, and possibly more. Only a brief summary of the clinical features of each condition would be required (perhaps between 5 and 20 lines of text). A list of the main symptoms in order of importance would occupy most of this space, and comments on differential diagnosis would follow. Guidance would be given as to how many and which symptoms might usually be required before a confident diagnosis could be made, but this would not be as rigid as in the research diagnostic criteria. Some of the problems about confidence of diagnosis or "goodness of fit" could be dealt with by providing an additional digit, to be coded according to the extent to which the clinical diagnosis fulfills the full set of Research Diagnostic Criteria (for instance: 1 = full set of RDC met; 2 = RDC not met but a confident clinical diagnosis can be made; 3 = provisional diagnosis only).

Research diagnostic criteria. In this document, the nomenclature and code numbers of the statistical classification would be accompanied by detailed diagnostic criteria suitable for use in research, as in DSM-III. Restrictive criteria that are potentially controversial, such as age limits or duration of symptoms, would be justified in preliminary comments upon each set of criteria. Different degrees of restriction could be specified for some conditions by the provision of extra codes. Extra codes for these and other purposes should pose no special problems for users of Research Diagnostic Criteria, since they are designed for use by workers with special time and interest who can master such additions at their leisure.

These comments pertain only to the classification of clinical disorders, as in ICD-9, and as in the first two axes of DSM-III. When a multiaxial classification of patients is presented, to provide the same three types of information for each axis would obviously be a great help to the users. If this can be achieved, a simple practical problem must be guarded against: Unless physically separate documents and handbooks are produced for each type of information, users will be overwhelmed by the sheer size and weight of the material. The present DSM-III handbook is already formidable, but contains only minimal information about Axes III, IV, and V.

WHAT TYPE OF CLASSIFICATION IS BEING PRESENTED, AND WHAT IS ITS STRUCTURE?

These questions refer to issues such as whether a classification (or an axis) is based upon etiology, or upon simple description, or upon varying mixtures of both.

The so-called combination categories that were a troublesome feature of ICD-7 (World Health Organization, 1955) and ICD-8 (World Health Organization,

1967), in which a description of a psychiatric disorder was combined with a physical cause codable elsewhere in the ICD, were purposefully omitted from ICD-9 (and were never a prominent feature of DSM versions). Nevertheless, both ICD-9 and DSM-III still contain sections in which psychiatric disorders are specified as having a known cause, sometimes physical (as in those disorders due to drugs, alcohol, or brain dysfunction), and sometimes psychological (as in the psychogenic psychoses, stress or adjustment disorders, and conversion disorder). To try to express both descriptive syndrome and cause in one statement or axis goes against the rules needed for the consistent and logical development of a number of axes that can then be joined in a comprehensive multiaxial system. A mixture or compromise of this sort is probably inevitable if a classification is to be attractive to clinicians. It seems likely that most clinicians have in mind a practically oriented, problem-solving classification of disorders in which etiology, when known, is given priority. Disorders recognized only as descriptive syndromes naturally take second place. Such an approach to classification may not be logically pure, but it works well enough in clinical practice. Not to be able to record etiology in a prominent fashion, when it is known, is probably too frustrating for most clinicians; so any single axis classification intended primarily for clinical use will need to represent compromises in these respects or run the risk of being unused.

The traditional order of psychoses, neuroses, personality disorders, and "the rest" has already been referred to; it does in fact represent a crude sort of structure for a classification, particularly if an additional traditional division of psychoses into organic and functional is also made. However, the historical sequence of development of concepts is probably not the best structure of those now available for the ordering of a classification. Other examples worth consideration are specificity of etiology, and the degree of development of the concept in relation to the hierarchy of disease-syndrome-symptom. None of these possibilities is likely to be ideal, but an attempt to use overtly some such system, or a combination of several, would be of great interest. If nothing else, it would involve a discussion of how many major and minor sections or subdivisions a classification should contain. For ICD-9, these decisions were dictated by the restrictions imposed as result of being only one part of a much larger statistical classification, with a restricted number of major categories. These restrictions have been relaxed for ICD-10, and many more options are now available for deciding the number and composition of both major and minor subgroups. DSM-III did not suffer from restrictions of this type, but the manual contains no discussion or justifications of the number and composition of its subgroups, other than the laudable but very general statement that these decisions "reflect the best judgement of the Task Force and its Advisory Committees that such subdivision will be useful. In this regard we have been guided by the judgements of those clinicians who will be making most use of each portion of the classification" (American Psychiatric Association, 1980, p. 7).

Apart from reflecting the conceptual basis of a classification, the number

Table 28.1. *Three grouping levels in a classification of psychiatric disorders*

Fifteen categories	Six categories	Three categories
1. Dementias 2. Transient and symptomatic organic disorders	1. Organic and symptomatic disorders	1. Severe psychotic mental disorders
3. Disorders due to alcohol 4. Disorders due to drugs	2. Disorders due to alcohol and drugs	
5. Schizophrenic disorders 6. Paranoid, acute, and other psychotic disorders 7. Affective disorders	3. Psychotic (functional) disorders	
8. Neurotic (anxiety) disorders 9. Somatoform disorders 10. Psychophysiological disorders 11. Stress reactions and adjustment disorders 12. Adult personality disorders 13. Other abnormalities of adult behaviour	4. Neurotic, stress and personality disorders of adults	2. Neurotic, stress, and personality disorders of adults
14. Disorders with onset usually in childhood or adolescence, and disorders of development	5. Disorders of childhood, adolescence, and development	3. Disorders of childhood, adolescence, and development
15. Mental retardation	6. Mental retardation	

of major subdivisions by means of which a classification is presented can also have important practical uses. More sophisticated users who have a great deal of information available about individual disorders and patients will be likely to use a complete and detailed form. In contrast, the use of a classification in conditions that do not allow the collection of much information will require the provision of simpler versions, particularly if the field-workers have had a comparatively brief and simple training. There is no need to devise fresh and different classifications for different users; it is sufficient to produce versions of one overall classification, but at different degrees of condensation.

Table 28.1 shows an example of this, based on both ICD-9 and DSM-III. The left-hand column shows a single axis, mixed-concept classification composed of 15 major groups that cover those disorders currently in both ICD-9 and DSM-III. Psychiatrists and professionally trained mental-health workers will recognize these groups, and information gathered in a country with well-developed psychiatric services would have many uses if expressed in these categories. The middle column shows the 15 categories condensed to only 6. These might still have plenty of uses for the publication of large-scale statistics designed, for instance, to show differences and similarities between different regions or countries, using rather diverse sources of information. The right-hand column shows a simple condensation to only three categories, which might be all that can be collected reliably in a region or country where mental-health information is collected by primary care workers with only brief and elementary training; such information would still be of use for the allocation of scarce personnel and limited resources.

THE USE OF A CLASSIFICATION FOR EDUCATION PURPOSES

The effort that went into the preparation of ICD-9 spanned several years and included psychiatrists from many countries and cultures. The Task Force that produced DSM-III in the United States of America also worked hard for several years, and consulted many subgroups and working parties. ICD-10 and DSM-IV will involve probably even more, rather than less, effort than their predecessors. Wide and detailed consultations such as these imply that the result must be of interest, even if not perfect. Any term or concept must have some virtues to survive the debates and tests which have gone on to produce an agreed classification, so the history and origins of the constituent terms and concepts of both ICD-9 and DSM-III are worthy of attention.

The educational value of these classifications has already been widely recognized, although admittedly as a secondary issue. DSM-III has probably had a bigger impact within the United States than has ICD-9 in this respect, because of the use of DSM-III by funding and insurance agencies if for no other reason. In addition, the provision of detailed diagnostic criteria has stimulated the use of DSM-III for research, thereby bringing it into prominence in many academic and teaching settings. One very simple approach that justifies some knowledge of a classification as part of psychiatry at all levels is to adopt the principles that

1. All psychiatric and mental-health workers should be familiar with at least one major classification.
2. They should understand it at a level of detail appropriate to their training and work.
3. They should know a little about what is wrong with it, in addition to knowing something about its virtues.

This last point is the key to the use of classifications in psychiatric education. The stultifying effect of the rote learning of a list of categories should be avoided, and attempts made to engage in a critical but constructive debate. This need for constant criticism (and therefore eventual improvement) of a classification is one reason why a multiplicity of national classifications should be avoided. Psychiatrists have difficulty enough listening to the ideas and concepts of colleagues at an individual level in the difficult field of psychiatric classification without having to cope, in addition, with the hazards of national pride and honor.

A study of any one classification in this way should inevitably include discussion of how it resembles and differs from other classifications, both past and present. In such a discussion, reference must always be made to the original purposes of each classification, and it is important to avoid a mechanical listing of differences and incompatabilities with no reference to their origins. In this regard, comparisons between ICD-9 and ICD-10 and DSM-III and DSM-IV need to be kept in context. ICD-9 and ICD-10 have to be produced so that the many and diverse member nations of the World Health Organization are satisfied by both the product and by the process of consultation. The product must be suitable for use by many different groups, and it must reflect as far as possible what is the common agreed core of international psychiatric terminology and concepts. This means that the ICD is always likely to be somewhat conservative in its content, since the World Health Organization cannot expect the whole world to accept recently developed ideas from any one particular group of workers or country; to obtain international recognition, research findings or new ideas must stand the test of time to some extent. This contrasts with the easier task of those preparing a classification aimed primarily at the psychiatrists in only one country. Even though the United States is unusually large and its psychiatrists numerous and diverse, they do share at least a common language, a scientific culture, and an administrative framework for health services, all of which have both direct and indirect effects upon the acceptability of a psychiatric classification.

The last decade or so has seen a marked upsurge of interest and activity in psychiatric classification, and there seems to be every prospect that it will continue. This must be a good sign for psychiatry, since it originates from the need to reexamine basic ideas and assumptions in the light of new knowledge about psychiatric disorders. To have one's pet assumptions and favorite terminological customs challenged can be uncomfortable and even startling, but this is the penalty we pay for progress.

REFERENCES

American Psychiatric Association. 1980. *Diagnostic and Statistical Manual of Mental Disorders, Third Edition, DSM-III*. Washington, D.C.
Spitzer, R. L., Endicott, J., and Robins, E. 1978. Research diagnostic criteria. *Archives of General Psychiatry* 35:773–782.
World Health Organization. 1955. *Manual of the International Classification of Diseases, Seventh Revision (ICD-7)*. Geneva.
World Health Organization. 1967. *Manual of the International Classification of Diseases, Eighth Revision (ICD-8)*. Geneva.

World Health Organization. 1977. *Manual of the International Classification of Diseases, Ninth Revision (ICD-9).* Geneva.

World Health Organization. 1978. *Mental Diseases: Glossary and Guide to Their Classification in Accordance with the Ninth Revision of the International Classification of Diseases.* Geneva.

29 *Priorities for the next decade*

ROBERT E. KENDELL (United Kingdom)

THE SIGNIFICANCE OF DSM-III

Attitudes toward psychiatric classification have been transformed in the last decade. The publication by the American Psychiatric Association (1980) of a new, third edition of its *Diagnostic and Statistical Manual* was undoubtedly the most important event of that 10-year period, but of course, DSM-III was not delivered overnight by a stork. It was the product of a slowly developing change in attitudes toward classification and, in particular, of a growing realization that the reliability and validity of the disorders recognized in our nomenclatures could only be improved significantly by radical changes in our whole approach to nosology. DSM-III incorporated three important innovations: a multiaxial format, operational definitions of nearly all of its two hundred syndromes, and a novel grouping of categories that involved discarding the traditional concepts of psychosis and neurosis, as well as many other time-honored terms.

These changes could have been introduced 20 years earlier, for none of them depended on any recent technological innovation or etiological insight. The low reliability of psychiatric diagnoses and the existence of serious international differences in the usage of key terms such as "schizophrenia" were already apparent in the 1950s. By 1960 the artificiality and limited usefulness of the distinction between neurosis and psychosis had been repeatedly exposed (Mapother, 1926; Bowman & Rose, 1951), the advantages of separate axes for syndrome and etiology had been cogently argued (Essen-Möller & Wohlfahrt, 1947), and the World Health Organization (WHO) had been asked by its own expert adviser to provide mental disorders with operational definitions (Stengel, 1959). But for a variety of reasons that were politically understandable, if not scientifically justifiable, we had to wait 20 years for such changes. The most important obstacle to progress was the psychoanalytic movement, not because it opposed any particular innovation but because it taught two generations of American and Canadian psychiatrists that defense mechanisms were more important than symptoms and that classification was of little importance because most varieties of mental disorder shared the same etiology and required the same treatment. Psychiatry, therefore, had to wait while the psychoanalytic tide

332

slowly receded and the crippling consequences of unreliable and unstable diagnostic labels became apparent to more and more persons.

One of the reasons DSM-III has had such a profound impact since its publication in 1980 is that the changes it introduced were long overdue. It facilitated developments in clinical research and psychiatric epidemiology that had been delayed for the best part of a generation and that gave a new impetus to the search for biological correlates. It has also provoked much valuable discussion about the implications of defining a syndrome in one way rather than another, about the relative merits of different ways of defining individual syndromes or of subdividing groups of related syndromes, and about how validity is to be established in the absence of any real understanding of underlying mechanisms.

Five years after the publication of DSM-III several things are clear. DSM-III has been accepted, albeit with varying degrees of enthusiasm, by the American Psychiatric Association's membership and is increasingly used, particularly for research purposes, in other parts of the world as well. Its fundamental innovations are widely accepted despite the uncomfortable changes in traditional attitudes and practices which they have involved. On the other hand, much of its detailed content – the identity and format of its five axes, the disorders it does and does not incorporate, and the precise ways in which many of these are defined – are the subject of much debate and criticism (see, for example, Spitzer, Williams & Skodol, 1983). It is also clear that the introduction of an influential national classification with a fundamentally different format from that of ICD-9 has weakened the role and raison d'être of the ICD as an international lingua franca. By its very existence it serves as a standing invitation to other national associations to produce their own national or regional classifications. For a variety of reasons, therefore, the coming decade will be a critical period.

This is, therefore, a well-chosen time to hold an international conference on classification, and we should be grateful to the World Psychiatric Association's Section on Nomenclature and Classification for taking this initiative and making possible an exchange of views, aims, and priorities for the coming decade. A revised edition of DSM-III (DSM-III-R) is already in an advanced stage of preparation, which probably means that the format of DSM-IV is already starting to be determined. ICD-10 is also beginning to take shape. Although this tenth revision is not due to come into use until 1992 or 1993, the revision conference is planned for 1989; and broad outlines for this revision will need to be agreed upon long before that.

ICD-10 AND DSM-IV

There is no realistic prospect of ICD-10 and DSM-IV being identical in the way that their predecessors ICD-8 and DSM-II were in the 1970s. The mental disorders section of the ICD is only one of the 17 sections of a comprehensive classification of all "diseases, injuries, and causes of death," while the underlying cause of some mental disorders such as brain injury and cerebral infections, for example, will be classified in other parts of the ICD. The American Psychiatric Association's *Diagnostic and Statistical Manual* is an isolated and self-sufficient classification of mental disorders. It is also concerned only with disorders commonly encountered in the United States, whereas the international classification has to be applicable to the wider range of disorders encountered in other parts of the world. Despite these fundamental differences, it is vital that DSM-IV and ICD-10 should be as similar as possible; they should share the same basic framework, and as far as possible the same diagnostic terms, the same groupings of syndromes, and the same definitions of individual disorders.

The draft proposals for the mental disorders section of ICD-10 produced by an "Informal Consultation" in Geneva in April 1984, provide a reasonable starting point for a common framework. They envisage the provision of "precise diagnostic criteria" or operational definitions for every disorder, at least for research purposes. Although the basic structure of the parent international classification will be a single set of alphanumerical categories, it is proposed that this should be accompanied by three additional "axes" dealing, respectively, with underlying or associated physical disorders, associated psychosocial and environmental factors, and the level of social adjustment or disability. They also suggest a terminology and grouping of syndromes similar to that of DSM-III, with all affective disorders and all psychoactive substance use disorders being brought together, as well as the adoption of American terms such as "somatoform disorder" and "paraphilia."

These are, of course, only draft proposals, and many detailed discussions and negotiations lie ahead; several increasingly detailed drafts will probably be produced over the next four years. In addition, it should be noted that the task force to produce DSM-IV has yet to be appointed. The relationship between the WHO and the American Psychiatric Association, and between the small groups of psychiatrists primarily responsible for designing these two classifications, will be crucial to the eventual outcome. If both teams accept the desirability of a common framework, are willing to make compromises to achieve this, and communicate with one another often, so that neither deviates unknowingly or unintentionally from the other, we may end up in the early 1990s with two classifications that are not only improvements on their predecessors but also closely related and easily translated, close cousins if not identical twins.

UNITY OR DIVERSITY

The subtitle of the World Psychiatric Association Conference on International Classification was "Unity and Diversity," and its opening session was devoted to a description of several national diagnostic systems with papers by French, Brazilian, Scandinavian, Egyptian, and Chinese psychiatrists describing their own particular approaches to classification. I fear, however, that we will have to choose between unity and diversity. Either we strive for a single international classification that we can all use, a lingua franca to enable us to communicate with one another as freely and accurately as possible, or else we cling to our separate cultural traditions and use them as a vehicle for our professional and national machismo. The latter course has many attractions, but we have been taught more than once in the last hundred years that it leads to chaos. It is worth recalling the observations made nearly 70 years ago by the committee appointed by the American Medico-Psychological Association (the forerunner of the American Psychiatric Association) to produce a classification for use throughout the United States. As the members of that committee said in their 1917 report:

The first essential of a uniform system of statistics in hospitals for the insane is a generally recognized nomenclature of mental diseases. The present condition with respect to the classification of mental diseases is chaotic. Some states use no well defined classifications. In others, the classifications used are similar in many respects but differ enough to prevent accurate comparisons. Some states have adopted a uniform system, while others leave the matter entirely to the individual hospitals. This condition of affairs discredits the science of psychiatry and reflects unfavorably upon our Association, which should serve as a correlating and standardizing agency for the whole country. (May 1922)

By 1968 the World Health Organization (WHO) had managed to get us out of that situation by persuading almost every country contributing to the psychiatric literature to use the International Classification. It would be regrettable if we were to revert to the chaos of 1917 on a global scale.

General agreement to use the ICD will only be achieved, however, or even be desirable, it two conditions are met. The first is that the international classification must become more truly international. At present there is a widespread view among African, Asian, and South American psychiatrists that ICD-9 and its predecessors have been based too exclusively on European and North American concepts and experience, that there are no suitable categories for many of their patients, particularly those with acute psychotic illnesses of good prognosis and others with multiple somatic complaints of varying kinds (Wig et al., 1985). Europe and North America must be prepared to listen attentively to their colleagues from the developing countries, particularly as that is where the majority of psychiatric patients are to be found. For their part, the developing countries must be prepared, as they are now doing with the help of the WHO, to mount adequate prospective studies of these "atypical" patients, as their symptomatology, course, and outcome must be known before they can be adequately classified. The second condition is that research workers, as opposed to national associations and the agencies responsible for official statistics, must be free to introduce novel categories and classifications or novel definitions of existing disorders whenever they wish to. Classifications can only be improved if alternative ways of defining syndromes and new ways of expressing the relationships between related disorders are explored and compared with existing methods.

UNRESOLVED ISSUES

Suppose for a moment that general agreement could be reached so that in the future we would aspire to have no more than two classifications, that of the World Health Organization and the American Psychiatric Association, that these two would be as similar as possible, and that both would have a multiaxial format and provide operational definitions for all their constituent categories. These would be invaluable achievements, but we would still be left with a daunting array of problems. We have not yet decided how many axes we want or need or how many disorders we wish to recognize. The way in which we group these disorders together – as neuroses, functional psychoses, somatization disorders, paraphilias, and the like – are all arbitrary, provisional, and unstable. The same is true of our present operational definitions of individual syndromes as none of these as of yet commands international approval. Perhaps the most fundamental issue of all is that we are still incapable of defining what we mean by mental disorder.

Our classifications, categories, and definitions are unstable not because psychiatrists are particularly argumentative, fickle, or indecisive, but because we do not yet understand the etiology of the majority of the disorders we study and treat, and because the clusters of symptoms that we identify as characteristic of different syndromes merge imperceptibly into one another. The difficulties we have in deciding, for example, how best to classify depressions or anxiety states, or in deciding whether or how to separate the two, are an almost inevitable consequence of our inability to demonstrate natural boundaries or "points of rarity" within the broad territory in question, and of our rudimentary understanding of the underlying mechanisms. In such a situation it is almost inevitable that there should be disputes between the protagonists of rival classifications, and that concepts and categories should change from time to time almost as capriciously as fashions in clothes. We could, however, reduce the confusion and the conflicting claims in our literature if we gave more thought to our criteria for accepting any given condition as a "disease entity," or for preferring one set of subdivisions to another. For at least the last 20 years any new treatment has had to prove by clinical trial that it was superior to existing therapies before being accepted for general use. There is much to be said for imposing the same requirement on new classifications, but first, of course, we would have to decide what criteria we would use to compare rival classifications.

One of the most important achievements of DSM-III is that it provides an operational definition for almost all its two hundred categories of mental disorder. Many of these definitions are entirely arbitrary; they were not derived from any empirical comparison of a range of alternative definitions; and they were simply drawn up, or invented, by a group of men and women sitting around a table. Indeed, in some cases the disorder itself was a new concept derived in similar fashion. But a start had to be made somewhere, and once categories are defined in operational terms the stage is set for empirical comparisons, and any existing definition is only likely to be supplanted by another that has been shown to be superior in some respect, more reliable perhaps, or more stable over time, or more homogeneous with respect to treatment response or long-term prognosis. The task force that produced DSM-III described its categories and definitions with admirable objectivity and humility as "one still frame in the ongoing process." One of our most important tasks in the next decade is to explore the implications of those two hundred operational definitions and to compare each with its neighbors and possible alternatives. In this piecemeal way we will slowly work our way toward a better and more useful classification. It is not, one has to admit, a very exciting form of research, but it does enable us to pull ourselves up by our bootstraps. The work that has been done in the last 10 years, exploring the implications of different ways of defining schizophrenia, illustrates the kinds of comparisons that could and need to be carried out across the whole range of disorders. Another important form of exploration is to use discriminant functions, as Cloninger and his colleagues have done for schizophrenia, in an attempt to demonstrate a natural boundary between individual syndromes and other disorders (Cloninger et al., 1985). Once a natural boundary or point of rarity has been demonstrated, the problem of where to put the fence demarcating the boundaries of that syndrome is largely solved.

Classification on the basis of symptom patterns, the exercise that psychiatry has been involved in for the past hundred years, is a difficult and frustrating business and in most other branches of medicine it has largely been replaced by classification at a more fundamental level. Addison's disease and Down's syndrome have given way to primary hypoadrenalism and trisomy 21, and Mediterranean anemia has been replaced by a bewildering variety of haemoglobinopathies. Already several generations of psychiatrists have expected to see the etiology of schizophrenia and manic-depressive illness elucidated before they retired but have been disappointed. The same may still happen to us, despite our anticipatory abandonment of the term "functional psychosis." Neurophysiology and neuropharmacology are now developing so rapidly, however, that our chances of living to see the promised land must be considerably better than those of our predecessors. But whether we have to wait 5 or 50 years our chances of finding "biological markers" and elucidating etiology will be greatly improved if we can succeed in drawing the boundaries between one syndrome and another at points which correspond with some more fundamental discontinuity. Better classifications will not only make it easier for us to choose appropriate therapies and predict outcome; they also increase our chances of identifying the underlying biological abnormalities that have eluded us for so long.

THE DEFINITION OF "MENTAL DISORDER"

I have deliberately left until last the issue of the definition of the term "mental disorder." In the past this problem has never been squarely faced. Indeed, medicine has never decided, or at least never adequately defined, what is meant by the term "disease." The current international Glossary of Mental Disorders (World Health Organization, 1978) makes no attempt to define the term "mental disorder," nor does ICD-9, from which it is derived (World Health Organization, 1977). What is more, the International Classification contains no definition either of disease or of any of the related terms it uses, such as, "morbid entity," "morbid condition," or "specific disease entity." At least the authors of DSM-III were more frank. They accepted that "there is no satisfactory definition that specifies precise boundaries for the concept mental disorder," and then went on to say that each of the mental disorders described in the manual "is conceptualized as a clinically significant behavioral or psychological syndrome; typically associated with either distress or disability" (American Psychiatric Association, 1980). They also added that the term "mental disorder" implies the presence of some "behavioral, psychological or biological dysfunction." But nothing was said about how these various dysfunctions were to be recognized or distinguished from normal reactions to stress or adversity, or how clinically significant syndromes were to be distinguished from those that were clinically insignificant. As a result, the crucial issue of which phenomena are to be regarded as disorders, and by what criterion, is not advanced, nor have any fundamental problems been resolved.

Most of the social scientists who have examined the concepts of health and disease have unhesitatingly concluded that the reason physicians, in general, and psychiatrists, in particular, have such difficulty defining what they mean by these terms, or alternatively are so reluctant to commit themselves to a definition, is that they are not scientific or biological terms at all. They are simply "evaluative" or "normative" terms that are applied, and can only be understood, in a particular social context and frame of reference (see, for example, Sedgwick, 1982). Put simply, their argument is that the term "disease" is simply a label used to denote any phenomenon that a particular culture decides is undesirable and then decides further is more likely to be dealt with effectively by physicians and medical technology than by alternative institutions such as the law or the church.

The instinctive response of most doctors to such views is to reject them. But they do provide a plausible explanation of why different societies have in the past, and to some extent still do, adopt such different views on the status of, for example, epilepsy; homosexuality; the habit of smoking tobacco, cannabis, or opium; or habitual stealing or fire raising. They also shed a new and rather revealing light on the behavior of the various parties involved in the long series of disputes about the status of homosexuality in DSM-II (Bayer, 1981) and about Russian treatment of political dissidents (Bloch & Reddaway, 1977). Whether or not Sedgwick and his fellow sociologists are correct, psychiatry will remain vulnerable to their arguments until it defines what it does mean by mental illness; particularly as it is part of the sociologists' argument that our failure to define the terms "disease" and "illness" is deliberate, a device, that is, for enabling such labels to be applied to a wide variety of phenomena whenever it is convenient to do so.

The architects of ICD-10 and DSM-IV have four basic strategies available to them in this situation. The first, which the WHO has always adopted in the past, is to ignore the problem, perhaps in the hope that others will do the same, and make no attempt to define the term "disease" or any of its analogues. The second, adopted by the task force responsible for DSM-III, is to provide something that looks like a definition but, in fact, is so vaguely worded that any term with medical connotations can be either included or excluded as contemporary opinion requires. (A subsidiary strategy, adopted by both the WHO and the American Psychiatric Association, is to refer throughout to mental disorders rather than diseases on the assumption that the [undefined] term "disorder" will be both less contentious and broader in scope than the [similarly undefined] term disease.) The third strategy, which has never yet been adopted, at least by a psychiatric classification, is to provide an operational definition of disease (or disorder) that provides unambiguous rules of application like those provided for individual disorders, and then to abide by the constraints imposed by that definition. Unfortunately, such a definition would almost certainly exclude some conditions we wished to see included or include some conditions we wished to see excluded, or both. The fourth strategy is to concede openly that psychiatric classifications are not classifications of either diseases or disorders, but simply of the problems psychiatrists are currently consulted about, and that the justification for including such categories as oppositional disorder or pyromania (in DSM-III) or specific reading retardation (in ICD-9) is simply that, in practice, psychiatrists are consulted by or about people with such problems.

I suggested elsewhere (Kendell, 1985) that this might be the best course, at least for the time being. It avoids the ambiguity and intellectual dishonesty of the first two options and the serious constraints of the third. It does, of course, leave unresolved the question of which of the conditions listed in our glossaries is a disease and which is merely a problem resulting in a psychiatric consultation; but the use of the term "mental disorder" does that anyway. Both ICD-9 and DSM-III implicitly reject this approach, for both include in their glossaries a list of "conditions not attributable to a mental disorder that are the focus of attention or treatment," the so-called V codes. Many people, of course, will be reassured to know that they can consult and even receive treatment from a psychiatrist without, thereby, being deemed to have a mental disorder. But dividing our patients into two groups, those with and those without a mental disorder, makes it all the more vital to have an adequate definition of this term and a reliable criterion for distinguishing between disorder and nondisorder; at present we have neither.

Perhaps I should apologize for raising so intently this unsolved issue. I am convinced, though, that we must start to think more deeply than we have in the past about what we really mean by the term "mental disorder," which we use so frequently and so readily, and why it is that we have such difficulty defining it adequately or perhaps are so reluctant to try.

REFERENCES

American Psychiatric Association. 1980. *Diagnostic and Statistical Manual of Mental Disorder*. 3rd ed. (DSM-III). Washington, D.C.

Bayer, R. 1981. *Homosexuality and American Psychiatry: The Politics of Diagnosis*. New York: Basic Books.

Bloch, S., and Reddaway, P. 1977. *Russia's Political Hospitals*. London: Victor Gollancz.

Bowman, K. M., and Rose, M. 1951. A criticism of the terms psychosis, psychoneurosis and neurosis. *American Journal of Psychiatry* 108: 161–166.

Cloninger, C. R., Martin, R. L., Guze, S. B., and Clayton, P. J. 1985. Diagnosis and prognosis in schizophrenia. *Archives of General Psychiatry* 42: 15–25.

Essen-Möller, E., and Wohlfahrt, S. 1947. Suggestions for the amendment of the official Swedish classification of mental disorders. *Acta Psychiatrica et Neurologica Scandinavica*, Suppl. 47, 551–555.

Kendell, R. S. 1985. What are mental disorders? In *Science, Practice and Social Policy: Issues in Classifying Mental Disorders*, ed. A. M. Freedman, R. Brotman, I. Silverman, and D. Hutson. New York: Human Sciences Press.

Mapother, E. 1926. Opening paper of discussion on manic-depressive psychosis. *British Medical Journal* ii, 876.

May, J. V. 1922. *Mental Diseases*, p. 246. Boston: R. G. Badger.

Sedgwick, P. 1982. *Psychopolitics*. London: Pluto Press.

Spitzer, R. L., Williams, J. W. B., and Skodol, A. E. 1983. *International Perspectives on DSM-III*. Washington, D.C.: American Psychiatric Press.

Stengel, E. 1959. Classification of mental disorders. *Bulletin of the World Health Organization* 21: 601–663.

Wig, N. N., Setyonegoro, R. K., Shen, Y.-C., and Sell, H. 1985. Problems of psychiatric diagnosis and classification in the Third World. In *Mental Disorders, Alcohol and Drug Related Problems: International Perspectives on Their Diagnosis and Classification*, pp. 50–60. Amsterdam: Excerpta Medica.

World Health Organization. 1977. *Manual of the International Statistical Classification of Diseases, Injuries, and Causes of Death*. Geneva.

World Health Organization. 1978. *Mental Disorders: Glossary and Guide to their Classification in Accordance with the Ninth Revision of the International Classification of Diseases*. Geneva.

PART V

Panel on ICD-10

30 An overview of the prospects for ICD-10

ASSEN JABLENSKY (World Health Organization, Switzerland)

The origins of the International Classification of Diseases (ICD) can be traced back to 1891, when the first International Classification of Causes of Death, designed by a committee chaired by the French statistician Bertillon, was introduced. Another milestone is the year 1938, when, for the first time, in the fifth revision of the International Classification, a rudimentary classification of mental disorders was introduced (Kramer et al., 1979). It is my opinion, however, that the modern history of the classification of mental disorders in the framework of ICD began in 1959, when the World Health Organization (WHO) requested Professor E. Stengel to review the field and make recommendations about future developments in classification.

THE STATE OF PSYCHIATRIC CLASSIFICATION BEFORE ICD-8

In his comprehensive and incisive review, Stengel (1959) concluded:

The lack of a common classification of mental disorders has defeated attempts at comparing psychiatric observations and the results of treatments undertaken in various countries or even in various centres in the same countries. One of the fundamental difficulties in devising the classification of mental disorders is the lack of agreement among psychiatrists regarding the concepts upon which it should be based. Diagnoses can rarely be verified objectively and the same, or similar conditions, are described under a confusing variety of names. This situation militates against the ready exchange of ideas and experiences, and hampers progress.

This statement gave rise to many developments that we are still discussing today.

In his inquiry, Stengel identified 38 different classifications in use. Each classification was associated with the name of an authoritative professor of psychiatry, or with the name of a particular clinic, university department, or other institution, and each reflected the worldview of its author more than it offered an empirically observable descriptive picture of the phenomena to be classified. In fact, the situation prevailing in the 1950s was hardly different in any respect from the state of the field 60 years earlier, a state of affairs about which Tuke remarked caustically that "the wit of man has rarely been more exercised than

343

in the attempt to classify the morbid mental phenomena covered by the term 'insanity.' The result has been disappointing" (Tuke, 1892).

Stengel also concluded that ICD-6, which was the official classification at that time, had failed to provide an antidote to the toxic effects of the proliferation of classificatory systems developed ex cathedra and recommended a "drastic revision of the ICD relevant to psychiatry." This was to be achieved through agreement on operational definitions. It is important to note that as early as 1959, Stengel recommended implementing a "shift from abstract theory to description and a close scrutiny of the reasons for the low reliability of psychiatric diagnosis" – all this under the aegis of the WHO.

STEPPING STONES FOR ICD-10

The quarter of a century that has elapsed since Stengel submitted his report to the WHO has brought about significant changes in the art and science of psychiatric diagnosis and classification. I would like to mention just four significant changes. The first results from efforts like the WHO Programme A, which covered the period 1965–72. Within the framework of this program, eight international seminars were held that ultimately resulted in proposals for the classification of mental disorders in ICD-8. This program and its product, ICD-8, were important not so much because of any major innovations within the classification itself but because of the first glossary of mental disorders that was designed to fit the rubrics of ICD-8 and later was incorporated into the body of the ninth revision of the International Classification of Diseases (World Health Organization, 1978).

A second type of endeavor that was gaining momentum simultaneously with this program was collaborative international research. The two early examples of such research are the US-UK Diagnostic Project (Cooper et al., 1972) and the International Pilot Study of Schizophrenia (World Health Organization, 1973, 1979). These studies introduced for the first time on a large scale standardized methods in international comparisons of morbidity and clinical features of major psychoses. The development of instruments such as the Present State Examination (Wing, Cooper & Sartorius, 1974) and the computerized diagnostic classification system CATEGO associated with it laid the groundwork for later studies such as the WHO project on the determinants of outcome of severe mental disorders, which collected data on the epidemiology of such disorders in geographically defined populations. An example of the types of questions that it became feasible to ask and attempt to answer as a result of this development is related to the incidence of schizophrenic disorders in different geographical areas (Sartorius et al., 1986). If a wider clinical diagnosis or a range of CATEGO classes is applied to their definitions, we obtain significant differences between the different study sites (Figure 30.1). The two areas that have the highest incidence are in India, one rural and one urban. It is also of interest to note the differences between the rates for Aarhus (Denmark), Dublin (Ire-

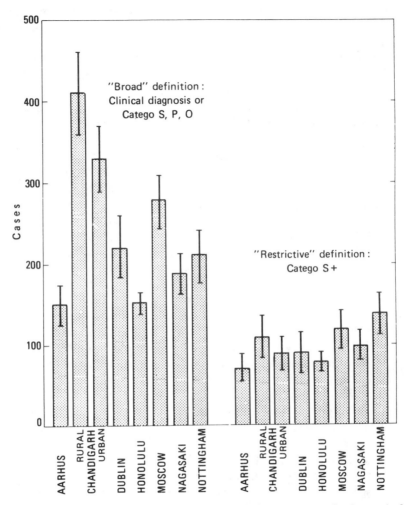

Figure 30.1. Incidence rates per million population age 15–54 (both sexes); for the "broad" and for the "restrictive" definition of schizophrenia

land), Honolulu (USA), Moscow (USSR), Nagasaki (Japan), and Nottingham (UK). The differences are significant. If, however, a standard definition based on the CATEGO program and its class CATEGO S+ – which was designed to pick up the so-called nuclear schizophrenic syndrome – is applied, then the significant differences between these very different populations as regards the incidence of schizophrenia disappear. The incidence is similar in different sites.

The third major development was the first multiaxial classification of psychiatric disorders specific to childhood, which was introduced by the WHO (Rutter, Shaffer & Shepherd, 1975).

The fourth development, which is of a general nature, was the universal revival of interest in diagnosis and classification and the many attempts to formulate explicit criteria, not only for international statistical purposes, but also for research and teaching. This has been evident in a number of countries, but undoubtedly some of the most significant developments have taken place in the United States. These have included, first, the St. Louis criteria (Feighner, Robins & Guze, 1972), the Research Diagnostic Criteria (Spitzer, Endicott & Robins, 1978), and, more recently, DSM-III (American Psychiatric Association, 1980), which have represented the most radical effort so far to redesign the classification of mental disorders.

The wide use of DSM-III, not only in North America, but also in an increasing number of countries, indicates that it has, indeed, filled a vacuum that existed at the time. It has met a demand that ICD-9, introduced earlier in 1979, was not in a position to meet fully. Such developments went hand in hand with clinical, epidemiological, and perhaps most significantly, biological research. Although such research has, up to now, produced relatively little with regard to the pièce de résistance of psychiatric classification, namely the major psychoses, it has greatly influenced other areas of clinical concern that had been for many years the quiet backwaters of classification. The dementias and other disorders of late life, the childhood disorders, and to some extent the neurotic disorders have become the focus of intensive and fruitful research.

More recently, the state of the art in the field of classification was reviewed in considerable breadth and depth in the context of the joint WHO/ADAMHA Project on Classification of Mental Disorder and Alcohol and Drug Related Problems, in which experts from more than 40 countries participated in various working groups, task forces, and a major international conference that was held three years ago in Copenhagen (World Health Organization, 1985). The conclusions of this broad review can be classified into seven major groups (Jablensky et al., 1983).

First, it provided evidence of a widely shared recognition that classification is an important epistemological and practical tool in psychiatry. In contrast to the 1960s, when reliability of diagnosis and classificatory categories were the main concerns, attention in recent years had gradually shifted to the validity of diagnosis.

The second major conclusion was that, although ICD-8 and ICD-9 had been widely accepted, this fact had in no way diminished the use and influence of so-called national or local classifications. The national classifications are alive and well and still being used for a variety of purposes. Of course, one would like to quote DSM-III as an example of national classification, but in the last few years, it has become, to a considerable degree, international.

The third conclusion was that the state of theory underlying current diagnostic concepts and classifications in psychiatry is unsatisfactory. There was a swing of the pendulum away from the previous psychodynamic reductionism in explaining mental disorders to models that recur to biological reductionism in explaining mental disorders.

The fourth conclusion was that developing-world psychiatrists have inadequate provisions; if it is taken into account that 75 percent of the population of the earth lives in developing countries, this means that the majority of the people who need good psychiatric care could not be served on the basis of planning linked to classificatory concepts that would be relevant to them. This was a major concern for psychiatrists in developing countries. Closely linked to this concern was the emphasis both developing and highly developed countries put on psychiatry as an element of primary health care, on extra hospital psychiatry, and on psychiatry within the context of the first contact care facilities.

The fifth conclusion concerns those areas of classification that, in the opinion of the participants in the project, remained wanting and underdeveloped. Quite a few areas could be quoted in this respect, but perhaps the following are the important ones: First, there was widespread dissatisfaction with the state of classification of the personality disorders. Second, it was emphasized that the existing classificatory provisions did not keep pace with clinical, epidemiological, and biological research in the area of alcohol and substance-abuse problems. The third area was that of the psychosocial problems, seen in the context of primary health care. And the fourth area was that of the problem of "nonpsychotic" disorders (referred to as such for want of a better common denominator). In the words of one participant in the project, "This is the group of conditions that still have to attract their Kraepelin" (Shepherd, 1985).

The sixth main conclusion concerned the strategy and methodology of classification. It was recognized that the chief obstacle to further improvements in classification is nothing more than the gaps in our knowledge about the nature of the phenomena to be classified. It became evident that there is increasing emphasis on the medical approach to classification, which relies on "clinical observation fortified by newer laboratory findings." This reliance on the knowledge base method, rather than on statistics, was somewhat in contrast to earlier approaches, which were based on expectations that the application of multivariate statistical methods would somehow help us to carve out natural entities of mental disorders. These expectations were never met, and in the view of the participants in the project, it seems we are back to the classical and well-tested method of clinical observation that can be supported by epidemiological and biological findings.

Last, it was unanimously concluded that there was a need for continued international collaboration on classification and diagnosis.

I should add here another important perspective that has emerged in some countries in recent years, although it was not discussed in the framework of the project I mentioned. This is the finding that classification is becoming increasingly linked to service-reimbursement schemes. For example, in the United States, there has been a lot of discussion about the so-called Diagnosis Related Groups and the prospective payment schemes and the ways in which these administrative innovations put a new type of demand on psychiatric classification. Whether this will be followed by other countries, of course, remains to be seen.

EPISTEMOLOGICAL, PSYCHOLOGICAL, AND UTILITY REQUIREMENTS OF A CLASSIFICATION

Before reviewing the mechanism for construction of the tenth revision of the International Classification and discussing the main ideas that may be reflected in its structure and contents, I should like to mention some general criteria that could be considered if we want to have an effective classification that performs well. I believe that there are three groups of criteria. First, there are epistemological criteria and requirements for classification. A classification should be able to articulate the universe of observations into meaningful units, and I am saying *meaningful*, not necessarily valid, because validity often comes later, once we have defined meaningful units. A meaningful unit should be a unit of observation that leads to some sort of purposeful action on the part of the users of the classification, be it research, treatment, or the management of patients.

A second epistemological criterion is that classification should be capable of generating new kinds of observations and questions that had not been possible with earlier versions of classifications or without that classification. Perhaps a distant analogy would be to the periodic table of the chemical elements, which brought together empirical facts that were there and were well known; but through a systematic ordering on the basis of an underlying principle, it allowed the making of new kinds of observations that had not been made before.

The third epistemological criterion is that the classification should be capable of increasing the reliability and the reproducibility of observations.

In addition to these epistemological criteria, there are also important psychological or cognitive criteria and requirements for classification. First, a classification should satisfy the need we all have for familiarity and comprehensibility and thus be in accordance with everyone's world map and the traditions of the place and culture in which one is working. It should be able to satisfy such needs in a variety of users, not in one culture, but in many, if it is going to be an international classification.

Another psychological criterion is that a classification should be easy to internalize and memorize because a system that is too complex in its structure and cannot be overviewed in a simple way is not likely to be practically useful.

A third group of criteria could be called utility criteria, which require that a classification should be adaptable to a variety of settings and cultures; that a classification should retain a measure of continuity with past classification schemes in order to facilitate the transition from one revision to another, as well as to reduce the costs of overhauling the entire administrative and statistical machinery of reporting after every revision of the international classification.

GENERAL FEATURES OF ICD-10

Against this background, I should like to mention the general features that have been adopted for the tenth revision of the International Classification of Diseases as a whole, not just the chapter on the classification of mental disorders. A number of meetings, including those of collaborating centers and expert committees, have agreed on the following general features for ICD-10: First, it will be open-ended and flexible. This means that it would be a classification that would allow additions in the course of time without a major revision, the aim being to postpone the eleventh revision of ICD as long as possible. In order to achieve this, the second feature proposed is the introduction of the so-called alphanumerical system of coding, in which the first symbol for an entry would be a letter of the alphabet and the second and third would be digits. This allows a considerable increase in the number of positions available in the classification. It is also envisaged that a certain proportion of those positions would be kept in the tenth revision, for additions that may become necessary as knowledge advances.

The next feature is that ICD will retain its basic uniaxial core structure. This should not be in conflict with multiaxial schemes and adaptations for special purposes, but the official document that will be adopted by governments will remain uniaxial.

The next feature is that the development of a *family* of documents will be encouraged, including adaptations, extensions, and classifications for special purposes that would include, of course, multiaxial systems that are of special concern to psychiatrists.

The next feature is that the three-character rubric will be the basic unit of classification, that is, the rubric defined by a letter of the alphabet and two digits. The appeal to all the special committees and groups that are developing the different sections of the classification is that they should try to identify at this three-character level the conditions, states, disorders, and diseases that are considered significant public-health concerns and need to be reported by most countries. Fourth-character codes can be added later, and there is no limit on adding further subdivisions for any kinds of special purposes or for national adaptations.

Another requirement is that the alphanumerical codes should be meaningful at every level. For example, at present – provisionally – the letter "F" has been assigned to the chapter on mental disorders, so that this letter already gives the heading of a chapter. The recommendation requires that the next digit reflect that the field of mental disorders is subdivided into meaningful areas. The same applies to the next digit. This requirement is too stringent, and when in the course of the past year, different working groups have met and tried to develop the specific contents of their sections, it became obvious that it is impossible to follow this recommendation to the letter. For that reason, a recent meeting of the ICD committee has relaxed this rule somewhat. Therefore, the present recommendation is that the classification should be meaningful at every level as far as possible, but it is acknowledged that this may not be feasible in all instances.

Finally, the so-called E and V codes, which refer to external causes of injuries and to psychosocial and other factors affecting the contacts of people with clinical services, will be retained and expanded, which means that we shall need a better classification of psychosocial factors underlying health behavior and contacts with the health services.

CONSIDERATIONS UNDERLYING THE CLASSIFICATION OF MENTAL DISORDERS IN ICD-10

Before outlining the structure of the proposals concerning Chapter F or 5, I should like to point to a few constraints on the classification of mental disorders in ICD because they will remain in force for the next revision. First, ICD is primarily a classification for statistical purposes. Only later in its development has the idea been introduced that it should also be a research, clinical care, and teaching instrument. But it remains in the eyes of the World Health Organization and the governments that make up this organization an important tool for statistical study and the reporting of disorders.

Second, ICD is a classification and not a nomenclature. This means that, to take the example of Chapter 5 or F, we have been allotted a certain number of "slots" in which we have to classify the entire universe of mental disorders. Therefore, the principles and the subdivisions have to be devised within these constraints. We cannot expand beyond these limits. Perhaps we can never achieve within the framework of ICD a true nomenclature of mental disorders, although steps in that direction are feasible.

The third constraint is that ICD is, and will remain, a classification of diseases and not a classification of people. Although any supplementary schemes for multiaxial recording would be closer to the idea of a clinical formulation – in which we describe an individual in many different respects – we should be reminded that the core of ICD will be a uniaxial classification of diseases and other conditions.

This raises the question of how radical the revision of Chapter 5 or ICD should be at this point. There are well-known shortcomings in ICD-9. For instance, it has limited clinical usefulness – especially when contrasted with DSM-III, which was designed with a different purpose in mind. Also, ICD-9 is the product of growth by accretion of new categories that have been added in subsequent revisions without any major restructuring of the basis on which it rests. It has retained its eclectic structure, although it conforms to some general principles.

The ideal Chapter 5 in the future revision of ICD should perhaps reflect to a greater extent than ICD-9 the recent advances in research and understanding of mental disorders that have taken place. It should also be capable of serving as a clinical manual, in addition to being a key for statistical reporting. It should be adaptable to the wider horizon of service settings that exist today; and also, perhaps, it should move one step farther toward an international nomenclature of mental disorders.

In order to meet these requirements, the following new features have been proposed. Chapter 5 in ICD-10 will be considerably expanded as far as the positions available for coding are concerned. It will contain a total of 100 rubrics instead of 30 as in ICD-9. No less than 25–30 percent of these rubrics, however, will be reserved for future use, and their categories will not be filled in in the process of the tenth revision. The core classification of mental disorders will be uniaxial, but in addition to the list of rubrics, it will include in the main body of the classification a revised glossary in which the present glossary definitions will be enlarged and supplemented in order to bring them closer to conceptual definitions of disorders indicating the nosological status of each group of conditions. A major innovation that has been proposed is the introduction of so-called clinical diagnostic guidelines. According to most of the experts consulted so far, these guidelines should be less stringent and less specific than those presented in DSM-II or in the Research Diagnostic Criteria. Nevertheless, they should provide guidance to the clinician as to the necessary and sufficient attributes of disorders that are required in the process of making clinical diagnoses and also should point to the conditions to be considered in the differential diagnosis of each disorder.

A "FAMILY" OF RELATED DOCUMENTS

The family of satellite documents around this core of Chapter 5 for ICD-10 will include research diagnostic criteria as an appendix. These criteria will not be in the main body of the classification but will be available to investigators. In addition to the ICD-10 operational criteria, it may be possible to include a selection from research diagnostic criteria from various sources. This appendix will not cover the entire field of classification, because there are large nosological areas in which it is unrealistic at present to draft research diagnostic criteria. We know too little in those areas, which, being too specific, may be counterproductive.

Second, there will be a key to multiaxial recording of diagnostic formulations. Third, there will be a separate classification of disabilities and handicaps that will be used in conjunction with this multiaxial key. A core classification of disabilities and handicaps is already available, but the revised version will be published together with ICD-10.

The next document will be an adaptation of the classification for primary health care. This means that special lists will be constructed of those conditions of particular importance in primary health care, and the definitions and criteria will have to be amended and adapted to serve the variety of users in such contexts. Another document will be the so-called crosswalk guide for comparisons between ICD-10 and ICD-9 and, possibly, selected parts of national classifications such as DSM-III-R.

Finally, there will be an appendix containing the Lexicon, a dictionary of psychopathological terms. A prototype dictionary has already been developed, and a version linked to ICD-10 will be prepared.

What is the mechanism for developing ICD-10? First, we already have a considerable knowledge base as a result of the project I mentioned earlier. The main work in constructing Chapter 5 will be carried out by panels of experts, each of which will be assigned to work on a particular subsection of the classification. A number of specific problems have already become evident in the process of consulting with many people who received drafts of ICD-10 with a request for comments and specific suggestions.

PROPOSED NEW FEATURES

The provisional list of categories for the mental disorders chapter of ICD-10 is given in the appendix to this chapter. The first new feature of the proposals for Chapter 5 is that there should be at least 10 major groups of disorders instead of the current major groups of ICD-9 – which are organic psychotic conditions; other psychoses; neurotic, personality, and other nonpsychotic disorders; and mental retardation. Instead of these four major groupings in ICD-9, it is envisaged that a larger number of categories will be introduced.

Another feature is that all the alcohol- and drug-related problems would be grouped together as substance-use disorders. In ICD-9 the different conditions related to alcohol and drugs were scattered throughout the classification.

A third feature is that all the affective disorders will be grouped together in accordance with the prevailing current view and also in order to stimulate further research.

A fourth feature is the suggestion that a new code be introduced along with a new category for acute nonschizophrenic and nonaffective psychotic disorders. This is particularly important to psychiatrists in developing countries who see a large number of such patients and find it difficult to accommodate their clinical observations to the straitjacket of the present classification of psychotic disorders.

Another possibility would be to introduce new categories for somatization disorders and for psychophysiological (psychosomatic) conditions. Also being considered is a new category for stress and adjustment-related disorders and a proposal to split the current personality disorders into two separate categories: the personality disorders proper and a group containing the so-called accentuated personalities or personality traits of psychiatric significance. The latter will allow the coding of morbid personality characteristics that may impinge on the prognosis of the disorder but that would not merit being classified as personality disorder. This would represent something like a separate personality axis of the classification.

Yet another feature is the proposal to split the current ICD-9 rubric for sexual deviations and disorders into two groups. One would include the gender identity disorders and the paraphilias, and the other would contain the sexual dysfunctions. These two groups actually represent very different disorders with regard to their clinical manifestations, treatment, prognosis, and so forth.

Further, there is a proposal to group together all disorders with onset specific to childhood and adolescence. The last point on this list is that the so-called culture-bound syndromes will be included in ICD-10 and probably will be distributed according to the predominant psychopathological features of their manifestations. This is a difficult area that was largely ignored in previous versions of the international classification.

QUESTIONS FOR FURTHER REFLECTION

In conclusion, I should like to enumerate a number of specific questions that have arisen and that cannot be answered without wise consultations. The first problem is the classification of dementias and their criteria. It seems that the field is developing so rapidly that the largest number of alternative proposals for classification concern this field. For example, it has been suggested that the dementias should be divided into cortical dementias, subcortical dementias, and mixed forms, which is an entirely novel classification proposed mainly by neurologists. Other proposals concern classification by etiology, age of onset, and so forth.

Another problem is the placement of the so-called endormorph syndromes associated with organic lesions to the brain. What should be done about the increasing number of findings in association with the diagnosis of schizophrenia, affective disorders, and more recently anxiety and other neurotic disorders, in which we find, for example, enlarged cerebral ventricles, borderline atrophy, and other organic characteristics? Although these are findings of great potential value, it would be difficult to allocate such disorders to the group of organic mental disorders. One proposal is to include within each major section – for example, the section on schizophrenia and related conditions – a special code for schizophreniform psychosis associated with demonstrable cerebral-organic findings, and to have the same device under the broad rubric of affective disorders and even within the group of neurotic disorders.

There is also the question where to place the alcohol and drug psychoses. Should they remain with the organic conditions, or should they be integrated with the other substance-use disorders and health problems?

Another issue is the subdivision of the schizophrenic disorders. Where should we place, for example, the schizotypal personality disorder that is more or less equivalent to the so-called latent or borderline schizophrenia? Should we place it within the personality disorders or within the classification of schizophrenia as a "disease spectrum" concept that would also include nonpsychotic manifestations?

Next is the issue of the acute psychotic episodes and their definition. Are there syndromes that are specific to these acute psychotic conditions? How robust are they cross-culturally?

Regarding the schizoaffective disorder, a question exists about its proper place: Should it be with the affective disorders or with the schizophrenic spectrum disorders?

Another quandary surrounds the so-called cycloid psychoses. There is evidence that the concept is being used increasingly outside the tradition that generated it. Is this concept suitable for inclusion in ICD-10?

Controversy also exists regarding the reactive or psychogenic psychosis. Is this an etiological or a descriptive concept? Many of the commentators on the draft raised the question, If we want to retain the descriptive character of the classification, does the inclusion of an etiological concept not conflict with this principle?

The next question is whether to retain or eliminate such terms as "neurasthenia" and "hysteria." The essay by Dongier included as Chapter 14 in this volume is a commentary on the complexities associated with the concept of hysteria.

Another issue relates to the classification of anxiety disorders. Should we identify in ICD-10 a separate subcategory of panic disorder in accordance with some recent publications? What is the relationship between the anxiety disorders and the obsessive-compulsive disorders? We have conflicting comments on this relationship.

A whole range of questions deal with the classification of the somatization disorders, the sexual disorders, the problem of homosexuality – whether it should even be mentioned in ICD-10 – and the problem of redefining and introducing new concepts in the area of personality disorders. Finally, the following question has been posed: "How to account, within the classification of childhood disorders, for parenting problems which may be more important in many cases than making a diagnosis of the child?" The above is just a sample of the many questions that have arisen and will have to be dealt with in due course.

COLLABORATION WITH WHO EXPERTS, NONGOVERNMENTAL ORGANIZATIONS, AND NATIONAL PROFESSIONAL SOCIETIES

Regarding the plan of action toward the development of ICD-10, the following should be mentioned: A collaborative agreement has been established between the World Psychiatric Association (WPA) and the WHO, according to which drafts of the conceptual definitions and diagnostic criteria will be sent by the WHO to the WPA, which will undertake the circulation of this document to national societies and their committees on nomenclature and classification. The WPA Section on Nomenclature and Classification will then analyze and digest the responses and communicate the main conclusions and recommendations back to the WHO. We are taking the same approach to professional societies that currently are not WPA members. At the same time, we will continue to work with a large number of WHO experts and panels on the range of documents that are associated with the new ICD proposal. An important question concerns the relationship between ICD-10 and DSM-III-R/DSM-IV. A working relationship has been developed between the groups responsible for the two classifications. It is obvious that a need for convergence is in the minds of all of us. How far this convergence can go is impossible to predict, but established formal consultations between the DSM and ICD groups will continue to explore in specific detail the extent to which this might be feasible. In an article published a few years ago, Kendell (1984) appealed to what he called the architects of ICD-10 and DSM-IV to try to sort out differences and get closer together. In his reply, Spitzer (1984) called for similar action but set forth modest expectations about the extent to which it would be possible.

To conclude on an architectural note, one thing about which we are sure is that ICD-10 will not look like a baroque monument. We hope that it will be a rather simple and utilitarian building like a railway station or a small airport from which flights will take off in different directions.

APPENDIX: PROVISIONAL LIST OF CATEGORIES FOR CHAPTER 5 ("F"), MENTAL, BEHAVIORAL AND DEVELOPMENTAL DISORDERS, IN THE TENTH REVISION OF THE INTERNATIONAL CLASSIFICATION OF DISEASES (1987 DRAFT)

F0 *ORGANIC, INCLUDING SYMPTOMATIC, MENTAL DISORDERS*

F00 *Dementia, not otherwise specified*

F01 *Dementia in Alzheimer disease*
- F01.0 Dementia in Alzheimer disease, senile onset (Type 1)
- F01.1 Dementia in Alzheimer disease, presenile onset (Type 2)
- F01.2 Dementia in Alzheimer disease, atypical or mixed type

F02 *Dementia in cerebrovascular disease*
- F02.0 Vascular dementia of acute onset
- F02.1 Multi-infarct (predominantly cortical) vascular dementia
- F02.2 Other (predominantly subcortical) vascular dementia
- F02.3 Mixed cortical and subcortical vascular dementia

F03 *Dementia associated with other disorders*
- F03.0 Dementia in Pick disease
- F03.1 Dementia in Creutzfeldt-Jacob disease
- F03.2 Dementia in Huntington disease
- F03.3 Dementia in Parkinson disease
- F03.8 Dementia in other specified conditions

F04 *Organic amnestic syndrome (Korsakov syndrome), other than alcoholic*

F05 *Delirium, other than alcoholic*
- F05.0 Delirium, other than alcoholic, superimposed on dementia

F06 *Other mental disorders due to brain disease, damage or dysfunction, or to physical disease*
- F06.0 Organic hallucinosis

F06.1   Organic catatonic state (stupor or excitement)
F06.2   Organic delusional or schizophrenia-like state
F06.3   Organic depressive state
F06.4   Organic manic state
F06.5   Organic anxiety state
F06.6   Emotionally labile or asthenic state
F06.8   Other
F06.9   Unspecified

F07   *Personality and behaviour disorder due to brain disease, damage, or dysfunction*
F07.0   Organic personality disorder
F07.1   Postencephalitic syndrome
F07.2   Postconcussional syndrome
F07.8   Other
F07.9   Unspecified

F08   *Other organic or symptomatic mental disorder*

F09   *Unspecified organic or symptomatic mental disorder*

F1   *MENTAL AND BEHAVIOUR DISORDERS DUE TO PSYCHO-ACTIVE SUBSTANCE USE*

F10 *Disorders resulting from use of alcohol*

F11 *Disorders resulting from use of tobacco*

F12 *Disorders resulting from use of opioids*

F13 *Disorders resulting from use of cannabinoids*

F14 *Disorders resulting from use of sedatives or hypnotics*

F15 *Disorders resulting from use of cocaine*

F16 *Disorders resulting from use of other stimulants (including caffeine)*

F17 *Disorders resulting from use of hallucinogens*

F18 *Disorders resulting from use of volatile inhalants*

F19 *Disorders resulting from use of other or unidentified substances*

4th- and 5th-character codes for specifying the clinical condition:
.0 *Acute intoxication*
.00 uncomplicated
.01 with trauma or other bodily injury
.02 with other medical complication
.03 with delirium
.04 with perceptual distortions
.05 with coma
.06 with convulsions
.1 *Hazardous use*
.2 *Harmful use*
.3 *Dependence syndrome*
.4 *Withdrawal state*
.40 uncomplicated
.41 with delirium
.42 with convulsions

.5 *Psychotic state*
    .50 schizophrenia-like
    .51 predominantly delusional
    .52 predominantly hallucinatory
    .53 mixed
.6 *Drug or alcohol induced dementia*
.7 *Drug or alcohol induced amnestic (Korsakov) syndrome*
.8 *Drug or alcohol induced residual state*
    .80 flashbacks
    .81 personality or behavior disorder
    .82 affective state
    .83 persisting cognitive impairment
.9 *Unspecified mental or behaviour disorder induced by drugs or alcohol*

F2   SCHIZOPHRENIA, SCHIZOTYPAL STATES, AND DELUSIONAL DISORDERS

F20 *Schizophrenia**
    F20.0 Paranoid schizophrenia
    F20.1 Hebephrenic schizophrenia
    F20.2 Catatonic schizophrenia
    F20.3 Undifferentiated schizophrenia
    F20.4 Post-schizophrenic depression
    F20.5 Residual schizophrenia
    F20.8 Other schizophrenia
    F20.9 Unspecified schizophrenia

F21 *Schizotypal states*
    F21.0 Schizotypal disorder (latent schizophrenia)
    F21.1 Simple schizophrenia (simple deterioration disorder)

F22 *Persistent delusional disorders*
    F22.0 Delusional disorder (paranoia)
    F22.8 Other persistent delusional disorders

F23 *Acute or transient psychotic disorders*
    F23.0 Acute delusional episode (bouffée délirante, cycloid psychosis)
    F23.1 Psychogenic (reactive) delusional disorder (psychogenic psychosis)
    F23.2 Schizophrenia-like episode
    F23.8 Other (undifferentiated) acute psychotic disorder

F24 *Induced delusional disorder (folie à deux)*

F28 *Other nonorganic psychotic disorders*

F29 *Nonorganic psychosis, not otherwise specified*

---

*Pattern of course:
F20.χ0 continuous
F20.χ1 episodic with progressive deficit
F20.χ2 episodic with stable deficit
F20.χ3 episodic remittent
F20.χ4 single episode, incomplete remission
F20.χ5 single episode, complete remission

F3   MOOD (AFFECTIVE) DISORDERS

F30 *Manic episode*

F31 *Depressive episode*
    F31.0   Severe depressive episode
    F31.1   Mild depressive episode

F32 *Bipolar affective disorder*
    F32.0   Bipolar affective disorder, currently manic
    F32.1   Bipolar affective disorder, currently depressed
    F32.2   Bipolar affective disorder, currently mixed
    F32.3   Bipolar affective disorder, currently in remission

F33 *Recurrent depressive disorders*
    F33.0   Recurrent severe depressive disorder
    F33.1   Recurrent mild depressive disorder
    F33.2   Recurrent depressive disorder, variable

F34 *Resistant affective states*
    F34.0   Cyclothymia
    F34.1   Dysthymia

F35 *Other mood (affective) episodes*
    F35.0   Other affective episodes
    F35.1   Other recurrent affective disorders
    F35.2   Other persistent affective states

F36 *Schizoaffective disorders*
    F36.0   Schizo-affective disorder, manic type
    F36.1   Schizo-affective disorder, depressive type

F39 *Affective disorders* not otherwise specified

F4   NEUROTIC, STRESS-RELATED, AND SOMATOFORM
    DISORDERS

F40 *Phobic disorder*
    F40.0   Agoraphobia
    F40.1   Social phobias
    F40.2   Specific (isolated) phobias

F41 *Other anxiety disorder*
    F41.0   Panic disorder (episodic paroxysmal anxiety)
    F41.1   Generalized anxiety disorder
    F41.2   Mixed anxiety and depressive disorder

F42 *Obsessive-compulsive disorder*
    F42.0   Predominantly obsessional thoughts or ruminations
    F42.1   Predominantly compulsive acts (obsessional rituals)
    F42.2   Mixed obsessional thoughts and acts

F43 *Reaction to severe stress and adjustment disorders*
    F43.0   Acute stress reaction
    F43.1   Post-traumatic stress disorder
    F43.2   Adjustment disorder

F44 *Dissociative disorder*

  F44.0–F44.4 Dissociative disorders of memory, awareness, and identity
  F44.0 Psychogenic amnesia
  F44.1 Psychogenic fugue
  F44.2 Psychogenic stupor
  F44.3 Trance and possession states
  F44.4 Multiple personality

  F44.5–F44.7 Dissociative disorders of movement and sensation
  F44.5 Psychogenic disorders of voluntary movement
  F44.6 Psychogenic convulsions
  F44.7 Psychogenic anaesthesia and sensory loss
  F44.8 Other dissociative disorder
  F44.9 Unspecified dissociative or conversion disorders

F45 *Somatoform disorder*
  F45.0 Multiple somatization disorder
  F45.1 Undifferentiated multiple somatoform disorder
  F45.2 Hypochondriacal syndrome (hypochondriasis, hypochondriacal neurosis)
  F45.3 Psychogenic autonomic dysfunction
  F45.4 Pain syndrome without specific organic cause
  F45.8 Other psychogenic disorders of sensation, function, and behavior

F48 *Other neurotic disorder*
  F48.0 Neurasthenia (fatigue syndrome)
  F48.1 Depersonalization-derealization syndrome

F49 *Unspecified neurotic, stress-related, or somatoform disorder*

F5   PHYSIOLOGICAL DYSFUNCTION ASSOCIATED WITH MENTAL OR BEHAVIORAL FACTORS

F50 *Eating disorders*
  F50.0 Anorexia nervosa
  F50.1 Bulimia nervosa
  F50.4 Normal weight bulimia
  F50.5 Obesity associated with other psychological disturbance
  F50.6 Vomiting associated with other psychological disturbances
  F50.8 Other eating disorder
  F50.9 Unspecified eating disorder

F51 *Sleep and arousal disorders*
  F51.0 Insomnia
  F51.1 Hypersomnia
  F51.2 Disorder of the sleep–wake schedule
  F51.3 Sleepwalking
  F51.4 Sleep terrors
  F51.5 Nightmares (dream anxiety)
  F51.8 Other sleep or arousal disorder
  F51.9 Unspecified sleep or arousal disorder

F52 *Sexual dysfunctions*
  F52.0 Lack or loss of sexual desire

F52.1   Lack of sexual enjoyment
F52.2   Failure of genital response
F52.3   Orgasmic dysfunction
F52.4   Premature ejaculation
F52.5   Vaginismus
F52.6   Dyspareunia

F53 *Psychological distress related to the menstrual cycle (including premenstrual tension syndrome)*

F54 *Psychological or behavioral factors associated with disorders or diseases classified elsewhere*

F6   ABNORMALITIES OF ADULT PERSONALITY AND BEHAVIOUR

F60 *Personality disorder*
F60.0   Paranoid personality disorder
F60.1   Schizoid personality disorder
F60.2   Dyssocial personality disorder
F60.3   Impulsive personality disorder
F60.4   Histrionic personality disorder
F60.5   Anankastic (obsessive-compulsive) personality disorder
F60.6   Anxious (avoidant) personality disorder
F60.7   Dependent personality disorder
F60.8   Other personality disorder
F60.9   Unspecified personality disorder

F61 *Personality trait accentuation*
F61.0   Paranoid
F61.1   Schizoid
F61.2   Dyssocial
F61.3   Impulsive
F61.4   Histrionic
F61.5   Anankastic
F61.6   Anxious (avoidant)
F61.7   Dependent
F61.8   Other

F62 *Enduring personality change, not attributable to gross brain damage or disease*
F62.0   Enduring personality change after catastrophic experience
F62.1   Enduring personality change after psychiatric illness

F63 *Abnormalities of gender identity*
F63.0   Transsexualism
F63.1   Dual-role transvestism

F64 *Habit and impulse disorders*
F64.0   Pathological gambling
F64.1   Pathological fire-setting (pyromania)
F64.2   Pathological stealing (kleptomania)
F64.8   Other habit or impulse disorder

F65 *Abnormalities of sexual preference*
F65.0   Fetishism
F65.1   Fetishistic transvestism

F65.2 Exhibitionism

F65.3 Voyeurism

F65.4 Pedophilia

F65.5 Sadomasochism

F65.6 Multiple abnormalities of sexual preference

F65.8 Other abnormalities of sexual preference

F66 *Psychological and behavioral problems associated with sexual development and orientation (hetero-, homo-, bisexual, uncertain, and prepubertal)*

F66.0 Maturational crisis

F66.1 Ego-dystonic sexual orientation

F66.2 Relationship problem

F66.8 Other problem or reason for referral

F66.9 Unspecified

F68 *Other abnormality of adult personality and behavior*

F69 *Unspecified abnormality of adult personality and behavior*

F7   MENTAL RETARDATION

F70 *Mild mental retardation*

F71 *Moderate mental retardation*

F72 *Severe mental retardation*

F73 *Profound mental retardation*

F79 *Unspecified mental retardation*

F8   DEVELOPMENTAL DISORDERS

F80 *Specific developmental disorders of speech and language*

F80.0 Simple articulation disorder

F80.1 Expressive language disorder

F80.2 Receptive language disorder

F80.4 Environmentally determined language disorder

F80.6 Acquired aphasia with epilepsy

F80.9 Other and unspecified developmental disorders of speech and language

F81 *Specific developmental disorders of scholastic skills*

F81.0 Specific reading disorder

F81.1 Specific spelling disorder

F81.2 Specific disorder of arithmetical skills

F81.3 Mixed disorder of scholastic skills

F81.9 Other and unspecified disorders of scholastic skills

F82 *Specific developmental disorder of motor function*

F83 *Mixed specific developmental disorder*

F85 *Pervasive developmental disorders*

F85.0 Childhood autism

F85.1 Atypical autism

F85.2 Childhood disintegrative disorder

F85.3 Hyperkinetic disorder associated with stereotyped movements

F85.4   Schizoid disorder of childhood
F85.9   Other pervasive disorder

F89 *Developmental disorder, not otherwise specified*

F9   *BEHAVIOURAL AND EMOTIONAL DISORDERS WITH ONSET
        USUALLY OCCURRING IN CHILDHOOD OR ADOLESCENCE*

F90 *Hyperkinetic disorder*
F90.0   Simple disturbance of activity and attention
F90.1   Hyperkinetic conduct disorder
F90.9   Hyperkinetic disorder, not otherwise specified

F91 *Conduct disorder*
F91.0   Conduct disorder confined to the family context
F91.1   Unsocialized conduct disorder
F91.2   Socialized conduct disorder
F91.9   Conduct disorder, not otherwise specified

F92 *Mixed disorder of conduct and emotions*
F92.0   Depressive conduct disorder
F92.8   Other mixed disorder of conduct and emotions

F93 *Emotional disorder with onset specific to childhood*
F93.0   Separation anxiety disorder
F93.1   Phobic disorder of childhood
F93.2   Social sensitivity disorder
F93.3   Sibling rivalry disorder
F93.8   Other emotional disorder
F93.9   Emotional disorder, not otherwise specified

F94 *Disorders of social functioning with onset specific to childhood or adolescence*
F94.0   Elective mutism
F94.1   Reactive attachment disorder of childhood
F94.2   Attachment disorder of childhood, disinhibition type
F94.8   Other disorder of social functioning
F94.9   Unspecified disorder of social functioning

F95 *Tic disorders*
F95.0   Transient tic disorder
F95.1   Chronic motor or vocal tic disorder
F95.2   Combined vocal and multiple motor tics (Tourette syndrome)
F95.9   Tic disorder, not otherwise specified

F98 *Other behavioral and emotional disorders with onset usually occurring during childhood*
F98.0   Enuresis
F98.1   Encopresis
F98.2   Eating disorder (other than pica)
F98.3   Pica
F98.4   Sleep disorder in infancy and childhood
F98.5   Stereotype movement disorder
F98.6   Stuttering (stammering)

F98.7 Cluttering

F98.8 Hypersomnolence and megaphagia (Kleine-Levin syndrome)

F99 *Unspecified behavioral or emotional disorder with onset in childhood or adolescence*

REFERENCES

American Psychiatric Association. 1980. *Diagnostic and Statistical Manual of Mental Disorders*. 3rd ed. Washington, D.C.

Cooper, J. E., Kendell, R. E., Gurland, G. J., Sharpe, L., Copeland, J. R. M., and Simon, R. 1972. *Psychiatric Diagnosis in New York and London*. Maudsley Monograph Series no. 20. London: Oxford University Press.

Feighner, J. P., Robins, E., Guze, S. B., Woodruff, Jr., R. A., Winokur, G., and Muñoz, R. 1972. Diagnostic criteria for use in psychiatric research. *Archives of General Psychiatry* 26: 57–63.

Jablensky, A., Sartorius, N., Hirschfeld, R., and Pardes, H. 1983. Diagnosis and classification of mental disorders and alcohol- and drug-related problems: A research agenda for the 1980's. *Psychological Medicine* 13: 907–921.

Kendell, R. E. 1984. Reflections on psychiatric classification – for the architects of DSM-IV and ICD-10. *Integrative Psychiatry* 2: 43–47.

Kramer, M., Sartorius, N., Jablensky, A., and Gulbinat, W. 1979. The ICD-9 classification of mental disorders. A review of its development and contents. *Acta Psychiatrica Scandinavica* 59: 214–262.

Rutter, M., Shaffer, D., and Shepherd, M. 1975. *A Multiaxial Classification of Child Psychiatric Disorders*. Geneva: World Health Organization.

Sartorius, N., Jablensky, A., Korten, A., Ernberg, G., and Cooper, J. E. 1986. Early manifestations and first-contact incident of schizophrenia in different cultures. *Psychological Medicine* 16: 909–928.

Shepherd, M. 1985. Contributions of epidemiological research to the classification of diagnosis of mental disorders. In World Health Organization (1985), *Mental Disorders, Alcohol- and Drug-Related Problems. International Perspectives on Their Diagnosis and Classification*. Amsterdam: Excerpta Medica/Elsevier, pp. 337–341.

Spitzer, R. L. 1984. Commentary on "Reflections on psychiatric classification" by Kendell, R. E. *Integrative Psychiatry* 2: 48–49.

Spitzer, R. L., Endicott, J., and Robins, E. 1978. Research Diagnostic Criteria. *Archives of General Psychiatry* 35: 773–782.

Stengel, E. 1959. Classification of mental disorders. *Bulletin of the World Health Organization* 21: 601–663.

Tuke, D.H. 1892. *A Dictionary of Psychological Medicine*. Vol. 1. Philadelphia: Blakiston, p. 229.

Wing, J. K., Cooper, J. E., and Sartorius, N. 1974. *The Measurement and Classification of Psychiatric Symptoms*. Cambridge: Cambridge University Press.

World Health Organization. 1973. *Report of the International Pilot Study of Schizophrenia*. Vol. 1. Geneva.

World Health Organization. 1978. *Mental Disorders: Glossary and Guide to Their Classification in Accordance with the Ninth Revision of the International Classification of Diseases*. Geneva.

World Health Organization. 1979. *Schizophrenia. An International Follow-Up Study.* Chichester: Wiley.

World Health Organization. 1985. *Mental Disorders, Alcohol- and Drug-Related Problems. International Perspectives on Their Diagnosis and Classification.* Amsterdam: Excerpta Medica/Elsevier.

31 *Panel discussion on ICD-10*

ERIK STRÖMGREN (Denmark),
LETTEN SAUGSTAD (Norway),
ROBERT L. SPITZER (USA),
P. C. MUSSERT (Netherlands),
JUAN E. MEZZICH (USA and Peru),
JOSÉ LEME LOPES (Brazil), PETER BERNER (Austria),
MAURICE DONGIER (Canada), HORACIO FABREGA
(USA), ROBERT E. KENDELL (United Kingdom),
MICHAEL GÖPFERT (Federal Republic of Germany),
FEDERICO ALLODI (Canada), FINI SCHULSINGER
(Denmark), CHARLES B. PULL (Luxembourg),
CARLOS ACOSTA (Cuba), COSTAS N. STEFANIS
(Greece), AND ASSEN JABLENSKY (World Health
Organization, Switzerland)

ERIK STRÖMGREN (Risskov, Denmark; panel chairman): Dr. Jablensky, through his overview of ICD-10 proposals, has provided us with an excellent and informative basis for discussion. This will start with comments presented by a group of scheduled discussants, which will be followed by some questions and comments offered by other participants in this symposium.

LETTEN SAUGSTAD (Oslo, Norway): The great problem with ICD-8 and ICD-9 has been that these revisions were internationally accepted, but not in official use. They were not effective. In only seven WHO member countries we found official admission statistics available since 1970 concerning psychiatric diagnosis. In only two of the countries the diagnoses were broken down according to separate ICD codes. More particularly, no information was available from any developing country. Evidently, the ICD-8 and ICD-9 are already too complicated for official statistical use in most countries. As Dr. Jablensky already mentioned, one of the main purposes of the ICD is to service public health and statistical work. Consequently, one of the first and most important aspects of the ICD-10 should be simplicity and practicality for general use. Secondly, international acceptance is clearly not enough to secure the usage of ICD-10 through its international collaborative projects currently in progress and particularly through contacts with the various national psychiatric societies and now also with the World Psychiatric Association.

Another point to be made is that the new revision should retain continuity with the previous classifications so that we can study time trends. This is a problem with regard to ICD-10. On the other hand, I am happy with the prospect of the ICD-10 reserving a great proportion of their numbers for incorporating new research, in particular biological research, so that it will not be necessary to change codes or make new revisions too quickly. I am also concerned about the introduced dichotomy resulting from placing the mood disorders, psychotic

365

or not, in one category, and reserving another category for schizophrenia and many other functional psychoses including acute psychotic episode, psychogenic or reactive psychosis, et cetera. Within this latter category certain depressive psychoses are included as well as acute depressions which really belong to the category of mood disorders. It remains to be seen whether these categories will be used, or whether the category of mood disorder will be considered the least stigmatizing and in practice the preferred diagnostic category.

This latter point is in agreement with the present international trend to use nonpsychotic diagnoses for admissions to psychiatric hospitals. In particular, there seems to be some preference for diagnosing mood disorders (depressive neurosis, depressions not elsewhere classified, et cetera), and concomitant reluctance to diagnose schizophrenia and other functional psychoses. In our recent studies of admissions, around sixty percent were classified as nonpsychotic, despite that the majority of them were nonvoluntary admissions. Dr. Jablensky gave me data from Bulgaria indicating that the incidence of schizophrenia was unchanged since 1972, but there was a marked rise in number of nonpsychotic admissions which now exceeds seventy percent. This is striking since the hospital population is steadily decreasing and one would think that, with so few beds available, the severity of the cases gaining admission is now even greater than before. It is therefore a question whether the official statistics really reflect true morbidity, or whether this confusing diagnostic situation reflects a lack of interest in diagnosis and classification and that clinical psychiatrists prefer the least stigmatizing diagnoses. The considerably greater complexity of the ICD-10 vis-à-vis the previous revisions, makes one wonder if it will be used more widely or more correctly. It may be useful to consider designing a truly simple and practical core classification which enhances comparability with previous revisions.

ROBERT L. SPITZER (New York, USA): Having spent so much of my own time in the last few years trying to achieve a consensus regarding nosologic issues within a single country, I can only have sympathy for Dr. Jablensky's task.

I am very glad to see that the rule regarding the ten major groupings is going to be applied flexibly. I think there are two different strategies that one can employ. At one extreme is the strategy we employed with DSM-III and its revision, namely, to start off with what are the basic clinical major diagnostic categories we want without worrying about digits and codes. The other extreme is that your statistical people present to you the codes and the number of categories that you can have. I think that, unfortunately, Dr. Jablensky, was presented, initially, with that second alternative. He was told, "You have ten codes for major categories, do the best that you can." I think that mental disorders do not fall very naturally into ten categories. Many of the initial ten categories were difficult to conceptualize because they combined a lot of different things. In DSM-III, we have about eighteen major categories, which seems useful. Major concepts reflected in such terms as mood disorders and anxiety disorders are very important and we need to treasure them.

As far as specific groupings, I share the views presented in Dr. Klerman's paper, in the sense that WHO would be making a very serious mistake not acknowledging the concept of panic disorder. Dr. Jablensky has stated that this concept has been noted in recent publications, which I suppose is an operational way of avoiding the issue of whether those publications actually represent research data. No one can disagree with the fact that there have been publications. Some people may disagree with whether those publications are sound or not, but it seems to me that there is an overwhelming amount of clinical and research evidence supporting the utility of the concept of panic disorder.

Regarding the issue of what is a mental disorder, it seems to me that the official classification has to list disorders and not just interesting things that one would like to code. It seems to me that those interesting things should be outside of a section on mental disorders and we generally use the V codes for that. Let me mention three examples. One is sibling rivalry, which can be a very troublesome problem, but I do not think that it should be regarded as a mental disorder. Similarly, "accentuated personality" may be something that one wants to note. In DSM-III, we encourage people to note personality traits on Axis II, but they are not given a code. I think you do want to distinguish personality disorder from nonpersonality disorder, and I do not see how you can justify coding nonpersonality disorder in a classification of mental disorders. Another example is malingering, which can also be a real problem, but is not a mental disorder. Dr. Jablensky has made reference to the spectrum concept, which often comes up – "Why don't you group schizotypal personality disorder with schizophrenia." It seems to me that it would be a very dangerous move for us to adopt the spectrum concept because we cannot adopt just one spectrum. If we adopt the spectrum concept, we have to look at all the spectrums and it seems to me the whole classification then falls apart. We then have to consider antisocial personality and alcoholism together, as clearly there is a relationship between them. What do we do about that? There are other spectrums and I think they should not be incorporated in the classification until there is a very clear, demonstrable, and compelling reason to link disorders which present in a very different way. Schizotypal personality disorder does not present ever with psychotic features, and in that way it is basically different from schizophrenia. We can certainly acknowledge that there may be a genetic relationship, but the clinical presentation of those disorders is different. I think that it would be a mistake to adopt the spectrum concept.

Regarding the phrase, "of psychogenic origin," frequently used in recent ICD-10 proposals, I think that is a serious mistake. For example, under sleep disorders of psychogenic origin and eating disorders of psychogenic origin, we classify conditions as mental disorders not because they are of psychological origin (whatever that means). We classify them as mental disorders because the presentation is in psychological symptoms or behaviors. I do not think we want to take the position that "of psychological origin" generally implies nonbiological origin. We do not have the data base to say that, for example, anorexia nervosa is of psychological origin. Anorexia nervosa is a disturbance in eating behavior.

This is the reason why it is classified as a mental disorder regardless of its etiology. Finally, I would like to comment on the classification of ego-dystonic homosexuality as a paraphilia. Our definition of paraphilia in DSM-III does not include ego-dystonic homosexuality, and I hope that this issue will be given more thought.

P. C. MUSSERT (Amersfoort, The Netherlands): I want to give ten short comments, and I hope not to fall into sibling rivalry with ICD-9 and DSM-III.

First, I agree that there is room for achieving better standards about occurrence and functional impairments in psychosis. ICD-9-CM suggests for this purpose the use of the fifth digit in categories 295 and 296. Further refinements are desirable, and should be standardized by investigating large groups of patients.

Second, symptom-orientated listing systems – for example, those found in DSM-III anxiety disorders – represent a denial of psychiatric tradition and knowledge about nosologic entities and about connections of symptoms with life events, other mental environments, life stages, and physical diseases and impairments. Although it would be appealing to have a theory-free classification, one has to note that in psychiatry, etiology, present state, diagnosis, prognosis, and therapy are strongly connected. It would, therefore, diminish our scientific thinking to separate diagnosis and classification from other fields of psychiatric knowledge.

Third, studies of patient careers in childhood and adolescence could probably give more insight in the specificity or nonspecificity of a diagnosis. What kind of patients have a career from (ICD-9 numbers) 309 (adjustment reaction) to 313 (emotional disturbance) to 300 (neurosis), or in another example, from 314 (hyperkinetic syndrome) to 312 (conduct disorder) to 301 (personality disorder)? Clinical studies should be conducted along with epidemiological studies, given that studies of the latter kind have recently shown incidences of certain disorders different from those obtained in patient studies. Paraphrasing the economic doctrine of money is what money does, one could perhaps say that psychiatry is what psychiatrists do and psychiatrists do only things for those that are referred to them.

Fourth, there is a great need of problem-intervention classification and registration systems that can be coded in a V-list. We need it especially in prevention projects and child mental-health care. There is a lack of comparable systems, and I hope ICD-10 will give solutions here.

Fifth, there is an important contrast between the developmental view of childhood disorders and the epidemiological and clinical research perspectives on child psychiatric classification, where disorders of children are listed as comparable to adult mental disorders.

Sixth, there is a great need for multiaxiality in child psychiatry classification as was pointed out in the 1960s at a WHO conference in Paris on childhood psychiatric classification. A five-axial scheme was later worked out in 1975. ICD-10 has to give the opportunity to find codes for all given axes – for Axes I through IV in Chapter Five or F, and for Axis V in the V-codes.

Seventh, there is a need for developmental differentiation. Categories such as 308 and 309, stress reactions, and adjustment reactions, do not have the same manifestations in childhood as in adults. The denial of the specificity of child psychiatry defaulted into the use of adult classification systems. In this respect, there should be diversity instead of unity.

Eighth, Chapter Five or F of ICD-10, therefore, could be divided into the five following sections:

1. Disorders of childhood
2. Disorders of adult psychiatry
3. Personality disorders (that should not be used below age 16)
4. Specific developmental disorders like those in Axis II of the Rutter-WHO five-axial system
5. Mental retardation, including possibility for coding intelligence levels above IQ seventy as are used in the European modification of Axis III of the Rutter system.

Ninth, perhaps there should be a larger representation for the field of child and adolescent psychiatry in the section on nomenclature of the World Psychiatric Association.

Finally, I would like to mention that more than twenty universities and clinics of child psychiatry from eight European countries have representation in the German-speaking Commission for Classification and Documentation of the European Society of Child and Adolescent Psychiatry. We work in connection with the Maudsley Institute of Psychiatry where Rutter and co-workers developed their well-known multiaxial classification system for child and adolescent psychiatry. Our committee is ready to cooperate in multinational studies that could lead to a well-shaped child and adolescent psychiatry component in the new ICD-10, with a useful multiaxial schema.

JUAN E. MEZZICH (Pittsburgh, USA): I would like to offer some comments about structural issues relevant to the design and construction of ICD-10. One has to do with the way disorders are defined. In recent ICD-10 drafts, it is mentioned that disorders should be defined as systematically as possible, which is often taken to mean that diagnostic criteria should be singly necessary and jointly sufficient to define a disorder. This reflects the classical approach to categorization which is not necessarily the most suitable to real situations. In fact, according to certain studies, the classical approach does not represent the cognitive processes of diagnosticians as well as the so-called prototypal approach does. The latter is characteristically polythetic, and allows for multiple disorders to be diagnosed. It is systematic and probabilistic. Consequently, the prototypal approach may be useful for both clinical guidelines and research criteria.

Regarding how the whole range of disorders are organized in an overall nosology, the concept of spectrum has been raised. To illustrate the complexity of this issue, one could consider the somewhat controversial idea of including schizotypal personality disorder within the group of schizophrenic and related disorders. A parallel could be drawn between this idea and the inclusion of cyclothymic personality disorder within the spectrum of affective disorders, which has been implemented in some well-known standard diagnostic systems and in some recent proposals. The degree to which schizotypal and cyclothymic disorders are genuine personality conditions as opposed to emergent, episodic, or progressive syndromes may be considered here. In any case, we face the challenge to be consistent in our application of the concept of spectrum.

In response to the widely perceived clinical usefulness of the multiaxial approach, it should be possible to offer a multiaxial schema in ICD-10 which complements rather than interferes with its core classification of mental disorders and which is presented for standard rather than for optional use.

Finally, I would like to refer to the subtitle of this conference: "Unity and Diversity." I think ICD-10 represents an opportunity for core uniformity in international communication, as well as for the possibility of incorporating some diversity originating from DSM-III and other national or regional approaches. The latter may be considered as complementary classifications or codings or as national adaptations that respect the essentials of the core international classification. This way, we may obtain enhanced communication across countries, as well as experience, at least in some parts of the world, with innovative schemas which may lead to future improvements in international classification.

JOSÉ LEME LOPES (Rio de Janeiro, Brazil): I am a representative of the Third World. I must say, first, that the International Classification is well received in my country. We have a long tradition of academic psychiatry and now from participating in this symposium, I have the impression that the ICD intends to be a system of conceptual definitions and a system of operational definitions, and that the ICD maintains a classical epistemological position. Dr. Jablensky said that ICD is a classification of diseases, not of individuals, but the diseases disappear behind the mental disorder.

Finally, I will make a point about delirium tremens. In the proposal there is delirium tremens within Alcohol Withdrawal States. I think there is also a delirium tremens *a potu nimio,* not only one *a potu suspenso.*

PETER BERNER (Vienna, Austria): First of all, I am not very happy with the title of the section on schizophrenic and other psychotic disorders, because this relates these other psychotic disorders too much to schizophrenia. I would reverse the titles "Psychotic Disorders including Schizophrenia" or even leave out schizophrenia and write just "Psychotic Disorders" and then list there schizophrenia. Another controversial point is that schizoid personality does not figure in that section. I agree it should not, but on the other hand, cyclothymic disorder is listed among the affective disorders although there are many arguments against considering cyclothymic personality as an affective disorder.

Another important issue seems to be the subdivision of schizophrenic disorders. I feel that in view of the catamnestic studies of Bleuler, Müller, and Huber, which just invalidated the classical distinction among paranoid, hebephrenic, and catatonic forms, one should at least question, whether it is worthwhile to keep this subdivision.

An important problem with schizoaffective disorders is where to place them.

I think it is extremely important how we define schizophrenia, how we define manic-depressive disorders, and how we handle Jaspers' hierarchical principle. Will ICD more or less stick to the classical Jasperian hierarchy or will it adopt an attitude which is closer to the American position giving more weight to manic-depressive disorders? I think this will determine what will be the appropriate place of schizoaffective disorders and cycloid disorders.

Some words about the glossary. I think the glossary and the conceptual definitions are of primary importance. I would suggest that the different aspects of each category be mentioned in the glossary, so that the users may know that there are wider and narrower concepts of the different categories, how these concepts are defined, and why they are so defined. The conceptual definitions should refer to the hypothetical assumptions, empirical reasons, and practical reasons underlying their development. Regarding the clinical diagnostic criteria, which apparently will be less stringent than those in DSM-III, there are basic options that have to be examined: whether to go in the direction of DSM-III or not.

A final point concerns the separate documents. I believe Dr. Jablensky indicated that there will be an appendix of research diagnostic criteria in ICD-10. Let me mention that we have published a set of such criteria within the framework of the WPA, and I think collaboration in this area would be very useful. My main question refers to the report on the 1984 Consultations on ICD-10 Proposals in Geneva, in which it was mentioned that there should be a list of documents of assessment. I am wondering if the plan is to develop an appendix containing research diagnostic criteria or assessment documents. Probably both would be interesting and worthwhile.

MAURICE DONGIER (Montreal, Canada): I classify my remarks into two categories: general issues and a special issue about the somatoform or hysterical disorders. First of all, should we, as in the bad example given by DSM-III, mix Greek and Latin in the words we create? Somatoform is a typical example of this, in which the first root comes from Greek and the second from Latin. The French Academy does not like very much this kind of thing, but maybe this is Gallic idiosyncracy. Second, in this category of somatomorphic disorders, I think as Dr. Spitzer does, that it is a very bad idea to use the word "psychogenic" in several subtypes. Psychogenic conversions is a case in point. Whoever has worked with epilepsy, especially psychiatrists, knows very well that many, perhaps most, epileptic seizures are in part psychogenic, namely triggered or facilitated by psychological events. This is typically the kind of problem that one meets again and again, especially in the field of conversion.

Another more general issue is how much the people working towards ICD-10 have been influenced by DSM-III and the attempt to expand the role of the new classification from a statistical purpose to a research and educational tool. Dr. Jablensky tells us that ICD-10 will include research diagnostic criteria, multiaxial aspects, a family of glossaries and appendices, manuals, and dictionaries, as DSM-III does. Moreover, they would turn to panels of experts, and that is somewhat of a problem. There is the risk of suffering from intellectual deprivation if we try to teach our trainees only empirically developed criteria accepted by committees of experts. One may wonder whether the best solution to improve the state of our science is to be strictly democratic, or to turn to the great geniuses of psychiatry, and whether people like Kraepelin, Bleuler, or Schilder would have been members of such committees. I believe people tend to forget (this happens only too often, particularly on the North American continent) that the development of psychiatry has taken place more through creative individual experience, intelligence, and intuition, than through empirically developed series of criteria and sophisticated statistics. That, as well as the excessive attention paid to reliability at the expense of validity, are the major pitfalls that the development of ICD-10 should avoid.

HORACIO FABREGA (Pittsburgh, USA): I think that Dr. Jablensky's overview of ICD-10 prospects was excellent, very thorough, very scholarly, and very comprehensive. Most of the changes that have been proposed are very positive. In the following comments I will be scrutinizing small things.

With Dr. Spitzer, I am puzzled by the absence of a definition of what a disorder is – whether the ICD-10 is addressed at disorders or at problems. With regard to that question, is distress, for example, sufficient for a definition of disorder? If it is, then it seems to me that sibling rivalry, in opposition to Dr. Spitzer, would constitute a disorder. Certainly, it can be squeezed under adjustment disorder. The definition of a stressor is very vague, very general, and when a stressor begins and or ends is very problematic. I suppose that sibling rivalry can be defined in relation to when certain maturational points are reached and the stressor of competition surfaces. I am carrying out this exercise to show the softness of some of the concepts that are brought into play in the definition of disorder. By the same token, you can say if impairment is a sufficient criterion for disorder, malingering certainly would constitute a disorder insofar as well-acted symptom profiles would include functional disturbance. So, that is one question that I have about the definition of disorder.

I was not too clear about the synopsis of culture-bound syndromes presented by Dr. Jablensky. From my perspective, an awful lot of what DSM-III or ICD-9 constitutes really are culture-bound syndromes, only they are Western culture, you see. Once you allow for schizophrenia and affective disorders and the like, which, I believe, are culture-bound in their manifestations, a certain kind of upbringing and level of literacy and other kinds of unusual cultural experiences account for the manifestations of these disorders as we have come to define them. That is a problem; there is a double standard built in here. Somehow, there seems to be the notion that the ICD-9 and DSM-III are the real, definitive or authentic classification schemes, whereas the culture-bound syndromes are somehow different. I would submit that they, in certain ways, are comparable.

I certainly am in favor of including open codes like the new code for acute psychotic condition not elsewhere classified. It seems to me that if you define these things properly and in a relatively abstract language, then you do away with an awful lot of the culture-bound syndromes. By the same token, many of these so-called culture-bound syndromes, which incidentally are very poorly understood, can be construed as adjustment disorders – unusual adjustment disorders. In other words, the content is conditioned by the culture of the person. So, the culture-bound issue is another question that I have.

With regard to my specific topic, namely the so-called marginal or transitional categories, I thought that the section of the ICD-10 draft was rather good insofar as it has expanded the category for stress and adjustment disorders. I found those useful and comprehensive and together with the various categories available for symptoms and behavioral disorders not elsewhere classified, disregarding the proviso about the definition of a psychiatric disorder, I thought that gave ample room for the coverage of marginal and transitional categories of illness.

ROBERT E. KENDELL (Edinburgh, UK): Because the success or failure of ICD-10 is going to depend largely on how useful and how acceptable it is in the Third World, it is vital at this stage that Dr. Jablensky and his colleagues know what psychiatrists working in those areas think of the draft proposals – how they react to them and whether they can see themselves using them in the future. ICD-10, compared with its predecessor, ICD-9, is a radically new classification incorporating some very major changes. The grouping of syndromes is completely different. The terms and the groupings of psychosis and neurosis have been abandoned. Several other hallowed terms such as "manic depressive psychosis" and "hysteria" have also been abandoned. There is a commitment to a multiaxial format, a commitment to the provision of operational definitions for all syndromes, et cetera.

I take the minimal comments made on these issues by other commentators to mean that they accept and approve, and, if that is so, I am delighted because I certainly regard these changes, most of which are derived from DSM-III, as major advances and very important improvements. To me, therefore, most of the comments made by previous speakers about whether or not panic disorder should be included, whether or not malingering should be included, where schizoaffective disorders should best be put, are trivial points of detail. They are not crucial to the framework of ICD-10. Of course, they are, at one level, important issues, but I would see them as trivial issues compared with the major ones which I hope are really being taken on the nod and accepted. If that is so, that is very good news.

I would like to make one trivial point of my own and that is that we must try to decide what it is that we are classifying. As Dr. Spitzer pointed out, there are going to be problems with terms like "malingering" and "homosexuality" even if it is dressed up with the adjectival phrase, "ego-dystonic." We are going to have innumerable problems like that unless we can openly admit that we are not classifying diseases and that we are not even classifying disorders. We are simply classifying the kinds of problems which psychiatrists currently deal with. It may be difficult to do that in the context of an international classification which is formally a classification of diseases, injuries, and causes of death. But, if we can have a preamble, at least to the separate publication of section F, to that effect, we will save ourselves many unnecessary arguments and battles.

Dr. Jablensky compared ICD-10 with the architectural structure of a small airport. I rather like that metaphor. I can commend Edinburgh Airport to him as a modestly sized and well-designed airport. Of course, flights come in and flights go out from airports; some of the incoming flights are going to be flights of fancy and I think it is one of Dr. Jablensky's important tasks to make sure that the flights of fancy are grounded and do not take off again.

MICHAEL GÖPFERT (Konstanz, Federal Republic of Germany): I want to make two comments with regard to the V codes. First of all, I want to go back to the issue of the culture-bound syndromes. The V codes, as I understand them, as they are defined currently, are very culture-bound to the Western society. I would like you to try to imagine what a marital conflict means, for example, in a Bangladeshi family as opposed to a family in downtown Montreal or in Berlin. Similar comments could be made about parent–child problems.

My second comment refers to a tendency to reserve the code "parent–child problem" for the use of child psychiatrists. Generally, V codes seem to be reserved for child psychiatrists. I am not sure whether I should state myself here as a child psychiatrist with interest in adults or as an adult psychiatrist with an interest in children, but I can assure you that I know of lots of parent-child problems, particularly from my work with schizophrenics, where the parent-child problem really is associated with the parent, not primarily with the child.

FEDERICO ALLODI (Toronto, Canada): I wonder how are we going to prevent that almost immediate plans be made for ICD-11. This may result from the process of preparing for ICD-10, which, as a definitional process, should involve many cultural points of view, including those of non-European cultures in the Third World. As Dr. Kendell said, the main issue is the compilation and categorization of problems rather than of illnesses. If we begin to decentralize the process of categorization we may find that the problems psychiatrists deal with (anxiety, homosexuality, et cetera) are seen very differently in various parts of the world.

So, when we consult with people from very different cultures, we might realize that the main problems they face in their clinical work have very little to do with what we are planning for the ICD-10. How can we prevent an onslaught on ICD-10?

FINI SCHULSINGER (Copenhagen, Denmark): I will pose only one question provoked by Dr. Spitzer's remarks in which he warned against including a spectrum concept of diseases in ICD-10. In DSM-III, there are things called major depressive disorder and minor depressive disorder. That is, of course, a spectrum. The question I would like to ask Drs. Jablensky and Spitzer is the following: What are the purposes of a classification? Should it reflect the state of the art? Should it have a pedagogical function among all psychiatrists, or, should it be something else? If there is good evidence that major and minor schizophrenic disorders have something to do with each other, should that be reflected in the classification system or not?

CHARLES B. PULL (Luxembourg, Luxembourg): I would like to come back to Dr. Kendell's final comments. ICD-10, as we see it now, seems to be quite a revolution. What is revolutionary in the outline of ICD-10 does not seem to be so much of a problem. Everybody seems to accept the need for diagnostic criteria, for some kind of multiaxial evaluation and for a different grouping of syndromes. All the discussion which has been going on here and elsewhere, always (it seems to me) concerns some peculiarities of this or that national school or some specific category like schizoaffective, which really seem to represent a rather small proportion of the patients we have to classify. What I would strongly advise regarding national schools which have some peculiarities (and representing the French, I know that the French do have some peculiarities) is that they should put those peculiarities into operational diagnostic criteria. When you do that, most of the differences just vanish or if there are differences that remain – and I don't think they will – they could be mentioned in the classification by some sort of bypath, pointing out where to classify those patients in ICD-10.

ROBERT L. SPITZER: I would like to try to answer Dr. Schulsinger's question. He asks if I believe that the classification should have some pedagogic use. Of course, it should. In fact, within the text of DSM-III, there is a statement indicating that there is evidence linking schizotypal personality disorder to schizophrenia. So, that evidence is not ignored, but it is not reflected in the classification itself. It has been said that DSM-III is inconsistent in that within the affective disorders we do have a spectrum concept because we include cyclothymia and dysthymic disorders with major depression and bipolar disorder. We have to agree on what we mean by spectrum, because I would say that the above case does not represent a spectrum concept. I would say that cyclothymic and dysthymia belong within affective disorders because the presenting symptoms of both of those disorders are disturbances in mood. On the other hand, the presenting symptoms of schizotypal personality disorder and schizophrenia are markedly different. The diagnosis of schizophrenia requires the presence of psychotic symptoms, as most people would agree, or, at least, in the way it is defined in DSM-III. So, to have schizotypal and schizophrenia within the same grouping, as would be suggested by the spectrum concept, would not be based on shared phenomenology. My point is that if you put those two disorders together, then you have to look at all of the other associations between disorders. I gave one example, antisocial personality disorder and alcoholism, which have a very high relationship. Are you going to bring those together? It seems to me that then the integrity and coherence of the classification system, unless we go into some kind of three-dimensional approach, will suffer greatly.

CARLOS ACOSTA (Havana, Cuba): For many years, we have been working with ICD-8, and ICD-9, and have made some modifications and contributions to Chapter Five. They have been published as the Cuban Glossary for the International Classification of Psychiatric Disorders. I have a question in relation to the category, disturbance of conduct not elsewhere classified, coded as 312. Cuban psychiatrists pondered deeply and discussed the use of this category.

The risk of failing to distinguish between disease and delinquency as well as the difficulty in clinically delineating the entities comprised in this category led to the elimination of its use. On the other hand, compulsive disorder of conduct coded as 300.3, and kleptomania coded as 307.9, were accepted. I would like to know the opinion of others in relation to the future of these categories.

COSTAS N. STEFANIS (Athens, Greece): I will come back to Dr. Kendell's last remark which I think is a fundamental issue in classification. What do we classify? Problems or complaints presented by persons visiting psychiatrists, or conditions that a person has and are diagnosed by the psychiatrist as mental disorders? This question has to be clearly answered because it determines the whole philosophy and the structure of the classification system. To me, it is only when we classify conditions reliably and by commonly adopted criteria as disordered mental states that we can proceed to establish credibility for the profession and provide a solid basis for psychiatry as a science. Psychiatric diagnosis may not, at present, be as precise and valid as we would wish it to be, but there is no substitute for enhancing its cogency and pragmatic usefulness. To construct a classification system based on the professional role of psychiatrists would be confusing and impractical. This is why I would oppose the introduction of a statement in the preamble of ICD-10 indicating that we classify complaints or problems that psychiatrists deal with. That would equate psychiatry with the social role of the psychiatrists, which may vary in different cultural settings.

Admittedly, we have to diagnose on the basis of the information obtained through observation and evaluation of behavioral phenomena presented by people. However, it is only when we are able to attach a categorical meaning to those multidimensional phenomena that we can claim scientific expertise and aspire for reasonable progress in the field.

ASSEN JABLENSKY (Geneva, Switzerland): I will make a few comments on the common themes which have emerged in many of the questions and remarks that have been made. Taking the last one about the definition of what is being classified. I would like to remind you that there is no WHO or ICD definition of disease in general. Therefore, it would be difficult to introduce a special definition for Chapter F. On the other hand, it is obvious that this question is likely to arise in one form or another and I would personally prefer that we point out the complexity of the issue in a preamble to Chapter F. I do not believe we can go beyond what many philosophers of science and great clinicians have done; and, therefore, perhaps, it would be futile to try to invent a definition of mental disorder for Chapter F. Perhaps we can supply this preamble with a few good references from people like Jaspers whose name was already mentioned. Also in this context, we should not forget that Chapter F is not for psychiatrists alone, but also for general practitioners as well as for health personnel who have no qualifications as physicians. In most of the developing countries, some of the users of the classification will be so-called medical assistants or other personnel with less extensive training than physicians. This is why we have to pay special attention to the other issue which was mentioned by several speakers and that is the relevance of this classification to the needs of developing countries. As I mentioned before, complementing the core ICD-10, there will be a special adaptation of the classification for non-psychiatric community settings especially in developing countries. I should like to mention that the first outline of what is being proposed was developed by an international conference in Jakarta, where eighty percent of the participants were psychiatrists from developing countries. We are taking special care to ensure the adequate representation of psychiatrists from the Third World in the various panels which are taking part in the development of ICD-10.

The next general issue was to what extent should ICD-10 reflect the state of the art in psychiatry? While the consensus of most of the meetings has been that it should reflect this to a greater extent than ICD-9 did, we should be mindful that an international classification must by necessity be somewhat conservative and probably follow one or two steps behind what is the latest development in research and rely more on findings which have already gained some currency and have been confirmed. But, the aim will be to make this classification more congruent with the present state of psychiatry which, actually, is very different from what it was over 25 years ago.

A number of specific questions were asked about the spectrum concept. I think that what we have in mind is a phenomenological spectrum rather than a genetic spectrum. I do not agree with Dr. Spitzer that there is no conflict between the logic of including cyclothymic personality in a group of affective disorders and the logic of including schizotypal personality together with the personality disorders and not with schizophrenia. I think that the basis for our current proposal for the classification of schizotypal personality is that it contains, in sort of a miniature or in a micro and abortive forms, all the basic schizophrenic disturbances. This is the only reason for the existence of this concept. It is a phenomenological spectrum to my mind, but of course, this is one of the issues which inevitably will continue to arouse controversy and discussion.

Regarding research criteria, we are going to present a collection of such criteria which can be recommended for wider use. In this process, we will make use of newer anthologies of research criteria as well as canvass the field for any other criteria which may deserve to be included.

The question about the disturbance of conduct not elsewhere classified will be discussed further by the panel which we have on childhood and adolescent disorders and it is difficult for me to predict what the future will show. I would certainly welcome specific suggestions for modifications in this area.

Regarding the V codes and the related question of the culture-bound syndromes, I would like to say that one of the main defects of ICD-8 and ICD-9 was that they ignored the cultural variation which exists in the manifestations of many disorders. We will try to make up for this lapse in ICD-10. Dr. Fabrega is perfectly right in that culture-bound syndromes should not be limited to those syndromes that occur south of the equator. Anorexia nervosa is also a culture-bound syndrome and this will be explicitly stated in the conceptual definition which will precede the description of this category, so that we have a broader view of culture-bound syndromes. But, there are syndromes which occur with great frequency in particular cultural groups. They cannot be easily subsumed under the existing major rubrics of classification. We are going to convene a special meeting in order to consider their classification; they will not be ignored in the tenth revision of the International Classification.

I am very grateful for the various remarks and suggestions. They will certainly be taken into account. I also feel rather encouraged by this discussion because there was no dispute of the general principles which underlie the proposals for ICD-10, although they depart very significantly from the framework of ICD-9. So, I take it as expressing that the state of the art of classification today does not conflict with the framework proposed for ICD-10.

ERIK STRÖMGREN (panel chairman): Thank you very much, Dr. Jablensky, for providing a solid foundation for our discussions. I think the session has been extremely constructive and rewarding.

World Psychiatric Association Section Committee on Nomenclature and Classification, 1983–1989

Michael von Cranach (FRG), Chairman
Ulysses Vianna Filho (Brazil), Vice-Chairman
Juan E. Mezzich (USA), Secretary
Amarendra N. Singh (Canada), Treasurer
John E. Cooper (United Kingdom)
Hanfried Helmchen (FRG)
Masaaki Kato (Japan)
Gerald L. Klerman (USA)
Morton Kramer (USA)
Javier Mariátegui (Peru)

Mogens Mellergård (Denmark)
Charles B. Pull (Luxembourg)
Darrel A. Regier (USA)
Letten Saugstad (Norway)
Shen Yu-cun (P.R. China)
Robert L. Spitzer (USA)
Erik Strömgren (Denmark)
Antonio B. Vieira (Portugal)
Narendra N. Wig (Egypt)
Hans U. Wittchen (FRG)

Index

abnormal singular reaction, 50
Achenbach Child Behavior Checklist, 288
Acosta, C., 375–6
adaptive functioning, 267, 292
adjustment disorder: admission statistics
and, 258, 261; classification revision and,
352, 369, 373; cultural variability and,
162–4; DSM-III revision and, 281; as transitional illness category, 157–62
admissions statistics, 366; adjustment disorder and, 258, 261; affective disorders and,
253, 254, 256, 257, 258; anxiety and, 259;
depressive disorders and, 256–9; developing countries and, 257, 259–60; functional
psychoses and, 253, 254, 261; intermediate psychoses and, 253, 254, 256; international classification standards analysis
and, 253–8; manic-depressive disorders
and, 253; organic disorders and, 261; paranoia and, 257, 259; reactive disorders
and, 253, 254, 259; revision of ICD and,
253, 254, 258–62; schizophrenia and, 253–
4, 256, 257, 259
affective disorders: admission statistics and,
253, 254, 256, 257, 258; bipolar disorders
and, 136–7; Chinese classification and,
74, 77; classification controversy and,
136–8, 140–1; DSM-III and, 84, 135, 138,
270; Egyptian classification and, 59–60,
62; Nigerian classification and, 67–8; revision and, 358, 370, 375
Africa: acute atypical psychosis and, 116;
cross-cultural mental health differences
and, 317–19; cultural differences and, 65,
67–8; see also Nigerian classification
age: autism and, 100–1, 109; CIDI and, 215,
217–18; DIS and, 209–10
agoraphobia, 84, 140, 270; epidemiology
and nosology and, 306, 310–14
Alcohol, Drug Abuse and Mental Health
Administration (ADAMHA), 18, 175;
CIDI and, 211–12; WHO and, 346
alcohol-related problems, 58, 62, 71, 74, 75,
76, 226, 229, 276, 317, 347, 352, 356, 357

Allodi, F., 374
American Medical Association Standard
Nomenclature of Diseases, 9
American Medico-Psychological Association, 335
American Psychiatric Association, 260, 263;
see also Diagnostic and Statistical Manual
amnesia (psychogenic), 148
Angst, J., 137
anorexia nervosa, 225, 367–8, 377
anxiety states, 354, 366, 368; admission statistics and, 259; classification controversy
and, 136, 138–41; diagnostic reliability
and, 230; DSM-III and, 84, 270–1, 279; Nigerian classification and, 70
Ash, P., 221
Asia, 116; see also Chinese classification system; Japan
Association for Methodology and Documentation in Psychiatry (AMDP) documentation system, 235; described, 181–2;
multiaxial classification and, 182–203
Astrup, C., 124
Asuni, T., 66
attention deficit disorder, 267
Australia, 254
autism, 284, 287, 291; age and, 100–1, 109;
assessment methods and, 106–7; behavioral studies and, 105–6; biological factors
and, 104–5, 112; Child Study Center and,
99–100; communication and, 101–4, 110,
112; definition problems and, 99; diagnostic criteria and, 110–11; diagnostic features and, 107–10; DSM-III and, 99, 100–
1, 111, 267; facilitation of classification
and definition and, 112; high- and low-
functioning, 109–10
"automatic mental activity," 43, 44

Baillarger, J., 37, 89
Barlow, D. H., 140
Bartko, J. J., 237
Bayle, A. L. J., 89
behavioral changes (illness definition), 154